Introduction to Health Information Management

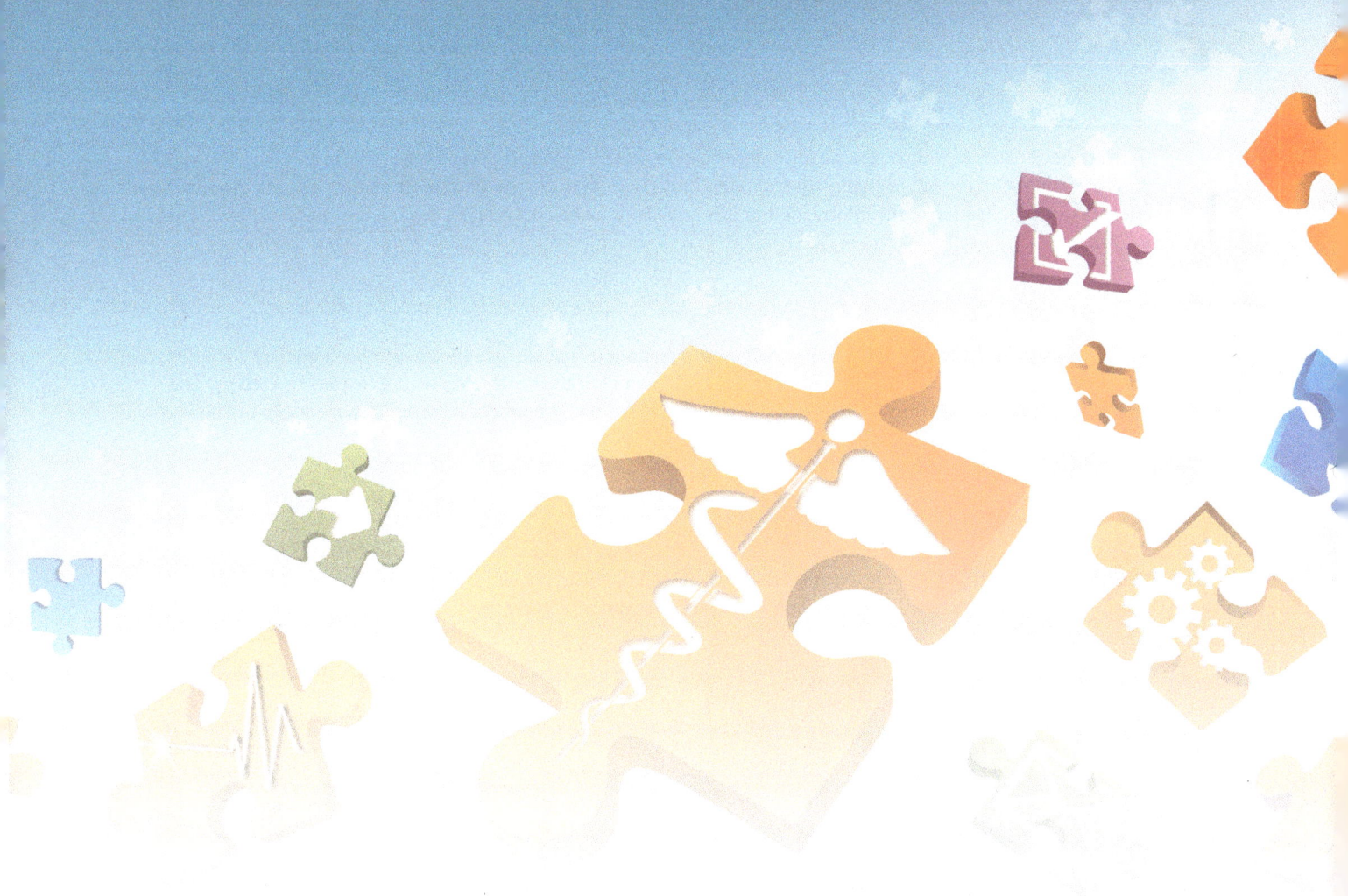

Sue Biedermann • Donna Olson

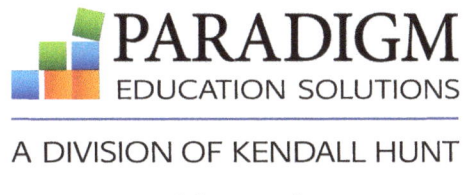

PARADIGM
EDUCATION SOLUTIONS

A DIVISION OF KENDALL HUNT

Minneapolis

Care has been taken to verify the accuracy of information presented in this book. However, the authors, editors, and publisher cannot accept responsibility for web, email, newsgroup, or chat room subject matter or content, or for consequences from application of the information in this book, and make no warranty, expressed or implied, with respect to its content.

Trademarks: Some of the product names and company names included in this book have been used for identifica-tion purposes only and may be trademarks or registered trade names of their respective manufacturers and sellers. The authors, editors, and publisher disclaim any affiliation, association, or connection with, or sponsorship or endorsement by, such owners.

Photo credits: Photo credits follow the Index on page 439. Cover photo: © VikaSuh/Shutterstock.com

We have made every effort to trace the ownership of all copyrighted material and to secure permission from copyright holders. In the event of any question arising as to the use of any material, we will be pleased to make the necessary corrections in future printings. Thanks are due to the aforementioned authors, publishers, and agents for permission to use the materials indicated.

ISBN 978-0-76386-071-4 (text)

© 2015 by Paradigm Education Solutions, a division of Kendall Hunt

7900 Xerxes Avenue S STE 310
Minneapolis, MN 55431-1118
Email: CustomerService@ParadigmEducation.com
Website: ParadigmEducation.com

All rights reserved. No part of this publication may be adapted, reproduced, stored in a retrieval system, or transmitted in any form or by any means, electronic, mechanical, photocopying, recording, or otherwise, without prior written permission from the publisher.

Printed in the United States of America

Brief Table of Contents

Preface ix

Chapter 1 Introduction to Health Information Management 1

Chapter 2 Healthcare Organizations 26

Chapter 3 Hospital Organization and the Medical Staff 52

Chapter 4 Health Record Purpose and Components 72

Chapter 5 Health Record Organization and Storage 108

Chapter 6 Information Technology in Health Care 132

Chapter 7 Electronic Health Records 156

Chapter 8 Legal Aspects of Health Information Management 198

Chapter 9 Classification Systems and Reimbursement 240

Chapter 10 Healthcare Statistics 272

Chapter 11 Quality Management and Data Collection 312

Chapter 12 Management 342

Appendix A Acronyms and Abbreviations 376

Appendix B Glossary 385

Appendix C AHIMA Code of Ethics: Principles and Guidelines 405

Appendix D Sample Medical Forms 411

Index 429

Table of Contents

Preface ix

Chapter 1 Introduction to Health Information Management 1

The History of Health Information 3
Health Information Management Roles 3
Where HIM Professionals Work 4
Essential Skills 4
   Critical Thinking 4
   Communication 4
      Written Communication 5
      Email Communication 5
      Verbal Communication 6
      Nonverbal Communication and Body Language ... 6
   Professionalism 7
      Manners and Common Courtesy 7
      Personal Appearance 8
Professional Organizations 9
Professional Credentials 10
Job Opportunities in HIM 12
   HIM Supervisor/Manager 12
   Positions That Report to the HIM Supervisor/Manager ... 12
   Hospital Medical Coder 12
   Clinical Documentation Improvement Specialist ... 13
   Cancer Registrar 14
   Medical Transcriptionist 14
   Medical Scribe 15
   Privacy Officer 15
   EHR Implementation Coordinator and Trainer ... 15
   Performance Improvement Coordinator 15
   Physician Office Manager 16
HIM versus HIT 16
The HIM Job Search 17
   Writing an Effective Résumé 17
   Job Search Tools 18
Ethics 19
Chapter Summary 20
HIM Review 21

Chapter 2 Healthcare Organizations 26

The Evolution of Health Care in the United States ... 28
   The 1920s 28
   The 1930s 29
   The 1940s–1960s 29
   The 1960s 29
   The 1970s–2010 30
   2010–Present 30
Health Insurance 30
Private Health Insurance 31
   Indemnity Plans 32
   Managed Care 32
Public Health Insurance 33
   Medicare 33
   Medicaid and CHIP 34
Healthcare Regulation 35
   Accreditation 35
   Licensing 36
   Certification 36
Healthcare Organizations 37
   Acute Care Hospitals 37
      Classification of Acute Care Hospitals 38
      Ownership of Acute Care Hospitals 39
      Governing Bodies 39
Other Healthcare Organizations 40
   Long-Term Acute Care Hospital (LTAC) 40
   Rehabilitation Care Facilities 40
   Ambulatory Care Facilities 40
      Outpatient Surgery Centers 40
      Emergency Departments 41
      Observational Services 41
      Diagnostic Clinics 41
      Physician Offices 42
   Home Health Care 42
   Long-Term Care 43
   Hospice 43
   Behavioral Health Care 44
Accreditation for Alternative Care Facilities 44
Healthcare Organizations and Associations 45
Chapter Summary 46
HIM Review 46

Chapter 3 Hospital Organization and the Medical Staff 52

Hospital Organization 54
   Hospital Departments 55
   Nursing 57
   Specialty Units 58
   Specialty Clinics 59
The Medical Staff 59
   Physician Designations 61
   Hospital Privileges 61
   Medical Staff Organization 62
   Medical Staff Departments 63
   Physician Employment 64
   Chief Executive Officer versus Medical Chief of Staff ... 64
Chapter Summary 66
HIM Review 67

Chapter 4 Health Record Purpose and Components 72

The Patient Record 74
Purpose of the Patient Record 75
   Primary Uses 75
   Secondary Uses 76
   Internal Uses 78
   External Uses 78

Forms/Information Included in the Patient Record ... 79
   The Hospital Record ... 79
   Acute Care Documentation ... 80
      Admission ... 80
      Medical History and Physical Examination ... 80
      Assessment, Plan, and Provisional
         Diagnosis ... 81
      Physician Orders ... 82
      Diagnostic Findings ... 82
      Patient Care Documentation ... 82
      Intake and Output ... 83
      Medication Records ... 83
      Restraint Logs ... 83
      Patient Care Notes ... 83
      Transfer Record ... 84
      Consultation Report ... 84
      Discharge Summary ... 84
   Additional Forms for Surgical Service Patients ... 84
      Consent for Surgery ... 84
      Anesthesia Report ... 85
      Recovery Room Report ... 86
      Operative Report ... 86
      Pathology Report ... 86
      Postoperative Evaluation and Follow-Up ... 86
   Additional Forms for Obstetric Patients ... 86
   Additional Forms for Newborn Patients ... 87
Organization of the Patient Record ... 87
   Problem-Oriented Medical Record ... 87
   Source-Oriented Medical Record ... 89
   SOAP Notes ... 90
      Electronic Health Record Organization ... 91
Required Documentation in the Patient Record ... 91
   Electronic Health Record Documentation
      Requirements ... 94
Forms Committee ... 95
   Document Design ... 96
   Authority/Responsibility for Documenting ... 96
      Timelines ... 96
      Signature Requirements (Authentication) ... 97
      Incomplete versus Complete Records ... 97
Information Governance ... 99
Clinical Documentation ... 100
   Clinical Documentation Improvement ... 101
Chapter Summary ... 102
HIM Review ... 102

Chapter 5 Health Record Organization and Storage   108

Paper Record Storage ... 110
   Health Record Numbering ... 111
   Record Filing Systems ... 113
   Off-Site Storage ... 116
   Microfilm and Digital Storage ... 116
   Hybrid Records ... 117
   Digital Imaging ... 117
   Electronic Health Records ... 117
Health Record Life Cycle ... 118
   Late or Loose Documentation ... 119
   Record Retrieval ... 120
   Release of Information ... 121
      Committee Requests for Records ... 122
   Purging Patient Records ... 122

   Destruction of Patient Records ... 123
   Disaster Recovery Planning ... 124
Chapter Summary ... 126
HIM Review ... 126

Chapter 6 Information Technology in Health Care   132

Information Technology Basics ... 134
   Hardware ... 135
   Software ... 135
Information Access ... 136
Networking ... 137
   Communicating over the Network ... 138
   Connecting to the Network ... 138
Information Storage ... 139
   Calculating Data Storage Needs ... 140
   Measuring Access Speed ... 140
Data Management ... 141
   Data Standardization ... 142
   Databases ... 143
Consumer Informatics ... 144
Data Security ... 144
   Data Threats ... 145
   Prevention of Security Threats ... 146
The Information Technology Department ... 147
Career Opportunities in HIT ... 148
Chapter Summary ... 150
HIM Review ... 151

Chapter 7 Electronic Health Records   156

EHR Functions ... 158
A System of Systems ... 159
   Core EHR ... 160
   Administrative ... 160
   Clinical ... 161
   Document Management ... 161
   Financial Systems ... 162
EHR Advantages and Disadvantages ... 162
   EHR Advantages ... 163
      Improved Patient Safety ... 163
      Faster Diagnostic Results ... 163
      Fewer Duplicate Tests ... 163
      Simultaneous Access ... 164
      Legible Documentation ... 165
      Elimination of Lost or Misplaced Records ... 166
      Enhanced Privacy and Security ... 166
      Paperless Referrals and Prescriptions ... 166
      Improved Patient Engagement ... 167
      Reduced Record Storage ... 167
      Data Sharing ... 167
   EHR Disadvantages ... 167
      Implementation Costs ... 168
      Extensive Training ... 168
      Documentation Quality ... 169
      System Output Usability ... 172
   Unintended Consequences ... 172
Evolution of the EHR ... 173
   Government Influence ... 174
   Meaningful Use ... 175
      Meaningful Use Incentives ... 175
EHR Security ... 176
   The HIM Department's Role in EHR Security ... 178

Access Control 179
EHR Selection and Maintenance............ 180
   Ensuring High-Quality EHR Documentation.... 180
   Other Healthcare Data Systems............. 182
      Master Patient Index................... 182
         Duplicate Records.................. 183
      Admission, Discharge, and Transfer System ... 183
      Scheduling Systems..................... 185
         Practice Management System 185
         Bed Control System 185
Disaster-Preparedness and Downtime
   Procedures............................ 185
Systems Used in HIM Departments 187
      Release of Information.................... 187
      Record Analysis 187
      Transcription and Speech Recognition 187
      Coding 188
      Cancer Registry (Tumor Registry)............ 189
      Changing Roles of HIM Staff 189
The Personal Health Record (PHR)............. 190
      Benefits of the PHR 190
      A PHR versus a Provider Record 191
      Electronic PHR Applications................ 191
Chapter Summary............................ 191
HIM Review................................. 192

Chapter 8 Legal Aspects of Health Information Management   198

The Legal System 201
   Sources of Law.......................... 201
   Federal, State, and Local Law 202
Ownership of the Health Record................ 204
The Legal Health Record...................... 205
   Confidentiality........................... 208
      Protected Health Information
         Documentation................... 210
      Documents Not Considered Part
         of the Legal Health Record 211
   Consents for Treatment 211
   Types of Consents 212
   Obtaining Consents 213
Other Legal Documents in the Health Record 213
   Advance Directives....................... 214
   Living Will 214
   Durable Power of Attorney for Health Care 214
   Do Not Resuscitate 214
The Health Insurance Portability and
   Accountability Act of 1996 215
Privacy and Security of Health Information....... 216
   Privacy Officer 217
   Business Associate Agreements 218
   Monitoring Disclosures.................... 218
   Security Processes and Monitoring 218
   Breach Notification....................... 219
Identity Theft 221
   Liability and Safety....................... 222
   Red Flags Rule.......................... 223
Release of Information 223
   Authorized Release of Information........... 224
   Fees for Copying and Other Records Services... 227
   Special Circumstances.................... 227
   ROI Restrictions 227

Outsourcing ROI............................ 228
   Outsourcing Advantages.................. 228
   Outsourcing Disadvantages 228
Releases for Legal Purposes................... 229
Ethical Issues in HIM......................... 231
Compliance................................. 233
Chapter Summary............................ 234
HIM Review................................. 234

Chapter 9 Classification Systems and Reimbursement   240

Clinical Terminologies and Nomenclatures 242
   Systematized Nomenclature of Medicine—
      Clinical Terms (SNOMED CT) 243
   Logical Observation Identifiers, Names,
      and Codes (LOINC) 243
Classification Systems 244
   International Classification of Diseases 244
      ICD-9-CM 245
      ICD-10-CM 245
      ICD-10-PCS 245
   *International Classification of Diseases
      for Oncology, Third Edition* 247
   Current Procedural Terminology............. 248
   Healthcare Common Procedure Coding
      System 248
   *Diagnostic and Statistical Manual of Mental
      Disorders, Fifth Edition* 249
   Comparing Nomenclature and
      Code Systems 249
Indices..................................... 250
   Master Patient Index 251
   Disease and Operations Indices............. 251
Other Activities Related to the Coding Function... 252
   Encoder Software........................ 252
   Computer-Assisted Coding 253
   Coding References....................... 253
Payment Methodologies 254
   Diagnosis-Related Groups................. 255
   Ambulatory Payment Classifications 255
   Health Insurance Prospective Payment
      System/Resource Utilization Groups 256
   Present on Admission..................... 256
Case Mix Index 257
Billing Processes and Procedures............... 258
Revenue Cycle Management 259
Compliance................................. 260
   Fraud 262
      False Claims Act 263
      Whistle-Blower 263
      Unbundling and Upcoding 263
Clinical Documentation Improvement............ 264
Chapter Summary............................ 265
HIM Review................................. 266

Chapter 10 Healthcare Statistics   272

Statistical Applications in Health Care 274
   Reliability and Validity..................... 275
   Common Healthcare Statistics.............. 275
Basic Statistical Terms and Calculations 276
   Measures of Central Tendency 276
   Measures of Frequency................. 277

Measures of Variation	278
Calculating Healthcare Statistics	279
Length of Stay	279
Average Length of Stay	280
Inpatient Census	281
Daily Inpatient Census	281
Inpatient Service Day	282
Average Daily Census	283
Percentage of Occupancy	284
Death Rates	286
Gross Death Rate	286
Net Death Rate	286
Fetal Death Rate	287
Maternal Death Rate	288
Anesthesia Death Rate	288
Postoperative Death Rate	289
Autopsy Rates	289
Gross Autopsy Rate	290
Net Autopsy Rate	290
Hospital Autopsy Rate	291
Other Statistical Calculations	292
Nosocomial Infection Rate	292
Consultation Rate	293
Data Display and Presentation	293
Data Table	294
Bar Chart	294
Histogram	295
Line Graph	295
Pie Chart	296
Analytics and Decision Support	297
Trend Analysis	297
Vital Statistics	298
Research	300
HIM's Role in Research	300
Basic Steps in the Research Process	302
Develop a Hypothesis	302
Review the Literature	302
Conduct the Research	303
Review the Data and Submit for Publication	303
Institutional Review Board and Compliance	303
Ethical Issues	304
Chapter Summary	306
HIM Review	307

Chapter 11 Quality Management and Data Collection — 312

Quality Management	315
Safety and Regulatory Standards	316
The Joint Commission	316
Hospital Performance Measures	317
Sentinel Events	318
Federal Quality Standards	319
Consumer-Based Quality Measures	319
Documentation Quality	320
Documentation Timeliness	321
Illegible Documentation and Abbreviation Use . . .	322
Inconsistent Documentation	324
Incomplete Data Components for the Condition . . .	324
Case Management	325
Risk Management	328

Databases for Reporting Purposes	329
Registries	330
Trauma Registry	331
Birth Defects Registry	331
Immunization Registry	331
Cancer Registry	332
Case Finding	332
Abstracting	333
oding and Staging	333
TNM Staging System	334
Follow Up	335
Chapter Summary	336
HIM Review	337

Chapter 12 Management — 342

Management and Leadership	344
Manager	345
Leader	346
Working in Teams	347
Building a Team	347
Stages of Team Development	348
Meetings	349
Using a Flowchart	350
Recognition and Rewards	352
Project Management	353
Simple and Complex Projects	353
The Project Management Process	354
Project Management Tools	354
Selecting and Evaluating Employees	355
Interviewing Potential Employees	355
Writing a Job Description	355
Telephone Screening	356
Interview Questions	356
Illegal Interview Questions	357
Prehire Assessments	357
Employee Feedback	358
Performance Evaluations	358
Motivation	359
Training	360
Training and Orientation	360
Cross-Training	361
Recognition and Reward	362
Policies and Procedures	363
Policies	363
Procedures	364
Budgeting	365
Operating Budget	365
Capital Budget	368
Productivity	368
Chapter Summary	371
HIM Review	372

Appendix A Acronyms and Abbreviations — 376

Appendix B Glossary — 385

Appendix C AHIMA Code of Ethics: Principles and Guidelines — 405

Appendix D Sample Medical Forms — 411

Index — 429

Preface

Introduction to Health Information Management provides students with an up-to-date, accurate, and accessible introduction to the dynamic and growing career field of health information management. This textbook is designed to give students entering the field a firm foundation in all of the essential knowledge areas, including transitioning from paper to electronic health records, healthcare law, reimbursement and classification systems, healthcare statistics, quality and case management, and healthcare management in all types of healthcare facilities.

This text is designed for students taking the course Introduction to Health Information Management, for those enrolled in a certified, accredited associate degree program, and for students planning to attain certification as a registered health information technician (RHIT). To get the greatest benefit from this text, students should have already taken and passed a course in medical terminology.

This book provides students with the opportunity to begin exploring Paradigm's live, web-based electronic health record application, the EHR Navigator. Based on the best features of many industry EHR systems, the EHR Navigator offers students hands-on practice and the freedom to explore this emerging technology at their own pace.

Chapter Features: A Visual Walk-Through

Each chapter contains several engaging in-text and in-margin features created to aid student learning. These features, as outlined below and on the following pages, challenge students to think critically, expand their knowledge through online research, explore ethical issues in healthcare, and test their mastery of chapter content. Designed to aid students of all learning styles, these features also highlight the importance of professionalism and soft skills.

Engaging two-page chapter openers immediately draw students into the chapter topics by piquing their interest with attractive graphics and fun facts. The chapter openers also offer helpful career and professionalism tips, historical background, and insights from industry leaders to supplement each chapter's core content.

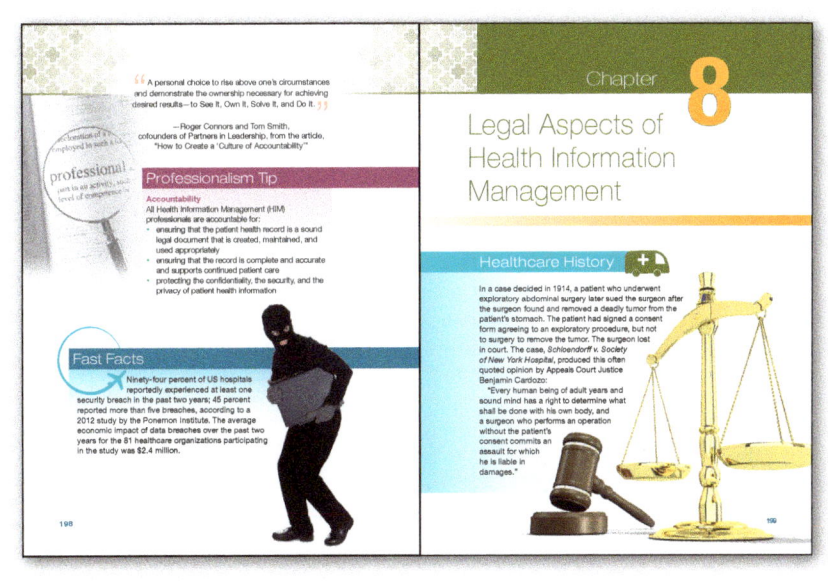

1 **Learning Objectives** establish a clear set of goals for each chapter and align with CAHIIM accreditation curriculum requirements for the HIM associate's degree.

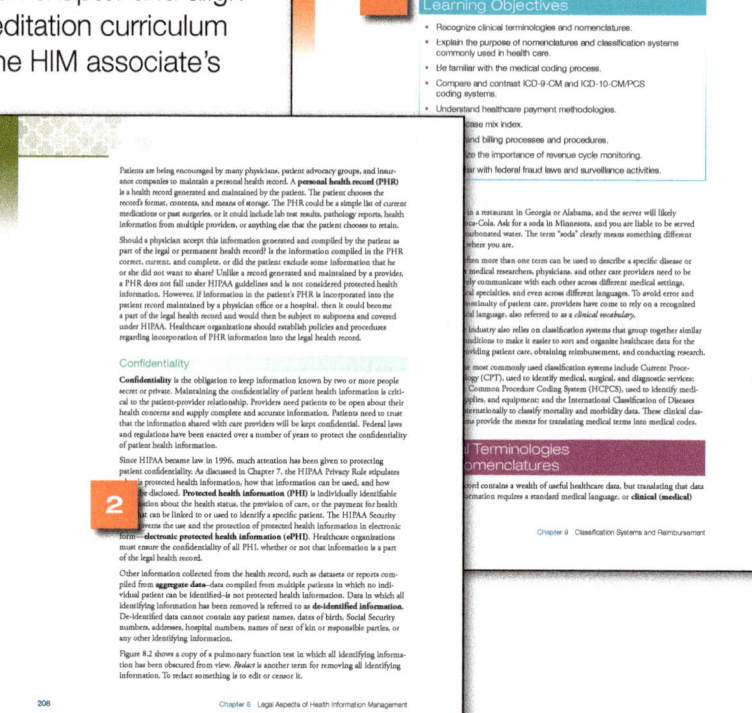

2 **Key terms** are set in bold and defined in the Glossary in Appendix B.

3 **Be Aware** margin feature alerts students to potential errors or complications.

4 **Expand Your Knowledge** margin feature speaks to today's digitally savvy students and integrates Internet resources and online learning opportunities.

x   Preface

5 **Think Ethics!** margin and in-text features highlight an ethical issue in brief.

6 **It Really Happens** provides students with real-world examples to promote critical thinking and increase awareness of legal and ethical issues they may encounter in the workplace.

7 **Take the Challenge** poses a critical thinking question or activity for students to consider on their own or for instructors to use as a starting point for in-class discussion.

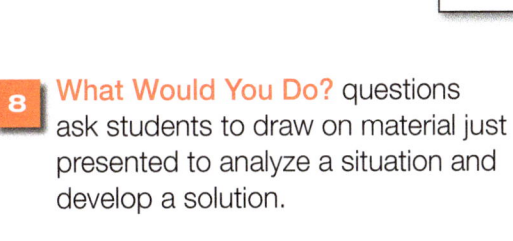

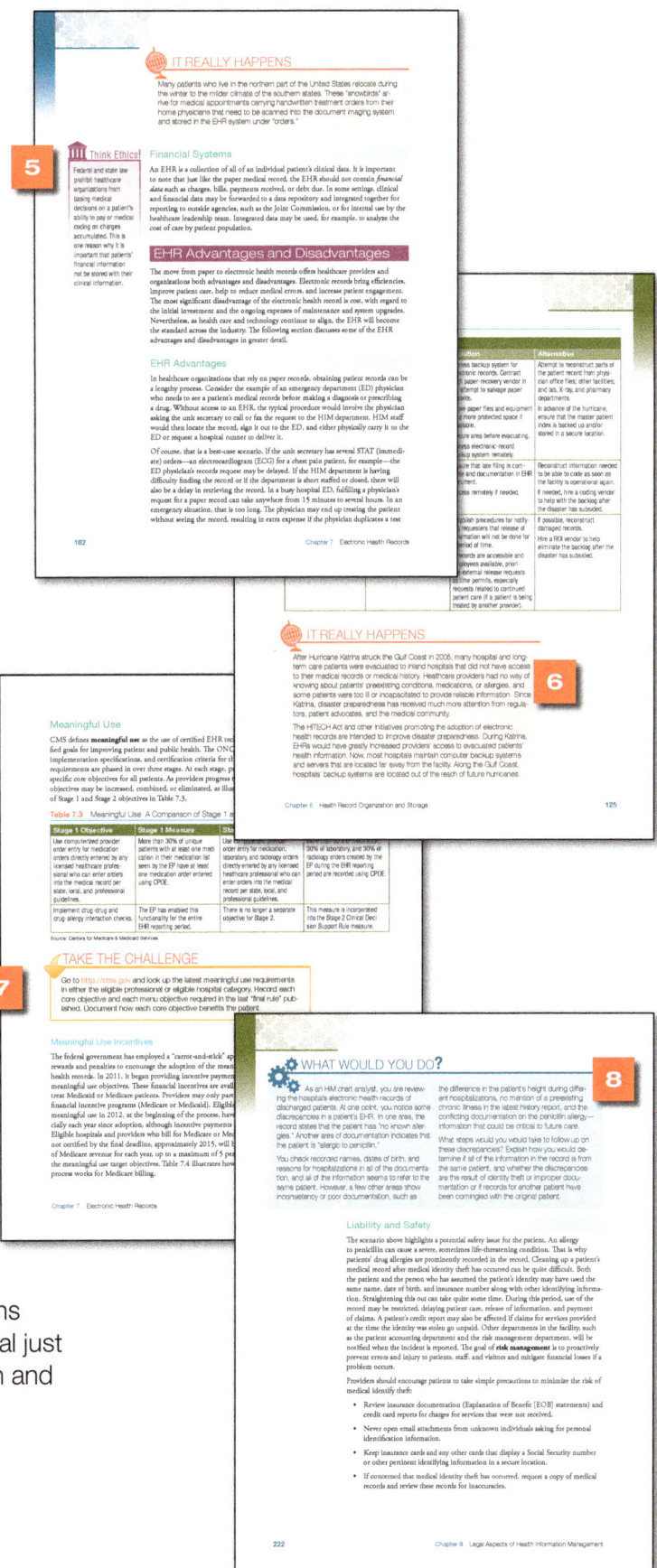

8 **What Would You Do?** questions ask students to draw on material just presented to analyze a situation and develop a solution.

Preface

xi

9 **Eye-catching photographs** reinforce the text and help students to visualize HIM concepts and real-world patient interactions.

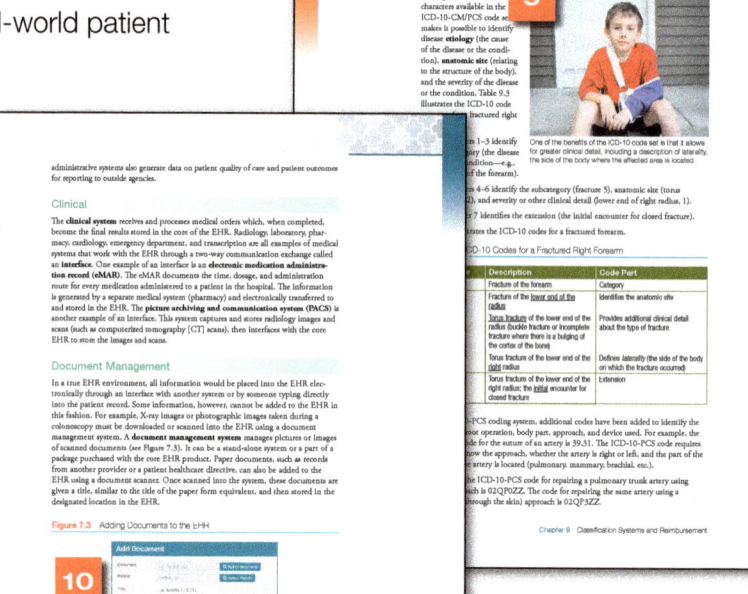

10 **Screenshots** from the EHR Navigator illustrate the key components of an EHR system as described in the chapter content.

11 **Clear and colorful charts** help students visualize in-text descriptions to better understand crucial concepts.

12 **Representative healthcare forms** provide additional detail and visual reinforcement of chapter topics.

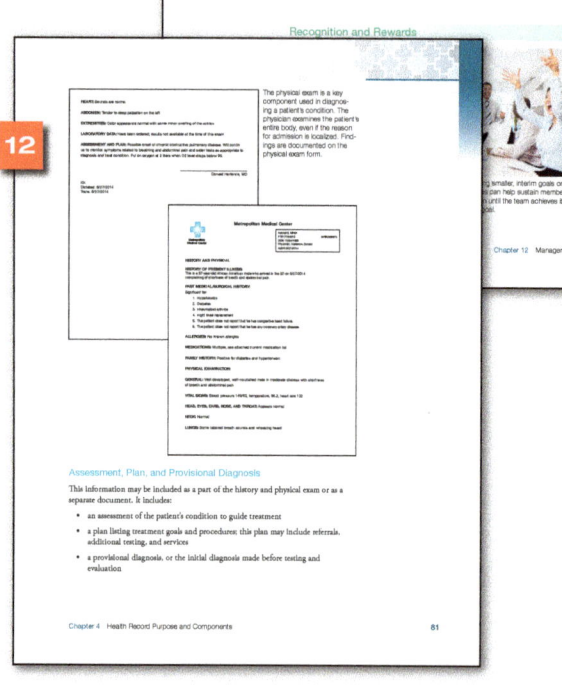

xii   Preface

13 **Tables** organize and encapsulate pertinent information related to the chapter and serve as a study aid.

14 **Examples of calculations** help students master commonly computed healthcare statistics.

15 **Chapter Summary** provides an overview of the key points of the chapter.

16 **HIM Review** provides multiple-choice and True/False questions, as well as critical thinking and practice-based assessments designed to give students a deeper understanding of the material.

17 **Navigator+** feature directs students to go online for more practice after they have completed the in-text exercises.

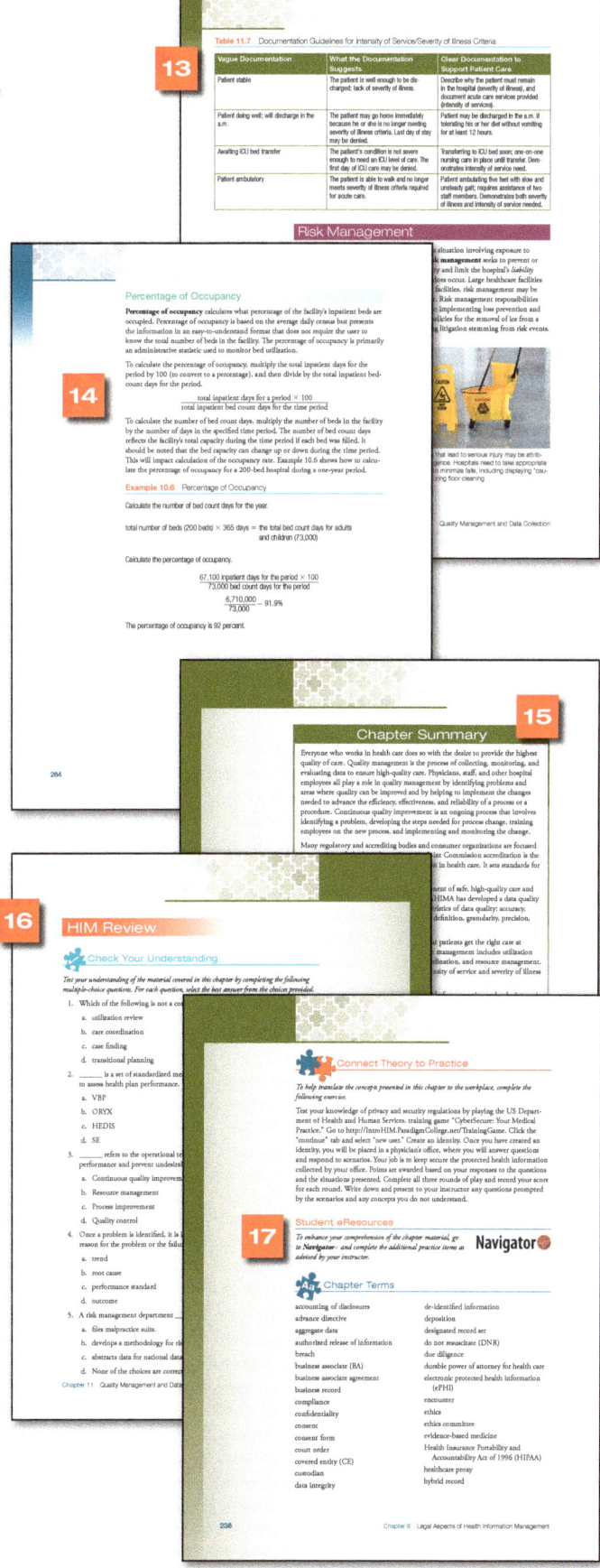

Preface xiii

Components

In addition to the many helpful in-text and in-margin features illustrated on the previous pages, *Introduction to Health Information Management* appendices and electronic resources enhance student comprehension and assist students of all learning styles in preparing for a successful career in health information management.

Appendices

Appendix A provides a useful reference of healthcare abbreviations and acronyms paired with their accompanying terms.

Appendix B contains a glossary of all boldface key terms in the text.

Appendix C puts the AHIMA Code of Ethics at students' fingertips.

Appendix D offers examples of the paper medical record documents that are referenced in the text and used in end-of-chapter and online activities.

Navigator+

Navigator+ is a learning management system that contains the *Introduction to Health Information Management* activities and assessments, as well as flash cards, quizzes, and other interactive learning opportunities designed to reinforce material presented in the textbook. Through the Navigator+ site at https://navplus.paradigmeducation.com, instructors can set up an Introduction to Health Information Management course. The Navigator+ site requires students to log in with the enrollment key provided by their instructor and the passcode provided with this textbook.

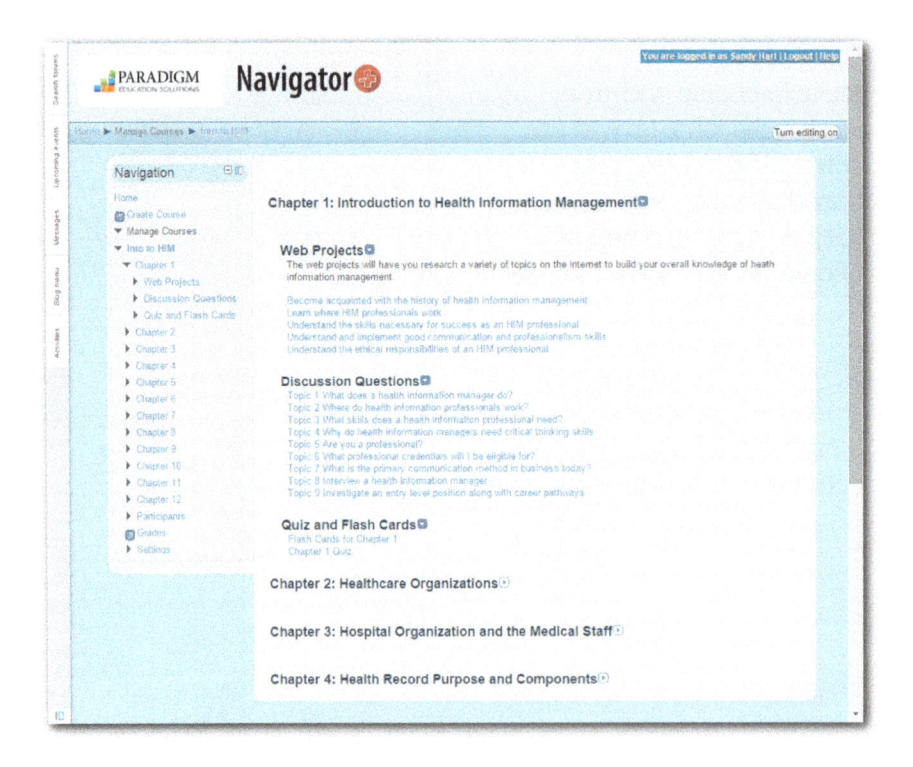

EHR Navigator

Access to Paradigm Education Solutions' EHR Navigator is included with this textbook. The EHR Navigator is a live software program that replicates professional practice and prepares students for today's workplace.

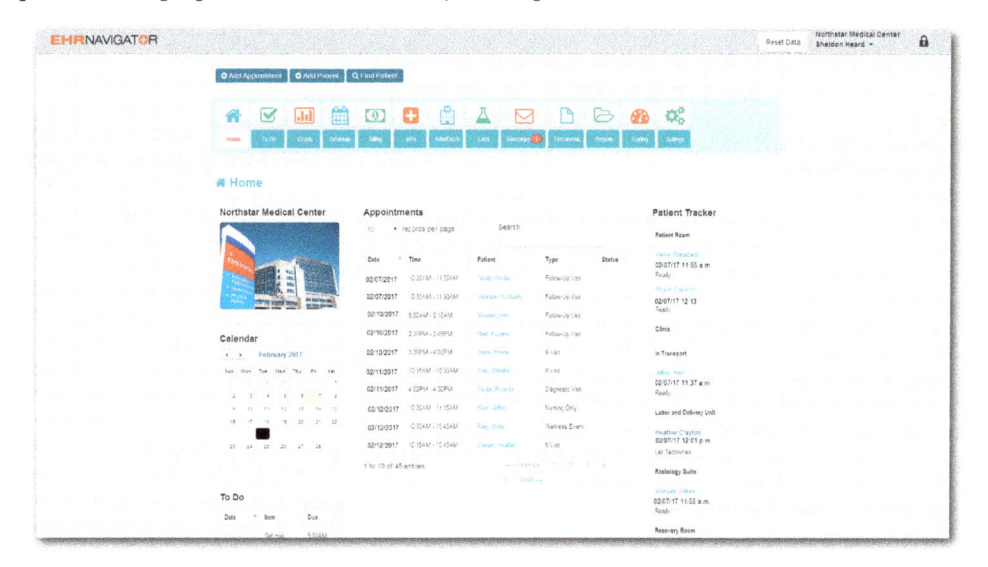

The EHR Navigator provides experience in all areas of EHRs—from adding and scheduling patient appointments, to adding clinical data to patient charts, to coding, to e-prescribing.

The interactive tutorials offer students practice in a variety of inpatient, outpatient, and personal health records activities, all within a format that is easy to navigate, colorful, and user friendly.

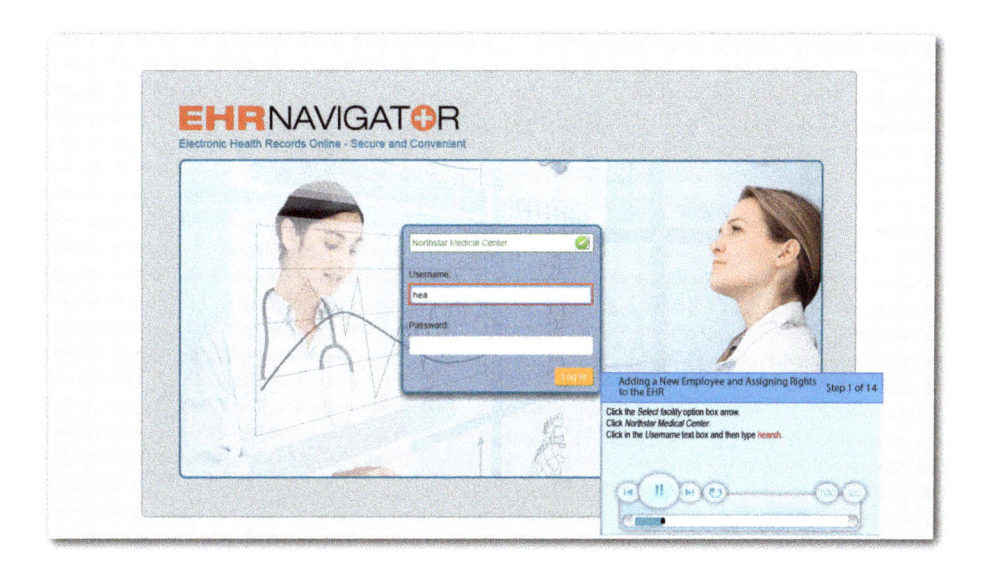

Ebook

For students who prefer studying with an ebook, this text is available in an electronic form. The web-based, password-protected ebook features dynamic navigation tools, including bookmarking, a linked table of contents, and the ability to jump to a specific page. The ebook format also supports helpful study tools, such as highlighting and note taking.

Additional Resources for the Instructor

Introduction to Health Information Management provides instructors with helpful tools for planning and delivering their courses and assessing student learning.

Instructor eResources

In addition to course planning tools and syllabus models, the Instructor's eResources provide chapter-specific teaching hints and answers for all end-of-chapter exercises. The eResources also offer PowerPoint® presentations as well as the ExamView® Assessment Suite. ExamView is a full-featured, computerized test generator that provides both print and online tests and the option for instructors to create customized tests using the chapter item banks.

Distance Learning Cartridges

Distance learning cartridges are available for this program.

About the Authors

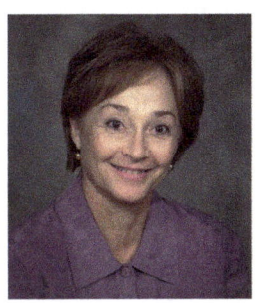

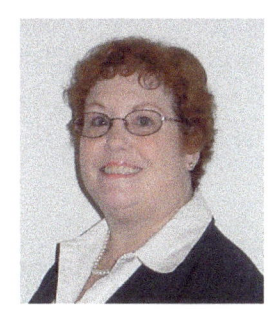

Sue Biedermann, MSHP, RHIA, FAHIMA

Donna Olson, MBA, RHIA

Sue Biedermann is an associate professor emeritus and a former department chair in the Health Information Management Department at Texas State University. She holds the American Health Information Management Association (AHIMA) certification of Registered Health Information Administrator (RHIA) and is a designated Fellow of AHIMA (FAHIMA). She has a bachelor's degree in medical record administration and a master's degree in health administration. Biedermann has taught in the HIM field for more than 35 years. Active in professional service, she has served on many AHIMA task forces, work groups, committees, and as a presenter at many healthcare conferences. She is past president and a former member of the board of directors of the Texas Health Information Management Association (TxHIMA). She has served on the advisory boards of several different HIT and HIA education programs. In 2009, she was awarded the AHIMA Foundation Educator Award.

Donna Olson is an associate professor at Collin College in north Texas where she teaches a variety of HIM courses. She also consults with hospitals and physician offices on work flow analysis, EHR, HIPAA, and meaningful use attestation. She has a bachelor's degree in medical record administration and a Master of Business Administration. During her 35-year career she has worked in a variety of healthcare settings as a coder, cancer registrar, HIM director and privacy officer, and corporate director of HIM services. Olson is an American Health Information Management Association (AHIMA) mentor and professional speaker and has served on the advisory board of several HIM publications. She has held a number of statewide and local leadership roles in HIM-related associations.

Authors' Acknowledgments

Thank you to Paradigm Education Solutions' management, editorial, and production staffs for supporting us through the challenges of creating this book. Thanks to all of my past students who have taught me so much about teaching. For their limitless support, thank you Jim and Amy.

Sue Biedermann

"With God all things are possible" Matthew 19-26.

It is through God's grace and his plan (not mine) that I was placed on a course to write this book, and for this, I am truly blessed.

I would like to express my gratitude to everyone who supported me during the process, especially my husband, Chip, and my daughter, Alicia, for their ongoing encouragement, for picking up the slack, and for understanding when work on the book took me away from them. I want to also thank my mother and father and my friends Sandra and Ken for listening patiently and sharing their experience and knowledge every step of the way.

It has been a joy to work with my co-author, Sue Biedermann. Her knowledge of the HIM field is extraordinary, as is her willingness to share that knowledge. Like the "Energizer Bunny," she just keeps going. I could not have asked for a better partner.

My thanks to Scott Charter, Chris Debrecht, and Denise Seguin for their guidance and expertise on the fast-paced and ever-changing world of information technology.

Lastly, thank you to all the hard working professionals at Paradigm Education Solutions for their patience and creativity. I had no idea how many people it takes to publish one book. Two staff members deserve my special thanks: Brenda Palo, Managing Editor for Health Careers, for standing by me throughout the entire process, and Developmental Editor J. Trout Lowen, who has handled the constant changes, demands, and deadlines without losing her sanity and who reminded me to always see things from the students' perspective.

To the "Bucket List": Check this one off!

Donna Olson

Acknowledgments

The quality of this body of work is a testament to the feedback we have received from the many contributors and reviewers who participated in the creation of *Introduction to Health Information Management*.

We would like to thank the following reviewers who have offered valuable comments and suggestions on the content of this textbook:

Hertencia V. Bowe, ABD-Ed.D, MSHA, RHIA
Fisher College
Boston, MA

Rhonda Houghton, MBA, RHIA
Collin College
McKinney, TX

Valerie Schmitt Prater, MBA, RHIT
University of Illinois at Chicago
Chicago, Illinois

We offer a special thank-you to:

Denise Seguin, Faculty, School of Information Technology at Fanshawe College of Applied Arts and Technology in London, Ontario, for her review of Chapter 6.

William Hervey, JD, LL.M., from Middle Georgia State College in Macon, GA, for his review of Chapter 8.

The ExamView and PowerPoint writers and testers.

An additional special acknowledgment of gratitude goes out to the members of the Paradigm Education Solutions Health Information Technology Board for sharing their thoughts and advice throughout the development of this text:

Catherine Bell, BS, RHIT, CCS
Milwaukee Area Technical College

Carmen Bellos, RHIT
WPC Healthcare

Ruth Berger, MS, RHIA
Chippewa Valley Technical College

Amy Bledsoe, MS, RHIA, CHPS, CHTS-PW, CHTS-IM
Spokane Community College

Jerrie S. Cleaver, MS, RHIA
Central Texas College

Angela Crouch, CPC
Daymar Institute

Darline Foltz, RHIA
University of Cincinnati—Clermont College

Carolyn Gaarder, MLA, RHIA
Minnesota State Community and Technical College

Misty Glasgow, MBA
Mercy Health

Kendra Hayes, RHIA, CTR
Longmont United Hospital

Lynnette Hessling, MSHI, RHIA, CHTS-PW, CHTS-TR
Ultimate Medical Academy

Karen Lankisch, PhD, RHIA
University of Cincinnati—Clermont College

Lorrie Laurin, BA, MT(ASCP)
Career Education Corporation

Ebony Lawrence, MHA, ABD-DrPH
AmeriTech College

Jorell Lawrence, BSHA, MSA-HR, CPC
Stratford University

Christy Lower, MS, RHIA
Davenport University

Yvonne Morrissey, BAS, CCS-P
Harrison College

Marla Phillips, MPH, RHIT
The Rehabilitation Institute of St. Louis

Sandra K. Rains, MPA, MBA, RHIA
DeVry University

Terri Randolph, MBA/HCM
Stratford University

Sabine Simmons, MSM, RHIA, CHPS, CPAR
Alabama State University

Diana Skarbek, MHA, RHIA, CCS
Brookdale Community College

Hard Work Beats Talent:
Six Simple Rules for Success

1. Get up early.
2. Focus on what matters. Each day.
3. Pay attention to detail.
4. Do more listening, less talking.
5. Develop yourself. Learn to use the tools around you.
6. Practice mental toughness.

(Source: Josh Bersin, principal and founder, Bersin by Deloitte. Read more about Bersin's six simple rules at http://IntroHIM.ParadigmCollege.net/RulesforSuccess.)

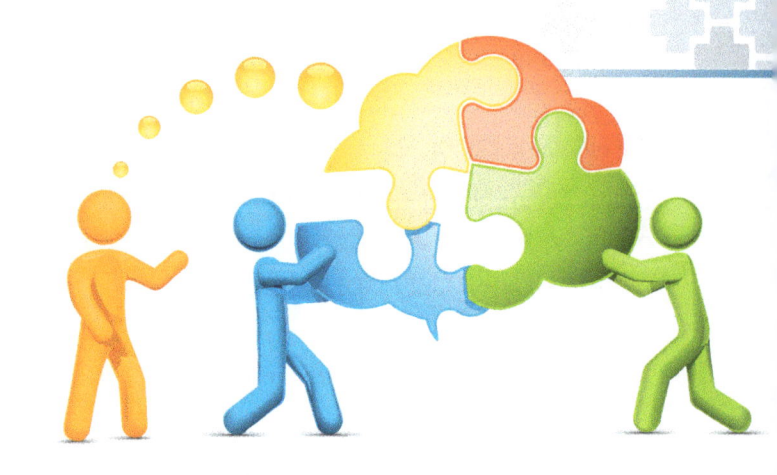

Job Outlook:

★★★ Good

Registered Health Information Technician (RHIT)

An aging US population means a rising demand for medical services, including tests, treatments, and procedures. This is good news for today's students entering the field of health information management (HIM). The federal Bureau of Labor Statistics projects that employment demand in the medical records and health information field is expected to grow faster than the average for all occupations through 2022 as more technicians are needed to organize and manage information in all areas of the healthcare industry.

The American Health Information Management Association (AHIMA) is the premier professional association of HIM professionals worldwide. AHIMA has 52 affiliated state associations and more than 71,000 members and is recognized as the leading source of HIM knowledge.

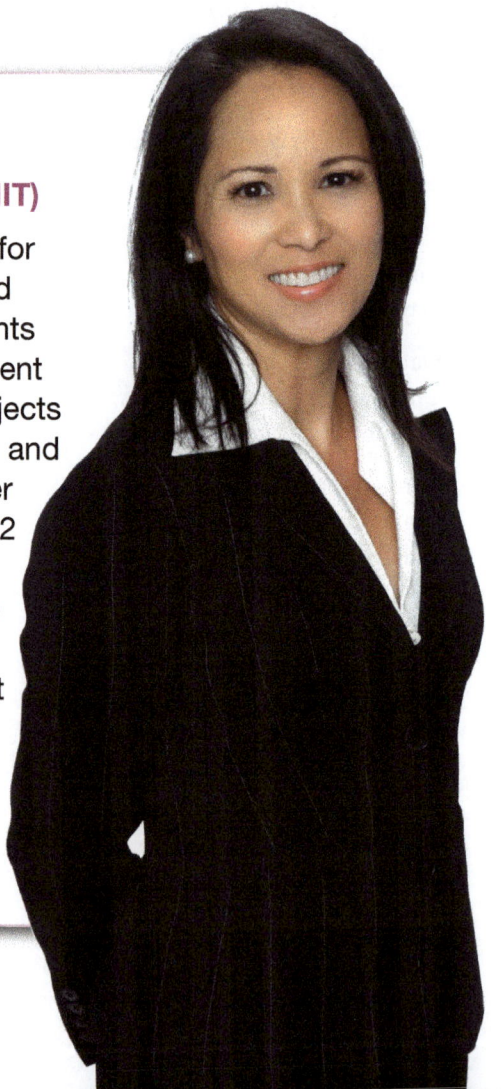

Chapter 1

Introduction to Health Information Management

> We have been through the decade of health IT—health information technology; we have now entered the decade of health IM—information management. The challenge of the coming years will not be the technology; it will be managing digital health information, including, but not limited to, the information content of electronic health records.
>
> —Linda Kloss, MA, RHIA, CAE
> Former chief executive officer, American Health Information Management Association

Fast Facts

Founded in 1928, the Association of Record Librarians of North America was created to improve the quality of medical records. The organization evolved to become the American Health Information Management Association.

Learning Objectives

- Be familiar with the history of health information management (HIM).
- Know where HIM professionals work.
- Describe the skills necessary for success as an HIM professional.
- Adopt good communication and professionalism skills.
- Recognize employment opportunities available to a registered health information technician.
- Describe the types of positions found in a health information department.
- Understand the difference between health information management and health information technology.
- Discuss the ethical responsibilities of an HIM professional.

Welcome to the world of health information management. Every time a healthcare provider assesses or treats a patient, the provider records the patient's medical information in a **health record**, also known as a *medical record*. **Health information management (HIM)** is the practice of maintaining, analyzing, and protecting confidential patient information contained in the health record. The HIM professional's most important duties are to ensure that patient information is accurate, meaningful, timely, compliant, and protected from unauthorized use. The HIM professional's diligence and attention to detail in record processing and medical coding are key factors in ensuring safe, high quality patient care and the financial health of the organization.

Numerous career opportunities are available to anyone entering the HIM profession, each with unique roles and responsibilities. HIM professionals:

- review patient records for timeliness, completeness, accuracy, and appropriateness of health data
- collect and maintain data for clinical databases and registries
- collect and analyze patient information for use in quality assessments
- review each patient encounter and assign clinical codes for reimbursement and data analysis
- implement, manage, and maintain health information storage, retrieval, and reporting systems
- protect the confidentiality of patient health information

The History of Health Information

In the early 1900s, health care was very different from what we know today. Whether providing treatment in a hospital or a patient's home, physicians recorded little about a patient's condition or the care provided. Physicians and hospitals were not required to keep track of lab results or to record signs, symptoms, operative procedures, or medications. Imagine how difficult it must have been to determine what treatments worked if there was no record of the result. If a physician could no longer treat a patient and another physician stepped in, the second physician would have no idea what the previous physician had diagnosed or what treatments the patient had received.

The **American College of Surgeons (ACS)** was established in 1913 to improve the quality of care for surgical patients. In 1918, the ACS set standards for hospital care. These included requiring hospitals to maintain an accurate and concise medical record for each patient. At a minimum, the patient record had to contain specific data elements such as name, date of birth, allergies, chief complaint, physical exam, and treatment plan.

Over time, these standards grew in importance, and it became apparent that hospitals needed a specialist who understood the intricacies of clinical documentation. In 1928, the ACS established the Association of Record Librarians of North America (ARLNA) to "elevate the standards of clinical records in hospitals and other medical institutions." In 1938, ARLNA changed its name to the American Association of Medical Record Librarians to better reflect its goal of improving the quality of the health record in all settings. The name changed again in 1970 to the American Medical Record Association as members' activities expanded outside of hospitals to other medical settings. In 1991, the organization changed its name to the American Health Information Management Association in recognition of the growing role of clinical data throughout the continuum of health care. Today, AHIMA is the premier professional association of HIM professionals worldwide.

Health Information Management Roles

A health information management professional is a college graduate with an expert understanding of both medicine and business. The HIM professional collects, analyzes, and displays medical data; provides the statistical information healthcare organizations need to make business decisions; and codes information in the health record to ensure that billing is accurate and compliant with all pertinent laws and regulations.

HIM professionals do not provide patient care. However, they do act as patient advocates, ensuring that patient health information is current, accurately recorded, and properly maintained in a secure environment that protects patient privacy.

To be successful as an HIM professional, it is necessary to have good computer skills and a strong ethical foundation. HIM professionals also need to remain current on healthcare laws and regulations. Many play a leadership role in their departments and organizations, acting as experts in the storage and release of protected health information (PHI) and supervising employees. All HIM professionals ensure the smooth day-to-day operations of their area of responsibility.

Throughout this course, you will learn about the roles and responsibilities of HIM professionals, the laws and regulations that govern the collection and use of health information, the roles and responsibilities of the medical staff, the adoption and implementation of electronic health records, and many other important aspects of this growing and dynamic career field.

Where HIM Professionals Work

An HIM professional with a two-year associate's degree has traditionally worked for a hospital or a large medical practice. A Pearson VUE analysis of registered health information technicians (RHITs) published in April 2011 found that hospitals are still the largest employers of HIM professionals. Other traditional employers include medical group/physician offices, HIM consulting firms, vendors, colleges, governments, and public health agencies.

Occasionally, HIM professionals can also be found working for insurance companies and in prisons, coroners' offices, and law offices. Insurance companies may need a health information technician with knowledge of healthcare coding to assist with claims processing. A law office may require someone with knowledge of medical terminology to read, interpret, and retrieve health information. As the health information field continues to evolve, HIM professionals will find new and unique opportunities for employment.

Essential Skills

Employers seeking HIM professionals are looking for candidates who exhibit excellence in critical thinking and communication, professionalism, and computer literacy. A student seeking to enter the HIM field should enjoy learning about business, science, medicine, statistics, and computer applications.

Critical Thinking

Critical thinking is the intellectually disciplined process of thinking that is clear, rational, open-minded, and supported by evidence. It involves analyzing, evaluating, and applying information gathered through observation, experience, reflection, and reasoning to guide one's beliefs or actions. In other words, critical thinking is not simply finding answers in a textbook and then memorizing the information. Having skill or knowledge (information retention) is not enough. A critical thinker does not see the lines that divide subject matter; he or she moves boldly forward using skills such as clarity, accuracy, consistency, relevance, sound reasoning, and fairness to solve problems and devise solutions. Developing critical thinking skills is a lifelong endeavor that must be practiced and nurtured. Are you a critical thinker?

Communication

Today's health information careers require individuals who can communicate effectively with all kinds of people in many diverse settings. During a single day, the health information professional may need to speak with a physician to accurately code a diagnosis for a medical condition and assist a patient who is filling out medical forms. The physician is highly educated and expects to converse in clear, professional, and accurately pronounced medical terminology. The patient may have a high school diploma and a limited knowledge of medical terms. Although these two situations are quite different, the HIM professional needs to adapt his or her style of communication to meet the needs of every individual.

Written Communication

An HIM professional is often expected to communicate in writing via memos, letters, policies and procedures, and, most frequently, emails. In all forms of written communication, some basic principles apply: keep it simple, stay focused on the topic, keep it brief, and make sure it is accurate.

To increase readability, use short paragraphs or bulleted lists. Avoid slang and instant-messaging abbreviations. Be careful not to overuse big words; it will not impress anyone and can actually frustrate the reader. Keep the tone positive, and always proofread the document to ensure there are no spelling or grammatical errors. When possible, it is a good idea to have someone else proofread the document with a fresh set of eyes, particularly if your spelling and grammatical skills are weak.

Email Communication

Email, the primary communication tool used in businesses today, requires some special consideration. In addition to the above guidelines, email should follow these standards:

- Do not put anything in an email that could not be published on the front page of a newspaper. Email is not a secure communication tool. Messages can be forwarded, copied and pasted, and printed, so be sure to use email wisely.

- Start and end each email message with a courteous greeting or closing.

- In email communication, your tone can be perceived as harsher than intended. If the subject matter is touchy or emotionally charged, do not discuss it in an email; instead, set up a face-to-face meeting.

- Never type in ALL CAPS; it is considered YELLING and it is rude. Repeated punctuation marks, such as !!! or ???, are also considered rude.

- Keep email professional (no jokes or innuendos).

- Unless specifically requested, do not "reply all"; reply only to the sender.

- Always acknowledge the receipt of an email in a timely manner, even if no response is expected. If you are unable to provide the requested information immediately, let the sender know when he or she may expect a reply.

- If you do not receive a response to your email right away, do not assume that the recipient is ignoring the message. There are many reasons the intended recipient may not have responded to the message. Follow up with a phone call to determine whether the email was received.

Verbal Communication

HIM professionals must be able to speak in a public setting as well as one-on-one with customers and other healthcare professionals. Some people become nervous when speaking with certain people or in a group setting, particularly when speaking to a large group. Even experts are sometimes nervous. The best way to calm these jitters is to be prepared. When making a speech or a presentation, jot down key points on a reference card in large, easy-to-read print. Keep it simple so that you can read the information at a glance. (Do not stand in front of a group and read a paper because everyone will fall asleep!) Practice your presentation out loud in front of a mirror or a trusted friend or a peer. Take a deep breath and relax; everyone is there to hear what you have to say. Remember to smile and use positive body language (e.g., stand up straight, make eye contact).

> **! BE AWARE**
>
> Common Mistakes to Avoid in Verbal Communication
>
> - *ain't* rather than *is not*
> - *aks* rather than *ask*
> - *gots* rather than *has*

Nonverbal Communication and Body Language

Body language is considered nonverbal communication because it sends a visual message to another person. How someone feels or what he or she is thinking can be communicated through posture, facial expressions, tone of voice, and gesture. Sometimes, body language can convey a person's mood or attitude more accurately than words. Is the person smiling or frowning, sitting up straight and leaning forward in conversation or slouching? Is the person maintaining eye contact or rolling his or her eyes? All of these examples demonstrate different feelings and attitudes conveyed through body language.

TAKE THE CHALLENGE

Describe what each person's body language is communicating in the photographs shown here.

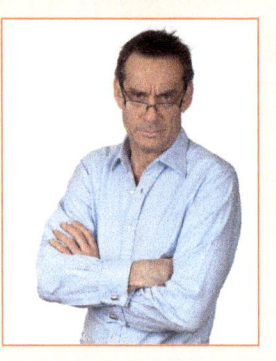

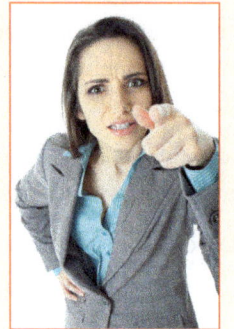

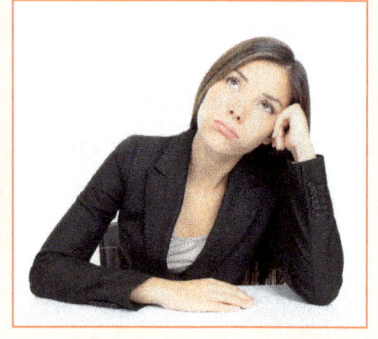

Professionalism

Professionalism is defined as the conduct, aims (aspirations and intentions), and qualities that characterize a professional person. Some of these qualities include demonstrating good manners and common courtesy, treating others with respect, dressing appropriately, having good personal hygiene, and practicing good communication techniques, such as those described earlier in this chapter.

The first step to behaving like a professional is to decide that you *are* a professional. Think of yourself as a professional, and you will be much more likely to act accordingly. Table 1.1 describes some of the key traits of a professional. Are you a professional?

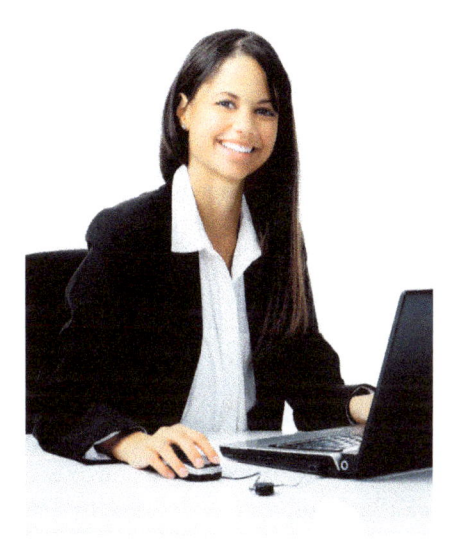

Actions you take or don't take in the workplace impact your professional reputation.

Table 1.1 Key Traits of a Professional

A Professional Does	A Professional Does Not
Set clear goals and priorities	Expect others to read his or her mind
Finish assignments early	Procrastinate and turn in work late
Accept challenges	Avoid difficult assignments
Recommend solutions to problems	Complain about problems
Keep commitments	Forget commitments
Maintain confidentiality	Gossip
Maintain financial balance and stay within a budget	Spend money without regard to budgetary parameters
Admit and correct mistakes	Hide mistakes and blame others
Give credit to all team members	Take all the credit
Embrace change	Resist or sabotage change

Manners and Common Courtesy

A professional always displays proper manners and courtesy. This has nothing to do with knowing which fork to use during an eight-course dinner; it is about practicing basic respect and civility when interacting with others. Think of each person as the most important person in the world, regardless of how that person looks or behaves or whether he or she has status in the company or community. Following a few basic rules can help to ensure that you display professionalism in every interaction:

- Say "please" and "thank you."

- Identify yourself: "Hello, this is Mary. How may I help you?"

- Allow others to go first—through a door or in conversation.
- Do not answer an email, the phone, or a text message while meeting with another person.
- Be on time.
- Ask, "Is this a good time?" before initiating a lengthy conversation.
- Try not to interrupt.
- If something upsets you, count to 10, take a break, or wait until the next day to respond.
- Never say or write something you may regret later.

Personal Appearance

Health information professionals are always making first impressions, each and every day. First impressions are based on how a person looks, stands, walks, and speaks. In the healthcare environment, it is important to appear approachable and professional. HIM professionals do not provide patient care, so they rarely wear scrubs or uniforms. Instead, HIM professionals dress in business attire. Business attire never includes:

- T-shirts
- sweatpants or sweatshirts
- jeans
- hoodies
- sportswear or gym wear
- tank tops
- halter tops or tube tops
- spandex
- capri pants
- sandals
- flip flops
- tennis shoes
- shorts
- skorts
- extremely high heels
- hemlines more than two inches above the knee
- low-cut blouses
- see-through clothing
- clothing with writing or logos

All clothing should be clean and wrinkle-free, with no tears, stains, or missing buttons. Jewelry should be simple (not excessively long or dangly); visible piercings should be on earlobes only. All tattoos should be covered. Nails should be clean and modestly manicured (not excessively long or loud in color). Makeup should be light and natural (you are going to work, not out on the town). Many healthcare organizations prohibit the use of perfumes and colognes, which can trigger an allergic or respiratory reaction in some patients. Use these products sparingly until you know your organization's policy.

TAKE THE CHALLENGE

Dressing professionally is an important part of the job. For each of the photos below, write a brief statement explaining whether the person in the photo is dressed suitably for a professional environment. Submit your assignment to your instructor or discuss in class.

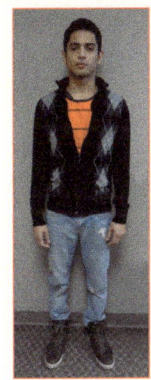

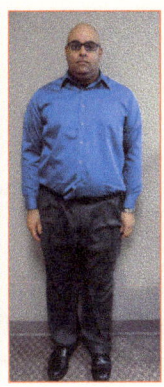

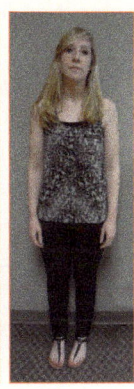

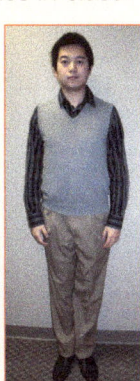

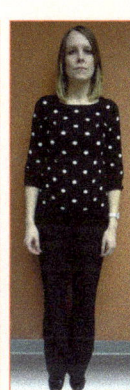

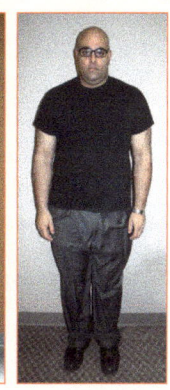

Professional Organizations

A professional organization is an association whose members share a professional or occupational status. The benefits of belonging to a professional organization include access to resources, professional training and certification, and opportunities to network with others in the same field.

The **American Health Information Management Association (AHIMA)** is the professional membership organization for individuals interested in or involved in the field of health information management. AHIMA offers members professional development opportunities, including an interactive career-mapping tool and an online job bank, continuing education courses for certification and recertification, and professional-practice standards (guidelines for best-practice policies and procedures for HIM interest areas). AHIMA also has an advocacy arm that actively petitions legal or membership interests, such as the adoption of electronic health records.

IT REALLY HAPPENS

Each year AHIMA's "Hill Day" brings advocacy leaders from each state to Washington DC to meet with members of the US Senate and the House of Representatives to discuss the issues and legal propositions important to the HIM profession. AHIMA members lobbied in support of the Genetic Information Nondiscrimination Act of 2008, which prohibits discrimination in health insurance or employment on the basis of genetic information.

AHIMA provides students with special benefits, such as discounted student memberships, scholarship opportunities, and mentorships. Access to AHIMA resources benefits students throughout their education and beyond. For more information, go to http://ahima.org.

Chapter 1   Introduction to Health Information Management

> **TAKE THE CHALLENGE**
>
> Go to http://IntroHIM.ParadigmCollege.net/AHIMAVideo and view the AHIMA video tour *Map Out Your Future*. After viewing the video, go to http://IntroHIM.ParadigmCollege.net/RHITCareerMap. Select an RHIT career and map your 10-year occupational goals using the Career Map tool. Share a screen capture of your career map with your classmates and your instructor.

EXPAND YOUR KNOWLEDGE

Each year on July 1, the AHIMA Foundation posts an application for its merit scholarship at http://IntroHIM.ParadigmCollege.net/Scholarship. Every student should apply for this wonderful opportunity.

The **AHIMA Foundation** is a separate, self-funded affiliate of AHIMA. The foundation offers a number of additional resources for research, education, and career development. These include:

- books, journals, and other publications
- the HIM Body of Knowledge (BoK), an online library of journal articles, government publications, practice briefs, white papers, and position statements
- scholarships
- research funding
- a faculty stipend program
- the Triumph Awards (HIM community-outreach awards)

Several other professional organizations offer healthcare-related information and resources as well:

- American Medical Informatics Association (AMIA), http://amia.org
- Healthcare Financial Management Association (HFMA), http://hfma.org
- Healthcare Information and Management Systems Society (HIMSS), http://himss.org

Professional Credentials

AHIMA also offers national certification exams. By taking and passing an AHIMA certification examination, a health information professional can become a credentialed registered health information technician (RHIT) or a registered health information administrator (RHIA). The AHIMA Commission on Certification for Health Informatics and Information Management (CCHIIM) oversees all certification-related matters. Certification provides HIM professionals with greater job opportunities and improved earning potential.

Practicing professionals may also obtain specialty certifications after meeting minimum educational and years-of-practice requirements. These specialty certifications include clinical health data analyst (CHDA), certified in healthcare privacy and security (CHPS), certified documentation improvement practitioner (CDIP), and certified healthcare technology specialist (CHTS).

Table 1.2 lists the AHIMA credentials available to an HIM professional and the educational requirements for each credential.

Table 1.2 AHIMA Credentials

Credential	Full Name	Educational Requirements	Focus	Continuing Education Hours Required
RHIT	Registered health information technician	Two-year associate's degree	Ensures quality of medical records. Uses computer applications and systems. Applies skills in coding diagnoses and procedures for reimbursement and research.	20
RHIA	Registered health information administrator	Four-year bachelor's degree	Expertly manages patient health information. Possesses a comprehensive knowledge of medical, administrative, ethical, and legal requirements and standards related to healthcare delivery and the privacy of protected patient information.	30
CCA	Certified coding associate	High school diploma or equivalent	Distinguishes him- or herself from entry-level coders by exhibiting commitment to the coding profession and by demonstrating coding competencies across all settings, including hospitals and physician practices.	20
CCS	Certified coding specialist	High school diploma or equivalent	Demonstrates mastery-level professional skill in classifying medical data from patient records, generally in the hospital setting. Recognized as an expert in health information documentation, data integrity, and quality.	20
CCS-P	Certified coding specialist-physician-based	High school diploma or equivalent	Distinguishes him- or herself as a mastery-level coding practitioner with expertise in physician-based settings such as physician offices, group practices, multispecialty clinics, or specialty centers. Recognized as an expert in health information documentation, data integrity, and quality.	20

Source: http://ahima.org/certification

The RHIT and RHIA certifications require attendance and graduation from a school accredited by the **Commission on Accreditation for Health Informatics and Information Management Education (CAHIIM)**, an independent accrediting organization that promotes and enforces accreditation standards for health information and health informatics education programs.

Students may take the RHIT exam during the last term of study or after all coursework has been completed. Students are encouraged to take the exam immediately after course completion. To learn more about the RHIT exam, go to http://ahima.org and click the Certification tab.

HIM professionals must complete **continuing education (CE)** training in the field every two years to maintain certification. The number of CE hours required depends on the credential or certification (see Table 1.2). Health information professionals are lifelong learners who strive to keep current with all of the changes that occur in the industry.

Job Opportunities in HIM

Job opportunities abound in the field of health information management. (Several of these positions are listed below, along with general descriptions of the qualifications required.) Job titles can be confusing, however. The same job title may have different responsibilities in different organizations, depending on the structure of the organization. An organization may designate a job title based on its business structure. A medical records supervisor at one organization may have the same duties as an HIM assistant director at another organization. Therefore, it is important to carefully review each organization's job description to understand the expectations for a particular position.

HIM Supervisor/Manager

An HIM **supervisor** or **manager** is responsible for human resource activities such as hiring, counseling, firing, and training staff. He or she is also responsible for budgeting and for developing and implementing policies and procedures to ensure the department's smooth operation. The HIM supervisor or manager is often a "go-to person" in the organization on whom others rely for expertise. A person with an RHIT credential is eligible to work as an HIM supervisor or manager in a small- to medium-sized hospital or as an office manager in a physician's office. In larger hospitals, this position usually requires a credentialed RHIA.

Positions That Report to the HIM Supervisor/Manager

A number of support positions report to the HIM manager. A high school diploma is required for some entry-level positions, although high school students may occasionally be hired for file/scanning positions. These positions require attention to detail, computer skills, and some knowledge of medical terminology.

The **vital statistics clerk** prepares birth and death certificates and submits the information to the appropriate state agency. This position involves direct patient contact, such as interviewing new mothers to obtain birth certificate information and required signatures. Many hospitals, particularly those that serve diverse patient populations, look for applicants who are bilingual.

HIM technician is the general name for a clerical staff member who performs a variety of duties in the HIM department, including record assembly and analysis, transcription processing and routing, physician completion activities, and release of information.

File/scanning and retrieval clerk is an entry-level clerical position. Duties for this position include preparing documents for final storage (filing paper records or scanning documents into the electronic health record system) and may include pulling paper records from storage or responding to customer requests for access to electronic records.

Hospital Medical Coder

A **hospital medical coder** reviews documentation in the medical record to determine which diagnoses and procedures to report. A hospital medical coder reviews all physician documentation, and diagnostic procedures (e.g., labs, X-rays, EKGs, and operative procedures), medications, and treatments provided. He or she then assigns each reportable diagnosis and procedure an alphanumeric code. The coder may use an *encoder* (computerized algorithm system) to assist in finding the appropriate codes and sequencing them according to coding rules. A hospital medical coder needs to be knowledgeable in three coding systems: the International Classification of Diseases, Tenth Revision, Clinical Modification (ICD-10-CM); the International Classification of Diseases, Tenth Revision, Procedure Coding System (ICD-10-PCS); and Current Procedural Terminology (CPT) codes. (These systems will be discussed in greater detail in Chapter 9.)

Based on the organization's needs, a coder may also abstract information into a database to collect additional details about a patient, such as discharge disposition, newborn birth weight, or number and types of transfusions. With experience, a hospital coder may take on advanced duties. Advanced coding roles include information retrieval and display (data analyst), quality assessments of coded information diagnosis related group (DRG) coordinator, staff training (coding trainer), auditing coded information for a vendor (auditor), and coding supervisor.

A registered health information technician may work as a **medical biller and coder** in a physician's office. This is not the same as a hospital medical coder. Table 1.3 outlines some of the differences between these positions.

> **BE AWARE**
>
> When looking at job advertisements for "coder," review the position description carefully. If the employer is not a healthcare organization, the position advertised may be for an information technology coder (someone who writes computer code).

Table 1.3 Hospital Medical Coder versus Medical Biller and Coder

Hospital Medical Coder	Medical Biller and Coder
RHIA, RHIT, CCS, CCA credentials	Certified professional coder (CPC) or CCS-P credentials
Works in a hospital or a hospital-based ambulatory care center. Numerous promotional opportunities in hospitals and outside the hospital environment.	Works in a physician's office or for a physician billing company. Limited promotional opportunities.
Uses books, reference materials, and a computerized encoder to code complex records.	Enters pre-coded information from a physician's charge ticket.
Challenging work. Always something new to code.	Repetitive work. Rarely sees new diagnoses.
Codes complex cases with up to 30 diagnoses and 20 procedures. Patient stays from 24 hours to a year or longer.	Provides data entry of codes preprinted on charge ticket. Usually two to four codes.
Uses all three coding disciplines.	Never uses ICD-10-PCS.
Uses CPT to code outpatient surgery.	May occasionally code an operative report using CPT.
Provides input for the CPT codes on hospital chargemaster (can be thousands of pages).	Provides input for the CPT codes on one-page charge ticket.
Is an expert on Medicare Severity Diagnosis Related Groups (MS-DRGs), Present on Admission (POA), and discharge dispositions.	Does not utilize Medicare Severity Diagnosis Related Groups (MS-DRGs), Present on Admission (POA), or discharge dispositions.
May code patient accounts totaling $2,000 to $2 million.	Bills patient accounts totaling $35 to $3,500.
Never handles a bill.	Produces and distributes bills.
Salary range: $17 to $35 per hour	Salary range: $12 to $18 per hour

Clinical Documentation Improvement Specialist

A **clinical documentation improvement (CDI) specialist** works with physicians in an acute care hospital setting to ensure that the documentation in the medical record supports all of the diagnoses and procedures provided to a patient. The CDI specialist works on the patient care unit with the physician to ensure that all documentation pertaining to a patient is captured and documented appropriately.

The CDI specialist also coordinates with the coding staff to ensure that all documentation needed for accurate and complete coding is in place. A CDI specialist should have inpatient hospital-coder experience, extensive diagnostic and treatment knowledge, and exceptional communication and interpersonal skills.

IT REALLY HAPPENS

Dr. Fahardo admitted a 72 y.o. patient with chief complaints of SOB (shortness of breath) and coughing. After an examination and diagnostic testing, Dr. Fahardo documented PNA (pneumonia) as the patient's diagnosis; no additional diagnoses were listed. Annette, the CDI specialist, reviewed the patient's record and found a chest X-ray positive for pneumonia; a sputum culture result showing growth of streptococcus, group A; and orders for respiratory therapy treatments and Vancomycin (a powerful and expensive antibiotic). Because PNA is viral and usually does not require hospitalization or antibiotics, Annette knew this was the more serious streptococcus pneumoniae. She also noted that the patient had type 2 diabetes, hypertension, and renal failure. Annette spoke to Dr. Fahardo and requested that he update the documentation to a more specific principal diagnosis and include the secondary diagnoses (additional reportable diagnoses).

Cancer Registrar

A **cancer registrar**, also referred to as a **tumor registrar**, reviews patient records for diagnoses and treatments related to cancer. Cancer-related data is then abstracted into a database. The information is maintained in the database in follow-up status for the life of the patient, and the registry staff tracks any change in cancer status. Most states have mandatory reporting requirements for cancer cases. A cancer committee provides oversight in accredited cancer treatment facilities, and a tumor board, a multidisciplinary group of physicians, reviews current cancer cases. The cancer registrar assists the committee chairperson in setting up meetings and records meeting minutes. A cancer registrar may become a certified tumor registrar (CTR) after fulfilling eligibility requirements and passing a national certification exam offered by the National Cancer Registrars Association (NCRA).

Medical Transcriptionist

A **medical transcriptionist**, also known as a *healthcare documentation specialist* or a *medical editor*, transcribes physician dictation into medical reports. A medical transcriptionist just starting out should be able to type a minimum of 80 words per minute and should have a solid grasp of anatomy, medical terminology, surgical equipment, radiology, and pharmaceutical terms. Transcriptionists may work in a physician practice or a hospital, as an independent contractor, or for an outside vendor. This occupation is one of the most popular work-from-home jobs in health care. The Association for Healthcare Documentation Integrity (AHDI) has established eligibility requirements and offers national exams for two credentials related to this position: registered healthcare documentation specialist (RHDS) and certified healthcare documentation specialist (CHDS).

Medical Scribe

A **medical scribe** is an unlicensed person who enters patient information into the electronic health record or the paper chart at the direction of a physician. This fairly new position is more often found in settings that have adopted the electronic health record (EHR). Scribes may also locate information in the EHR, such as test results, for the physician to review. The skills for this position include knowledge of medical and pharmaceutical terms, EHR computer proficiency, health information knowledge, and critical thinking.

Privacy Officer

The federal Health Insurance Portability and Accountability Act of 1996 (HIPAA) requires every healthcare practice and facility to have a **privacy officer**. In a small practice or healthcare facility, the privacy officer's responsibilities are often combined with another position, such as the physician office manager or the director of HIM. The privacy officer (who works with or who may also be the facility's security officer) establishes policies and procedures to protect the confidentiality of PHI, educates all facility personnel on the HIPAA Privacy Rule, audits PHI access, handles complaints related to privacy, and produces reports for internal use and governmental agencies. This position requires excellent communication and computer skills as well as investigative and problem-solving abilities. AHIMA has established eligibility requirements and offers a national certification exam for the credential of certified in healthcare privacy and security.

EHR Implementation Coordinator and Trainer

The **EHR implementation coordinator and trainer** is a relatively new position in health information. This key role assists in the selection and implementation of the EHR product, develops training materials, and trains users. On an ongoing basis, this individual assesses the needs of the changing healthcare environment and updates the system as necessary. This position requires exceptional computer, communication, and organizational skills as well as an in-depth knowledge of healthcare operations and medical terms.

Performance Improvement Coordinator

This position facilitates and provides technical and analytical support for quality and performance improvement (PI) initiatives and medical peer-review activities. The **performance improvement coordinator** usually reports to the quality improvement department. Job responsibilities include medical-information collection and review, medical-staff meeting preparation and minute taking, accreditation and survey preparation, and information reporting to designated regulatory agencies. The skills needed for this position include knowledge of healthcare operations, medical terminology, and regulatory and accrediting standards; proficiency in Microsoft Office applications; experience in quality and data management; effective interpersonal and communication skills; and strong organizational, computer, and information management skills.

Physician Office Manager

The **physician office manager** is responsible for the overall operations of the medical office, including hiring, assessing, and training staff; negotiating insurance contracts; preparing and monitoring budgets; paying invoices; and monitoring billing and accounts receivable. The office manager also prepares physician-credentialing information and ensures that all compliance requirements are in order. This position requires strong leadership and management abilities and sufficient knowledge of healthcare laws and regulations, medical terminology, medical billing, financial planning, and computers.

HIM versus HIT

Health information management and health information technology (HIT) are two separate career paths. However, these terms are often used interchangeably in college curriculums and employment advertisements, creating confusion for students and job seekers. Table 1.4 outlines the similarities and differences of these two career paths.

Table 1.4 HIM versus HIT Career Paths

	HIM	HIT
Education	Two- or four-year degree in health information management	Two- or four-year degree in information systems
Knowledge set	• health data content • privacy • anatomy/medical terminology • medical coding • health information applications	• computer programming • security • networks • software applications • databases
Reports to	health information department	information technology (IT)/systems department
Credentials	RHIT or RHIA AHIMA offers certification exams for credentials as a certified healthcare technology specialist.	None AHIMA offers certification exams for credentials as a certified healthcare technology specialist.
Job roles	• medical coder • cancer registrar • privacy officer • consultant • data analyst	• clinical analyst • technical applications coordinator • security officer • data resource manager
EHR roles	• selection and implementation specialist • workflow redesign specialist • trainer	• selection and implementation specialist • workflow redesign specialist • trainer

As healthcare facilities continue to move from paper records to electronic records, the responsibilities of the HIM and IT departments have evolved and created a need for exceptional collaboration between the two departments. Professionals in these departments must work hand in hand to ensure success in EHR implementation and maintenance.

The HIM Job Search

A healthcare organization should have a detailed job description for every position that outlines the skills and the qualifications required. Most employment ads also list the skills, the education, and the qualifications required for a particular position. Some ads specify a required number of years experience (e.g., "must have five years of inpatient coding experience at a large teaching facility"). However, many employers will consider a candidate who has less experience or other related types of experience. For the position mentioned above, for example, an employer would likely consider an individual with three years of inpatient coding experience at a small acute-care facility and four years of outpatient coding experience at an ambulatory-care facility.

To optimize your search for an HIM position, search online using a variety of job titles. (As discussed earlier, organizations may use different job titles for similar positions.) Start the search by using a keyword and then consider other words that may be synonymous. The following list demonstrates the different titles used in advertisements for a cancer registrar position:

- cancer registrar
- tumor registrar
- cancer data specialist
- cancer data analyst
- certified tumor registrar
- cancer registry coordinator
- oncology chart abstractor
- quality analytics registrar
- cancer registry conference coordinator
- medical abstractor

All of these job titles have the same hiring requirements and similar job duties.

Writing an Effective Résumé

A **résumé** is a marketing tool that a job seeker uses to promote his or her skills and value to an organization. Generally, an employer may take just 10 to 15 seconds to glance at a résumé and determine whether to consider an applicant. A résumé should be no more than one page, if possible. It should be concise, well organized, grammatically correct (all tenses should agree), and accurate. Use descriptive action words; do not use abbreviations or acronyms.

A résumé should display three skill types. **Adaptive skills** are behaviors and daily living skills that demonstrate the job seeker's ability to fit into the organization's culture. **Job skills** are skills gained through paid or volunteer work—including those skills

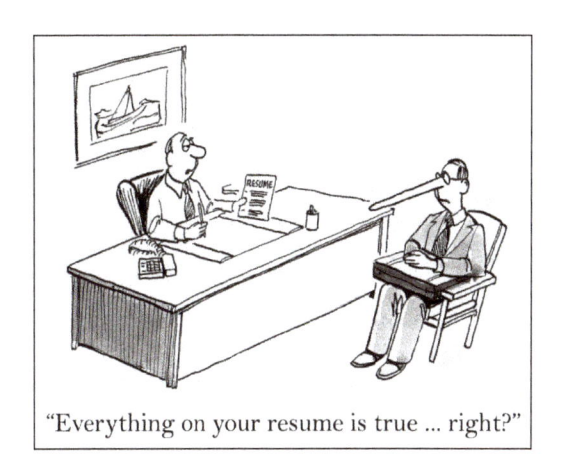

"Everything on your resume is true ... right?"

developed and sharpened at home or in school. **Transferable skills** are skills that can be transferred from one occupation to another. Table 1.5 lists skills in all three areas that are necessary for success in the HIM field.

Table 1.5 Skills to Include on a Résumé

Adaptive Skills	Job Skills	Transferable Skills
punctual	Microsoft Excel®	recording and classifying data
honest	ICD-10-CM	editing
dependable	Microsoft Outlook	team building
organized	encoder software	identifying equipment needs
mature	money management	problem solving
self-confident		
hardworking		

Of the skills discussed here, transferable skills are sometimes the most challenging to define. Still, these skills are the most important to have when entering a career field for the first time or when changing careers.

> **BE AWARE**
>
> A single typo may be enough to send your résumé to the trash bin. Always have someone else review and edit your résumé.

Job Search Tools

Many employment resources are available for RHIT job seekers, including:

- AHIMA's Career Assist Job Bank (membership required): http://careerassist.ahima.org

- State chapters of AHIMA (state HIMAs). A list of state organizations is available at http://IntroHIM.ParadigmCollege.net/StateAHIMA

- *For the Record*, a magazine covering the health information management industry: http://IntroHIM.ParadigmCollege.net/ForTheRecord

- Allied Health Careers (AHC), a health careers employment website: http://IntroHIM.ParadigmCollege.net/AlliedHealthCareers

- Indeed.com, a general employment website: http://indeed.com

For more information on résumé writing and to view sample résumés, visit the Student eResources section of Navigator+.

TAKE THE CHALLENGE

Gina, a student in an HIM program, is developing her résumé and preparing to search for a position in the HIM field. Although she has no work experience in health care, Gina has worked for more than eight years as a prison guard. Identify at least five transferable skills that Gina can include on her résumé.

Ethics

Working in health care requires strong moral values and a willingness to do the right thing every time. Working as a registered health information technician requires the highest personal and professional ethics. **Ethics** are standards of behavior based on moral values. To help guide its members and others working in health information management, AHIMA has developed a code of ethics.

The ethical principles enumerated in the AHIMA Code of Ethics are based on the organization's core values. The principles enumerated in the code apply to all AHIMA members and credentialed persons. Each principle is further illustrated by supporting guidelines that provide a noninclusive list of behaviors and situations. These examples can assist members in understanding how to apply these principles to real-world situations. The guidelines are not, however, intended to be a comprehensive list of all of the situations that may occur.

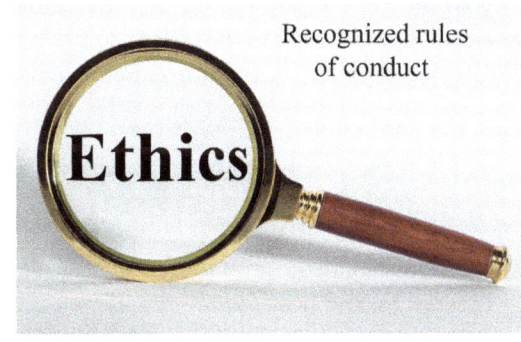

The AHIMA Code of Ethics promotes high professional standards and provides guidelines for ethical conduct.

The AHIMA Code of Ethics:

- promotes high standards of HIM practice
- identifies core values on which the HIM mission is based
- summarizes broad ethical principles that reflect the profession's core values
- establishes a set of ethical principles to be used to guide decision making and actions
- establishes a framework for professional behavior and responsibilities when professional obligations conflict or ethical uncertainties arise
- provides ethical principles by which the general public can hold the HIM professional accountable
- mentors new practitioners on the mission, values, and ethical principles of HIM professionals

The AHIMA Code of Ethics is reprinted in Appendix C of this book. Additionally, ethical issues are highlighted throughout this text in a feature titled *Think Ethics!* that appears both within the body of the text and in the margins. This feature is intended to draw attention to the ethical challenges that HIM professionals may face in the field, particularly in the areas of coding, legal release of information, and staff management. When faced with an ethical decision or issue, consider the following questions:

- Is this illegal?
- Am I being dishonest?

- Does this request make me feel uncomfortable?
- Is this the wrong thing to do?

If the answer to any of these questions is "yes," then the decision or the action may be unethical. Stop immediately and seek additional guidance from a supervisor, an ethics hotline, the facility's ethics and compliance officer, or a trusted mentor or friend. If you are asked to do something unethical and cannot find support or cannot identify an alternative course of action, the best solution may be to leave the employer. Although leaving is a difficult choice, it may be the best choice in the long run.

Chapter Summary

Since 1928, allied health professionals (called *medical librarians, medical record technicians,* and now *health information managers*) have provided expertise in the content and maintenance of health information. Today, the HIM role has expanded beyond the acute care hospital to all areas of health care. Data analysis, patient confidentiality, information maintenance and security, and quality assessment of patient care are the foundations of the HIM profession. HIM's future holds many new opportunities as healthcare organizations continue their transition to the electronic health record.

The health information profession offers a number of employment opportunities for credentialed experts in hospitals and physician offices, with vendors, and as educators. To succeed as an HIM professional requires excellent critical thinking and communication skills, knowledge of medical terminology and procedures, good people skills, and a commitment to the highest personal and professional ethical standards. A graduate with a two-year associate's degree from a CAHIIM-accredited HIM program who takes and passes the national exam will become credentialed as a registered health information technician. Students may take the exam as soon as they begin their last semester of coursework or after graduation.

HIM Review

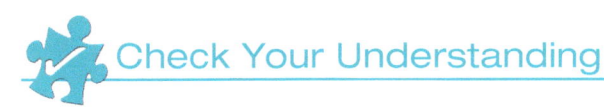

Check Your Understanding

Test your understanding of the material covered in this chapter by completing the following multiple-choice questions. For each question, select the best answer from the choices provided.

1. What is the primary method of communication used in business today?

    a. verbal

    b. written

    c. email

    d. public speaking

2. Which of the skills listed is not required for a job in health information management?

    a. critical thinking

    b. mathematics

    c. communication

    d. computer literacy

3. _____ is an example of good manners.

    a. Making sure you go first

    b. Interrupting others

    c. Being tardy

    d. Saying please and thank you

4. An individual who earns a two-year associate's degree in HIM is qualified to take the national certification exam to become a credentialed _____

    a. RHIT.

    b. RHIA.

    c. CHDA.

    d. CDIP.

5. An EHR coordinator _____

    a. purchases the EHR system for the organization.

    b. does not create an implementation plan.

    c. installs all of the hardware for the EHR system.

    d. develops training materials for the EHR system.

6. _____ collects and reports birth certificate information.

    a. A vital statistics clerk

    b. An HIM supervisor

    c. A privacy officer

    d. An HIM technician

7. A CDI specialist _____

    a. does not need to know coding applications.

    b. works with physicians to ensure documentation reflects the correct diagnoses and procedures.

    c. works closely with the respiratory therapy department.

    d. works in all healthcare settings.

8. When sending an email, always _____

    a. type in all caps.

    b. check spelling and grammar before sending.

    c. a and b

    d. None of the choices are correct.

9. _____ is not a professional quality.

    a. Being in charge of others

    b. Being on time

    c. Common courtesy

    d. Good communication

10. _____ initiated hospital standards of care in 1918.

    a. AMA

    b. AMRA

    c. ACS

    d. AHIMA

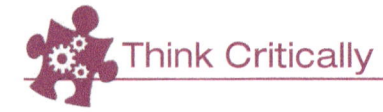

Think Critically

Consider the following real-world scenario and draft a response.

Write a paragraph explaining why health information managers need critical thinking skills. Discuss how these skills help them to succeed when knowledge is not enough.

Sharpen Your Comprehension

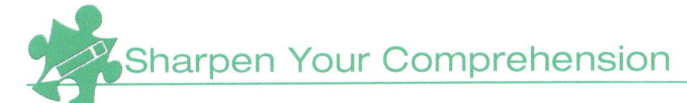

Complete the following matching exercise by selecting, from the list provided, the answer that best matches each of the numbered statements. For each statement, only one answer is correct.

a. AHIMA Foundation
b. adaptive skills
c. computer literacy
d. RHIT
e. privacy officer
f. body language
g. CDI specialist
h. written communication
i. vital statistics clerk
j. hospital medical coder

1. _____ Ensures that every patient's health information is kept completely confidential

2. _____ Communicates with the physician on a patient case that requires additional information

3. _____ Prepares birth and death certificates

4. _____ Provides as an online resource the HIM Body of Knowledge (BoK)

5. _____ A credentialed health information professional with a two-year associate's degree

6. _____ Includes memos, letters, policies and procedures, and email

7. _____ Behaviors and daily living skills that demonstrate a job candidate's ability to fit into an organization's culture

8. _____ One of the skills and talents employers seek in an HIM professional

9. _____ Communication style exhibited by a person crossing his or her arms or sighing loudly

10. _____ Reviews documentation in the medical record to determine which diagnoses and procedures to report and then translates each into an alphanumeric character

Connect Theory to Practice

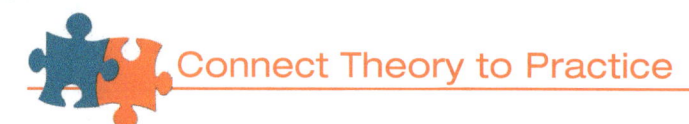

To help translate the concepts presented in this chapter to the workplace, complete the following exercise.

To successfully complete this exercise, you will need to interview an HIM professional who is RHIT certified.

1. Develop 10 to 15 questions to ask this person about his or her job.
2. Submit your questions to the instructor for feedback and approval.
3. Arrange a meeting at the HIM professional's workplace.
4. Meet and interview the HIM professional, using the list of approved questions. Remember to practice the professional skills discussed in this chapter, including courtesy, good communication, and proper attire.
5. Type a one-page summary of your meeting that includes the person's name, place of work, email address, date and time you met, and responses to your questions. Summarize your interview by documenting what you did and did not like about the position, and discuss why you would or would not consider applying for a similar job.

Student eResources

*To enhance your comprehension of the chapter material, go to **Navigator+** and complete the additional practice items as advised by your instructor.*

Chapter Terms

- adaptive skills
- AHIMA Foundation
- American College of Surgeons (ACS)
- American Health Information Management Association (AHIMA)
- body language
- cancer registrar/tumor registrar
- clinical documentation improvement (CDI) specialist
- Commission on Accreditation for Health Informatics and Information Management Education (CAHIIM)
- continuing education (CE)
- critical thinking
- EHR implementation coordinator and trainer
- ethics
- file/scanning and retrieval clerk
- health information management (HIM)
- health record
- HIM technician
- hospital medical coder
- job skills
- medical biller and coder
- medical scribe
- medical transcriptionist
- performance improvement coordinator
- physician office manager
- privacy officer
- professionalism
- résumé
- supervisor/manager
- transferable skills
- vital statistics clerk

> "I am interested in getting people to use the healthcare system at the right time, getting them to see the doctor early enough, before a small health problem turns serious."

—Donna E. Shalala,
Secretary of the US Department of Health
and Human Services (1993–2001)

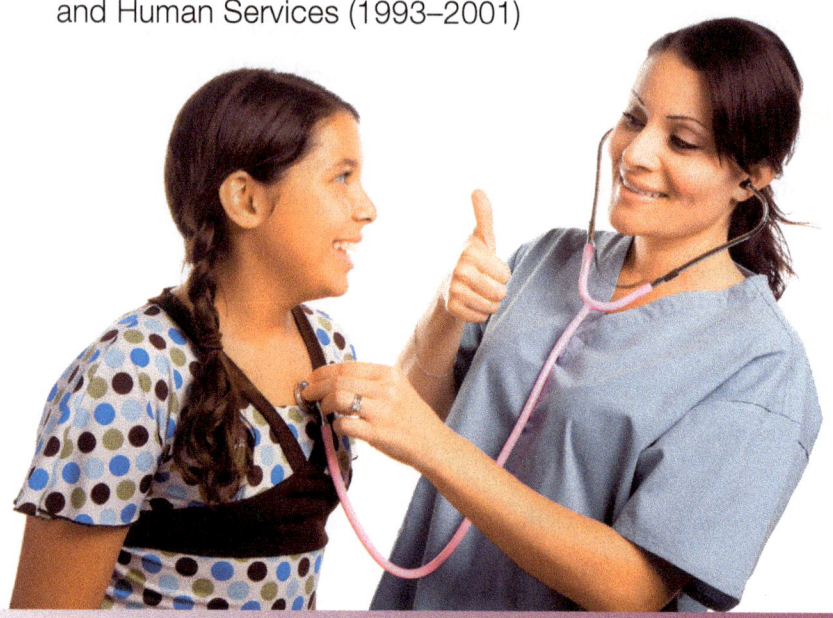

Top 10 Reasons People Go to the Emergency Department

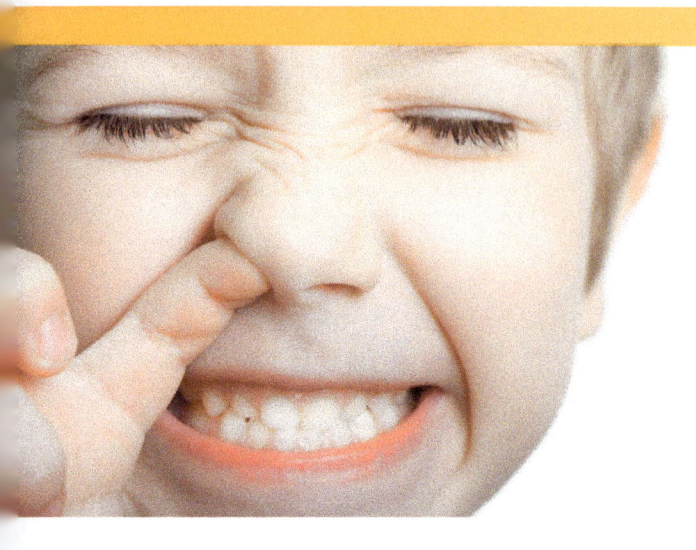

1. Headache
2. Foreign objects in the body
3. Skin infection
4. Back pain
5. Cuts and contusions
6. Upper respiratory infection
7. Sprains and broken bones
8. Toothache
9. Abdominal pain
10. Chest pain

Source: http://health.howstuffworks.com/medicine/10-common-reasons-for-er-visit9.htm

Chapter 2

Healthcare Organizations

The Provision of Health Care

The delivery of health care in the United States has changed significantly over the last century. To better understand our healthcare system today, we should consider the changes that have taken place throughout the years.

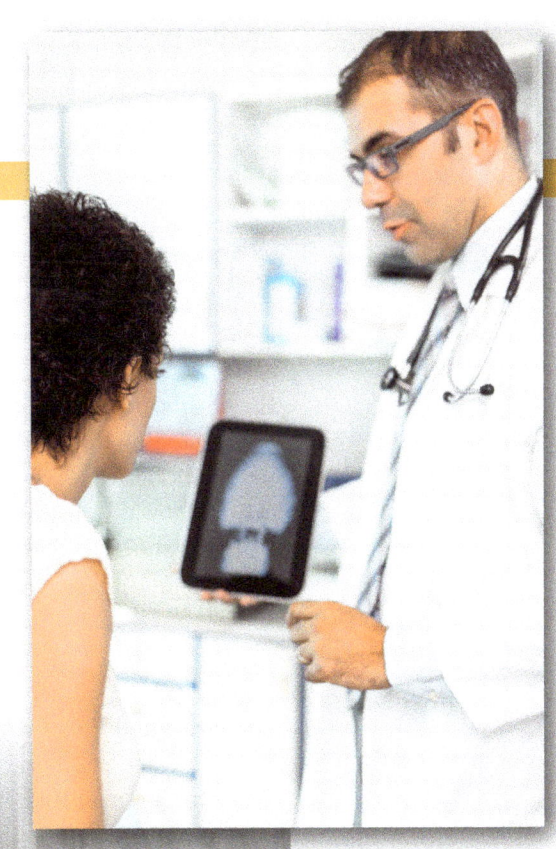

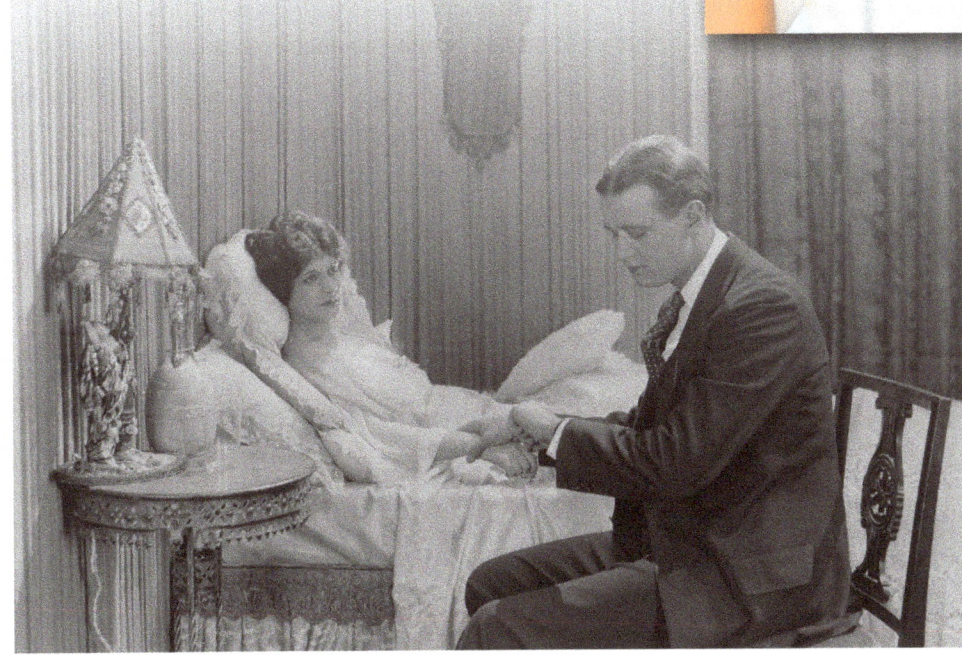

Learning Objectives

- Discuss the evolution of health care.
- Identify different types of health insurance.
- Describe healthcare regulation as it relates to health information management.
- Explain the role of acute care hospitals in the delivery of health care.
- Compare health care provided in acute care facilities to health care provided in alternative settings.
- Understand the role of regulatory bodies in the delivery of health care.

The Evolution of Health Care in the United States

The healthcare system in the United States is complex and like no other in the world. Understanding the development of this system requires a historical perspective. The way medical care is provided and paid for, the government's role in health care, and attitudes toward the provision of care have all changed through the years. Understanding the evolution of US health care is essential to understanding the state of the healthcare system today and many of the issues that impact it.

The 1920s

- Prior to the 1920s, medical "cures" were based less on science and more on folk remedies, trial and error, treatments found in books, and elixirs such as the Snake Oil Liniment sold by traveling medicine men/entertainers. Doctors did not know enough about diseases to be able to offer adequate treatment.
- Very few people had health insurance. Only a few large employers provided some type of hospital insurance for their employees. Everyone else traded, bartered, or paid for health care out of pocket.
- Doctors treated most patients at home.
- Hospitals were more like poorhouses where indigent patients went to die.
- Americans spent, on average, $5 per year on health care, which would be about $100 today.
- As doctors learned more about diseases and effective treatments, fees for their services started to rise.
- Increasingly, treatment shifted to hospital settings as physicians sought to take advantage of new technology (e.g., ultracentrifuge, refined techniques for X-rays, and drug purification and analysis).

- The rise in physician fees, the increase in hospital-based care, and the financial impact of the Great Depression put health care out of reach for many people—both those with health insurance and those without.

The 1930s

Blue Cross (BC) emerged as one of the first formal prepaid health insurance programs in the United States. Baylor Hospital in Dallas, Texas, created Blue Cross as a way to address a patient's inability to pay his or her hospital bills. **Blue Shield (BS)** was developed later to include payments to physicians.

The Blue Cross Blue Shield (BCBS) model charged all customers the same regardless of age, gender, health status, or preexisting medical conditions. BCBS soon became a model for other health insurance plans, and its success later played a significant role in shaping the development of Medicare and Medicaid.

The 1940s–1960s

In the wake of BCBS's success, other insurance companies sprang up. The federal government also began to provide tax incentives to companies that offered health insurance to their employees.

Insurers began to move away from the BCBS model and set different prices for insurance policies based on a variety of factors, including age, gender, health status, and preexisting medical conditions. This change resulted in a market in which the healthiest people were more likely to be insured.

President Harry Truman calls on Congress to create a national health insurance plan. In response, the **American Medical Association (AMA)**, the professional association for physicians, used its powerful lobbying strength to oppose the plan. The AMA feared that government-imposed limitations on insurance reimbursement for specific conditions would impact physicians' willingness to treat those conditions.

Advances in medical equipment and the availability of more treatment options led to an increase in the use of health care. New equipment and treatments resulted in more tests and treatments, increasing the cost of care.

With the government's encouragement, more companies began to include health insurance as an employee benefit. However, many people still had no health insurance, including the poor, the unemployed, those working part-time or temporary jobs, the self-employed, and employees at small companies that did not offer health insurance. When employees retired, their health insurance was terminated.

The 1960s

As health care became more available and the cost of care increased, the concept of national health insurance began to gain acceptance. The government moved slowly, first introducing a form of national health insurance for the elderly.

In 1965, two federal health programs were signed into law: Medicare, a health insurance program for the elderly, and Medicaid, health insurance for the poor and indigent.

The 1970s–2010

Healthcare costs continued to escalate throughout the end of the twentieth century and into the beginning of the twenty-first century due to:

- continued advances in medical technology
- increased competition between hospitals
- large employers choosing to self-insure employee health care rather than contract with private insurers
- rising medication costs
- an increase in lawsuits against providers that pushed up the cost of malpractice premiums for physicians

2010–Present

Many Americans continue to be unable to afford health insurance.

With rapid advances in medical technology, many types of surgical and other procedures that previously required a hospital stay can now be done on an outpatient basis.

Advances in pharmaceutical research and development are simplifying treatment for complex diseases, including HIV and cancer.

In 2010, the federal **Patient Protection and Affordable Care Act**, commonly referred to as the **Affordable Care Act (ACA)** and *Obamacare*, was signed into law. The law was intended to improve the quality and lower the cost of health care, to improve consumer protections, and to expand consumer access to health plans.

The ACA's major provisions include the following:

- Insurers can no longer refuse coverage to individuals with preexisting conditions.
- Young adults can remain on their parents' health insurance policy through age 26.
- Insurers can no longer terminate coverage without a reason.
- Patients have the right to appeal denied claims.
- Patients can use emergency care outside of the plan's network.
- Insurers can no longer set lifetime limits on coverage.
- Cost increases in insurance premiums are now subject to review.
- Individuals without health insurance may be fined.

The ACA also encourages consumers to become more informed and actively involved in their health care through the use of patient portals and personal health records.

> **EXPAND YOUR KNOWLEDGE**
>
> Watch the video *Information Technology Experts Talk about the Next Big Healthcare Apps* at http://IntroHIM.Paradigm College.net/HealthcareApp to learn about the potential of smartphone and tablet applications to increase patient engagement.

Health Insurance

Health insurance is a type of insurance coverage that pays for all or a portion of an individual's healthcare expenses. Individuals can purchase health insurance from a for-profit company, nonprofit company, or government entity, either on their own or through an employer. The insured (an individual) pays the insurer a specific dollar amount annually. In exchange, the insurer agrees to pay for some or all of the insured's medical and surgical expenses. Most often, the insurer makes payments directly to the care provider. A **provider** is an individual or an institution that provides direct patient care. Direct care providers include hospitals, clinics, physician offices, physicians, laboratories, and pharmacies. Depending on the individual's policy, the insurer may cover all of the cost of care, a portion of the cost, or pay for some procedures and not others. In most cases, the patient is required to pay a portion of the cost of care. Payment may take one of several forms or include a combination of payment types. Payment types include the following:

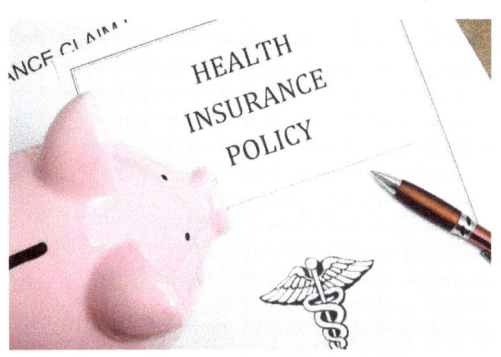

According to Congressional Budget Office estimates, 24 to 25 million Americans will obtain coverage each year through state and federal health insurance exchanges.

- A **copay** is a flat fee paid by the insured at the time services are provided.
- **Coinsurance** requires the insured to pay a share of the cost of care, usually a percentage (rather than a flat fee), after services are provided.
- A **deductible** is the amount of out-of-pocket costs the insured is responsible for each year. The deductible is usually a percentage of the cost of care and must be paid in full before the insurance company will pay a claim.

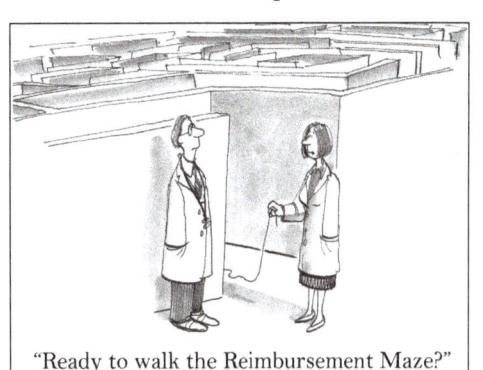

"Ready to walk the Reimbursement Maze?"

BE AWARE

Reimbursement rates for the cost of care vary considerably depending on the insurer, the plan, and/or the contract negotiated between the third-party payer and the care provider.

As the number of insurers and the variety of health insurance plans and options have continued to increase, the insurance marketplace has become more competitive. The introduction in 2013 of federal and state **health insurance exchanges** continued that trend. Authorized under the ACA, health insurance exchanges are government-run insurance marketplaces that are intended to foster competition and improve the quality and affordability of health insurance by lowering premium costs and expanding choice.

Private Health Insurance

Health insurance can be divided into two main categories: private insurance and public insurance. **Private health insurance** is purchased from for-profit entities or nonprofit organizations. Individuals pay a **premium** (a set amount paid monthly or annually) to cover the cost of insurance. Individuals may purchase private insurance through an employer as part of an employee benefits package, or they may purchase it independently. Insurance costs vary depending on the type of plan, the amount of the deductible, and the services covered. In some areas of the country, the insurance market is highly competitive, with many insurers offering a wide variety of plans. In other areas, only a few insurers offer coverage.

Indemnity Plans

Traditional **indemnity plans** reimburse either the patient or the provider for healthcare expenses when they are incurred. These plans are also referred to as **fee-for-service** plans. Individuals pay a predetermined percentage of the cost of services provided, commonly from 15 to 20 percent, and the insurer pays the remaining cost. Indemnity plans allow individuals greater freedom to choose their own physician or hospital than other plan types and may not require participants to select a primary physician or obtain a referral before seeing a specialist.

Managed Care

Managed care is a general term used to describe insurance plans that require participants to use a specific network of physicians, providers, and hospitals in exchange for lower premium costs. There are different types of managed care insurance plans; some offer fewer services and these are often less expensive. One hallmark of managed care is that these plans promote and cover the cost of preventive care more than many other types of plans. This is an effective strategy for reducing the overall cost of care because preventive care is less expensive than treating diseases and illnesses that could have been prevented or treated more effectively if detected early. Since the adoption of the ACA, coverage of preventive care is becoming more prevalent. There are three types of managed care plans, usually referred to by the acronyms *HMO*, *PPO*, and *POS*.

A **health maintenance organization (HMO)** provides health care to its members through its own network of physicians and hospitals. HMO plans may cover only a limited number of visits, tests, or treatments per year. Many HMOs require plan members to designate a **primary care physician (PCP)** for preventive and sick care. The PCP is sometimes referred to as a **gatekeeper** whose role is to authorize access to medical care within the scope of the plan. HMOs use gatekeepers to control costs by limiting patient care to designated provider(s) and necessary services. HMOs also monitor and compare the performance of network physicians on measures such as time spent with patients and services ordered in order to maximize physicians' financial contributions to the HMO.

Preferred provider organizations (PPOs) are similar to HMOs. PPOs contract directly with specific healthcare providers, referred to as *preferred providers*. PPO plans pay a higher percentage of the cost when a preferred provider delivers care. Unlike HMOs, PPOs also pay a portion of the cost for care when a member uses an out-of-network provider.

A **point of service (POS) plan** is a health insurance plan that includes elements of both HMO and PPO plans. Members of POS plans are required to select a network physician as their PCP. This physician is the member's "point of service" and he or she is responsible for monitoring all healthcare services provided to that individual. In a POS plan, the PCP is permitted to refer a patient to an out-of-network specialist or facility, although the insurer will pay less of the cost of care. POS plans lower healthcare costs by limiting patient choice.

Public Health Insurance

Public health insurance refers to health insurance offered by state and federal governments to individuals who meet specific criteria, such as age or income. Public insurance programs also provide health insurance to individuals who cannot obtain insurance in the private market. Public insurance should not be confused with publicly funded health care, which is health care that is subsidized by the government. The primary public health insurance programs that are federally funded are Medicare, Medicaid, and the Children's Health Insurance Program (CHIP). Other public insurance programs exist for individuals who do not qualify for Medicare, Medicaid, or CHIP. These are managed by individual states, and the availability of plans and coverage varies by state.

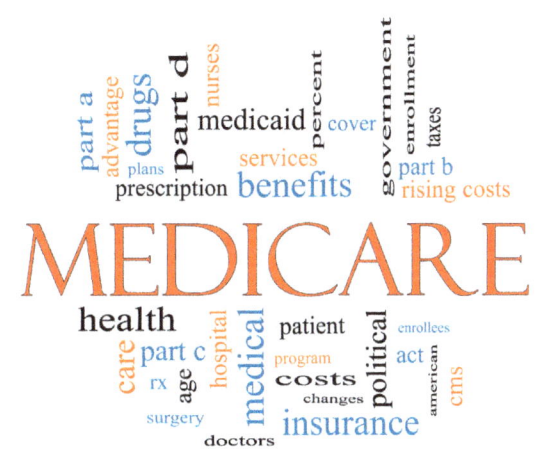

Medicare is not a single health insurance program, but a group of related programs.

Medicare

Medicare is a federal health insurance program, administered by the **Centers for Medicare & Medicaid Services (CMS)**, that primarily serves elderly Americans. Medicare was signed into law in 1965 to provide healthcare coverage to people age 65 and older. Over time, Medicare eligibility has expanded to include some individuals receiving Social Security disability payments and those diagnosed with end-stage renal disease or Lou Gehrig's disease. Medicare coverage is broken down into two main categories (the Original Medicare Plan and the Medicare Advantage Plan) and four parts. Parts A, B, and D relate to what is covered. Part C is specific to how insurance is provided.

Medicare Part A is a hospital insurance plan. It covers inpatient care provided in a skilled nursing facility, a critical access hospital, or another type of hospital. Hospice and some home health care may also be covered under Part A if certain criteria are met.

Medicare Part B covers outpatient care, physician services, physical and occupational therapy, and additional home health care.

Medicare Part C, also known as the **Medicare Advantage Plan**, is Medicare coverage provided by a federally approved private insurance company. It includes both Parts A and B.

Medicare Part D consists of a menu of prescription drug plans. Each plan includes a specific list of covered medications, called a **formulary**. Individuals choose the plan that best supports their needs based on drugs they are prescribed.

The federal government continues to manage the **Original Medicare Plan**, which consists of Medicare Parts A and B (hospital and medical insurance, respectively). Plan

Think Ethics!

According to the World Health Organization (WHO), every person has the right to timely, acceptable, and affordable health care, regardless of ability to pay. But not everyone agrees that health care is a basic right. What do you think? Read more about the right to health care at http://IntroHIM.ParadigmCollege.net/WHO.

Chapter 2   Healthcare Organizations

participants have the option of adding a standalone Part D plan that covers prescription medications. The Original Medicare Plan is a fee-for-service plan that includes a deductible and a copay or coinsurance. An individual who qualifies for Medicare is automatically enrolled in the Original Medicare Plan unless he or she selects the Medicare Advantage Plan, Part C.

Some individuals also choose to purchase a **Medigap policy** from a private insurer to help cover out-of-pocket expenses that are not covered under Medicare. This policy is sometimes referred to as a *supplemental insurance plan*. Items covered by a Medigap policy include copays or coinsurance, deductibles, and other similar expenses that are not covered by Medicare or Medicare Advantage.

Accountable care organizations (ACOs) are groups that come together for the primary purpose of providing coordinated care to Medicare patients, especially patients who suffer from chronic illnesses. These voluntary groups are comprised of physicians, hospitals, and other direct care providers. Care coordination is intended to improve the quality of care while reducing medical errors and duplication of services. Care coordination is also intended to reduce costs by delivering high-quality care in the most cost-effective manner.

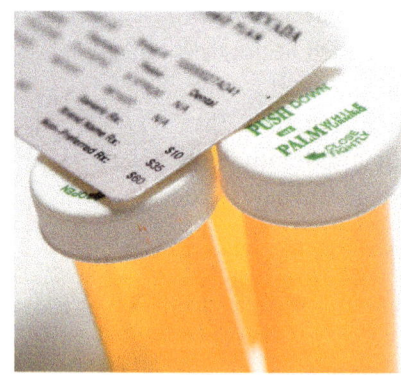

Most Medicare prescription-drug plans have a coverage gap, also called a *donut hole*. After a Medicare patient has spent a specific dollar amount on covered drugs in a given year ($2,850 in 2014), the patient must pay additional out-of-pocket costs for prescription drugs until he or she reaches Medicare's yearly spending limit for out-of-pocket expenses. Under the ACA, however, the gap is shrinking and is expected to close by 2020.

Medicaid and CHIP

Medicaid is a health insurance program for low-income Americans. It is a jointly funded state and federal program administered at the state level. Eligibility for Medicaid is determined by income and family size. Each state designs its own Medicaid program in terms of eligibility, application process, access to care, and services provided.

The **Children's Health Insurance Program (CHIP)** is a Medicaid program specifically for children whose families earn too much to qualify for Medicaid but not enough to afford private insurance. CHIP currently provides health insurance for more than 8 million children in the United States.

TAKE THE CHALLENGE

Look up the Medicaid program for your state. Identify the eligibility requirements and application/enrollment procedures. Also look at the Medicaid/CHIP state plan amendments (SPAs) to view recent changes in your state's plan.

Workers' compensation is insurance that covers employees injured on the job. It provides some wage replacement and medical benefits. An employee who accepts workers' compensation relinquishes the right to sue an employer for negligence related to the injury. Plans vary by jurisdiction. Workers' compensation is a state-administered program, but some federal funding is provided to offset the cost to the states.

Healthcare Regulation

Health care is heavily regulated. Healthcare facilities and providers are regulated at the federal, state, and local levels on matters such as the provision of care, care settings, the licensing of healthcare professionals, the privacy and the security of patient information, and the protection of patients' rights.

Healthcare organizations and providers are also subject to oversight by nongovernmental organizations through accreditation processes that evaluate and monitor performance based on best practices and other criteria.

Accreditation

Accreditation is granted to an organization that has met a set of predetermined standards following a peer review process conducted by an impartial, external accrediting organization. Accreditation is a private, voluntary activity. Healthcare facilities seek accreditation as a way to assess and improve the care they provide. Accreditation also communicates to the public that the organization has met or exceeded standards that reflect best practices in health care.

The **Joint Commission** is one of the most comprehensive and well-known accrediting organizations in health care. The Joint Commission accredits more than 20,000 healthcare organizations and programs in the United States, including hospitals; ambulatory, rehabilitation, long-term, and behavioral healthcare facilities; health plans; home health providers; laboratories; and other services.

The Joint Commission is an independent, nonprofit organization. Although accreditation by the Joint Commission is voluntary, it is recognized nationally as a symbol of quality that demonstrates an organization's commitment to meeting performance standards. To maintain Joint Commission accreditation, a healthcare facility must undergo on-site inspection by a Joint Commission survey team every three years. Without Joint Commission accreditation, a healthcare organization may not be eligible to receive Medicare funding or may be required to undergo a separate Medicare review process.

Other accrediting organizations in health care are specific to the type of care provided. The **Commission on Accreditation of Rehabilitation Facilities (CARF)** is one example. As its name implies, CARF accredits a wide variety of rehabilitation facilities and programs, including medical, behavioral health, and aging services. All accrediting bodies perform essentially the same function: evaluating an organization or a program against best practices and attesting that it meets or exceeds the standards set by the accrediting body.

An organization may choose to be accredited by more than one accrediting body. Each accreditation offers different benefits. An organization that has been accredited by

CARF, for example, has met the strict accreditation standards for the provision of rehabilitative care. Some managed care organizations require that a facility be accredited by CARF as a condition of reimbursement. The same facility may also choose to seek accreditation from the Joint Commission, which provides a comprehensive quality review of the entire facility rather than just its rehabilitative care services.

Licensing

All hospitals and healthcare facilities are required to have a license. Healthcare licensing is carried out by a governmental agency, usually at the state level and most commonly by the state department of health or the state department of public health. A **license** grants a healthcare facility the authority to operate and grants a healthcare provider the authority to practice within its scope of care. Licensure helps to ensure that facilities and providers meet minimum standards of quality and competency. A medical or facility license must be renewed periodically, just like a driver's license. For facilities, licensing often involves an on-site inspection and documentation of activities and outcomes. A healthcare facility may have its license revoked temporarily or permanently if it fails to meet the conditions required for licensure. Criteria for licensing and revocation vary by state. Table 2.1 provides a sample of licensing requirements issued by the Oklahoma Department of Health that pertain to health information management.

Table 2.1 Oklahoma Department of Health Licensing Requirements

Topic	Requirement
310:667-19-3. Maintenance	(a) A medical record shall be maintained for every patient admitted for care in the hospital. Such records shall be kept confidential.
310:667-19-6. Centralization of reports	(a) All clinical information pertaining to a patient's stay shall be centralized in the patient's record.
310:667-19-8. Content	(a) The medical record shall contain sufficient information to justify the diagnosis and warrant the treatment provided.
310:667-19-12. Outpatient medical records	(a) Outpatient medical records shall be maintained and correlated with other hospital medical records.
310:667-19-14. Retention and preservation of records	(a) State retention requirements. Medical records shall be retained a minimum of five (5) years beyond the date the patient was last seen or a minimum of three (3) years beyond the date of the patient's death. Records of newborns or minors shall be retained three (3) years past the age of majority.

Source: Oklahoma Department of Health

Certification

Healthcare organizations can also obtain **certification**. To receive payment from Medicare and Medicaid, healthcare entities must be certified by the CMS. Certification requires a healthcare entity to demonstrate its compliance with the health and safety standards spelled out in the CMS **Conditions for Coverage (CfCs)** and **Conditions of Participation (CoPs)**.

The following is just one example of a CoPs regulation related to the patient health record:

> A medical history and physical examination be completed and documented for each patient no more than 30 days before or 24 hours after admission or registration, but prior to surgery or a procedure requiring anesthesia services. The medical history and physical examination must be completed and documented by a physician (as defined in section 1861(r) of the Act), an oral maxillofacial surgeon, or other qualified licensed individual in accordance with State law and hospital policy.

To be in compliance with this requirement, a facility must have the appropriate policies, procedures, and monitoring in place and must educate physicians about the requirement, if necessary.

Healthcare Organizations

Health care is provided in many different types of facilities, which are often distinguished by the level or the intensity of services provided, the type of care provided, or the patient population served.

For example, a hospital designated as a **level one trauma center** has an emergency room equipped and staffed to care for the most severely injured or ill patients. Smaller **community hospitals** are equipped to treat some critically ill patients in certain circumstances; however, these hospitals primarily provide basic diagnostic services and treatment for less severe conditions.

Some facilities specialize in providing care for specific patient populations—children or veterans, for example. Other facilities provide care to patients suffering from a particular type of illness, such as a psychiatric condition or a chronic illness that requires long-term care.

Acute Care Hospitals

An **acute care hospital** treats patients in the acute phase of an illness. An **acute illness** is an illness or an injury with a rapid onset that is severe in nature but short in duration. A patient may stay in an acute care hospital for a few hours or a few weeks. Acute care hospitals also provide outpatient services, such as diagnostic testing (labs and X-rays), treatment, and emergency care, both to ensure patients have access to these services and to more fully utilize the equipment and the personnel within the facility. A stay in an acute care hospital is usually less than 28 days, but the average stay is two to four days. A woman giving birth commonly stays in the hospital for one to two days, a patient with extensive surgery may stay one to

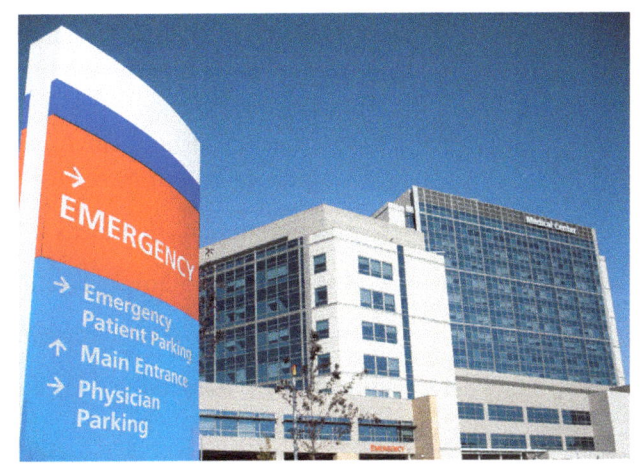

According to the American Hospital Association, in January 2014 there were 5,723 registered hospitals in the United States and 920,829 staffed hospital beds.

two weeks, and an acute psychiatric patient may stay up to four weeks. Other patients (e.g., major trauma patients, premature infants, patients waiting for a transplant) may stay much longer than 28 days.

Acute care facilities are staffed by highly skilled providers and offer sophisticated diagnostic testing and equipment that are only available in that environment. Some of the most common conditions treated at an acute care hospital are myocardial infarction (heart attack), traumatic injury, childbirth, and appendicitis. Surgeries for tumor excision and other conditions are also commonly performed.

Acute care hospitals also treat patients suffering from chronic illnesses who may require short-term hospitalization for pain or symptom management. A **chronic illness** is a long-developing, persistent illness that may have residual effects, such as persistent shortness of breath. Common chronic illnesses that may require hospitalization include exacerbation of chronic obstructive pulmonary disease, congestive heart disease, and chronic renal failure. Patients with chronic illnesses experience periods of time when the condition and its symptoms are well controlled. At other times, the condition becomes acute, and the patient may experience severe and possibly life-threatening symptoms that require hospitalization.

Because the level and the intensity of services available in an acute care facility are not available in other types of healthcare facilities, patients may move from one type of facility to another, depending on the level of service needed. A patient in a long-term care facility (nursing home) who develops pneumonia may be transferred to an acute care hospital for more intensive monitoring and nursing services and for diagnosis and treatment.

Classification of Acute Care Hospitals

There are many different ways to categorize hospitals, such as by size or kind of care provided, but hospitals are most commonly classified as urban, rural, teaching, or osteopathic. Medicare classifies a hospital as either urban or rural based on the metropolitan statistical area it serves. Hospitals can, however, be reclassified from rural to urban if they meet certain criteria.

Rural hospitals are located in small cities and rural areas at some distance from critical access hospitals. Rural hospitals typically offer basic health care. Patients with complex or serious medical issues may be stabilized at a rural hospital before being transferred to a larger medical facility. The American Hospital Association (AHA) defines a *rural hospital* as a hospital that meets one or more of the following criteria:

- 100 or fewer inpatient beds
- 4,000 or fewer admissions annually
- located outside of a metropolitan statistical area

A **critical access hospital (CAH)** is a small facility that provides limited outpatient and inpatient hospital services. CAHs are most often located in rural areas but may be located in nonrural areas under a special provision that allows qualified hospital providers to be treated as rural for the purpose of becoming a CAH.

Urban hospitals are located in large and midsized cities. These facilities tend to provide a higher level of care than rural hospitals because of the availability of sophisticated diagnostic equipment and a highly trained workforce. Medicare reimbursement is higher for patients in urban hospitals because these facilities provide a more advanced level of care and, as a result, have higher per-patient costs.

Teaching hospitals are affiliated with medical schools and provide medical students, interns, and residents with opportunities to observe and acquire hands-on training in comprehensive healthcare facilities that have patient populations with a wide variety of illnesses, injuries, and conditions. Teaching hospitals also train other healthcare professionals, including nurses and allied health workers.

In an **osteopathic hospital**, doctors of osteopathic medicine (DOs) provide the majority of care. This is consistent with the philosophy of osteopathic medicine, which emphasizes the whole person, rather than the treatment of specific symptoms or conditions, and the relationship of one body system to another. It places less emphasis on the use of pharmaceutical treatments and surgical interventions. The number of osteopathic hospitals is declining, however, as more and more DOs begin practicing at traditional acute care hospitals.

Ownership of Acute Care Hospitals

Acute care hospitals are commonly defined by ownership. The majority of these hospitals are either nonprofit or government owned; a smaller percentage are for-profit hospitals, also referred to as *investor-owned hospitals*. Ownership should not affect the quality of care or a facility's ability to become licensed, accredited, or certified.

A **for-profit/investor-owned hospital** is owned by private investors or public shareholders. These facilities can realize a profit by providing efficient care at lower costs. Over the last 20 years, the number of for-profit facilities in the United States has increased significantly with the growth of large national hospital chains.

A **nonprofit hospital** is a partially or fully tax-exempt organization that provides care to patients regardless of their ability to pay and provides charity care and community benefits in accordance with state and federal guidelines.

Military hospitals are designated for use by active duty and retired military personnel, military dependents and survivors, and other groups under special circumstances. These hospitals are run by the Department of Defense (DOD) or the Department of Veterans Affairs (VA). The DOD also operates the TRICARE health insurance program that serves both active and retired uniformed service members and their families. TRICARE offers both managed care and fee-for-service plans. Healthcare providers working in military facilities may be military personnel or civilian contractors.

Governing Bodies

A **governing body** is a group of individuals who are legally responsible for the operation of a hospital. Many times the governing body is composed of community and business leaders as well as representatives from the hospital administration and the medical staff (physicians with admitting privileges at the hospital). Governing body roles and responsibilities are defined by both Joint Commission accreditation standards and Medicare Conditions of Participation.

Other Healthcare Organizations

Healthcare services are provided in many nonacute-care hospital settings. These are often referred to as *alternative care sites* or simply *nonacute care sites*, and they include long-term, rehabilitative, and behavioral settings as well as outpatient facilities.

Long-Term Acute Care Hospital (LTAC)

Long-term acute care hospitals (LTACs) treat patients who are no longer in need of the diagnostic and treatment services available in an acute care setting but who are still too ill or injured to be discharged home or to a skilled nursing facility. Patient stays at LTACs average more than 25 days, rather than the two- to four-day average stay for patients in an acute care facility. LTAC patients commonly receive pain management, comprehensive rehabilitation services, intravenous antibiotic administration, wound care, and ventilator weaning. The cost of care in a LTAC facility is lower than in an acute care facility equipped with more-expensive diagnostic equipment and a more highly trained staff. Patients are often moved to a long-term acute care hospital when Medicare or Medicaid will no longer pay for acute care.

Rehabilitation Care Facilities

Rehabilitation is the process of restoring an individual's health and/or quality of life through therapy and education. Rehabilitation facilities treat patients who have an illness or injury that limits their ability to function. The goal of rehabilitation is to improve function, to increase independence, and to improve the patient's quality of life. Rehabilitation care can be provided either on an inpatient or outpatient basis and is used to treat many different type of conditions, from brain injury to knee replacement surgery.

Rehabilitation facilities are accredited by the Joint Commission and CARF. Facilities that treat Medicare and Medicaid patients must also follow the Conditions of Participation for **comprehensive outpatient rehabilitation facilities (CORFs)**, which provide diagnostic, therapeutic, and restorative services for the rehabilitation of injury, disability, or sickness.

Ambulatory Care Facilities

Ambulatory care includes a wide spectrum of services delivered in a number of different settings. **Ambulatory care** is outpatient care delivered during a single day with no overnight stay. It may involve a visit to a physician office, lab tests, outpatient or day surgery center, the emergency department (without hospitalization), outpatient cancer treatment, or some other procedure or treatment.

Outpatient Surgery Centers

Outpatient surgery is also known as *day surgery, ambulatory surgery*, or *same-day surgery*. The number of surgical procedures performed on an outpatient basis has been rising as advances in medical technology permit the use of less invasive surgical techniques. For example, a routine appendectomy is now performed using endoscopic instruments that allow a surgeon to make a very small incision. In the past, this surgery usually required a 3- to 5-inch incision and a few days in the hospital, but now patients can go home the same day. Improvements in anesthesia and pain control have also contributed to the rise of outpatient surgeries. Common surgical procedures performed in an ambulatory setting include tonsillectomy, hernia repair, some cosmetic surgeries, cataract surgery, and gallbladder removal. Diagnostic procedures commonly performed in an outpatient surgery setting include diagnostic endoscopy exams such as bronchoscopies, gastroscopies, and colonoscopies and many types of tumor and bone marrow biopsies.

Emergency Departments

The **emergency department (ED)** in a hospital is one of the most active areas in ambulatory care. Conditions treated in the ED range from minor illnesses and injuries, such as broken bones and fevers, to critical conditions like myocardial infarction and traumatic head injury. ED staff will assess the severity of the condition to determine whether the patient needs to be admitted for inpatient diagnostic testing and treatment or transferred to another facility for treatment. Patients may be observed for a period of time to determine if hospitalization is needed.

Observational Services

As mentioned previously, there may be times when a patient needs to be hospitalized temporarily for observation, particularly if the patient's condition could deteriorate quickly. Most often, these are patients admitted through the ED. In these instances, observation is considered outpatient for billing purposes. The patient may be held in the ED for observation or moved to a hospital room. Generally, the care team must determine within 24 hours if the patient should be admitted or discharged.

Diagnostic Clinics

There are many types of ambulatory diagnostic clinics. Some are part of a hospital and others are freestanding. Some of the most common types of outpatient diagnostic clinics are described here.

Laboratory clinics   Outpatient laboratory clinics perform a variety of complex diagnostic tests on bodily fluids and tissues for physician offices that do not have lab capabilities. Outpatient lab clinics are convenient for patients and cost-effective for physicians. Some hospitals also provide outpatient laboratory testing as a way to increase utilization of their laboratory services.

Radiology   An outpatient radiology clinic performs computerized tomography (CT) scans, magnetic resonance imaging (MRI), ultrasounds, and X-rays for physician practices that do not provide these services. Physicians trained to interpret the scans review the images and provide a written summary of findings to the ordering physician.

Cardiology   Most often located within a hospital, outpatient cardiology clinics provide consultation and management of chronic diseases, diagnostic testing (e.g., ultrasound, Holter monitoring, and stress testing), interventional procedures (e.g., placement of pacemakers and defibrillators), and cardiac rehabilitation, including preventive education and medically supervised exercise programs. Some clinics may also provide preoperative risk assessments. Cardiology clinics offer many services that are not available in any other setting.

Endoscopy   The general term for a procedure that uses a scope to look inside the body. Common endoscopic exams include the stomach exam (gastroscopy), the esophagus exam (esophagoscopy), and the colon exam (colonoscopy). In addition to these screening exams, endoscopy clinics specialize in the evaluation and the treatment of digestive and abdominal tract conditions. These clinics can be located within a hospital or as a stand-alone facility.

Other types of outpatient clinics include mental or behavioral health centers that provide substance abuse treatment and mental health services, physical therapy clinics, and chemotherapy and radiation therapy centers that specialize in cancer treatment.

Physician Offices

Physician offices are another type of ambulatory care setting—one that most people are quite familiar with. Some physicians work as solo practitioners while others work together in a small practice or in a group medical practice, defined as 25 or more eligible professionals in the same practice. The scope of practice for a physician office is somewhat dependent on the specialties of its physicians. Many practices see patients for routine physical exams and to treat minor illnesses and injuries. Other specialty practices may perform medical procedures such as biopsies and endoscopic examinations.

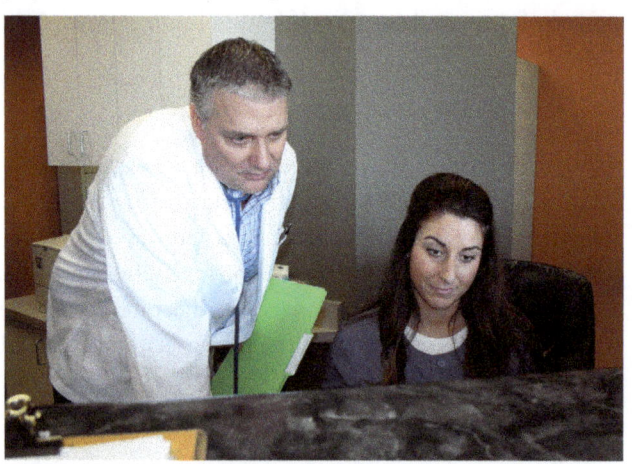

A primary care practice is usually the patient's first point of contact with the healthcare system. Primary care practices provide health promotion, disease prevention, health maintenance, counseling, and patient education, as well as diagnosis and treatment of acute and chronic illnesses.

Home Health Care

The term **home health care** refers to a wide range of healthcare services provided to a patient at home or another place of residence. Some nursing home patients receive home health care, such as oxygen therapy, if such services are not provided by the nursing home. The use of home health care is increasing as it becomes possible to provide more types of advanced care at home and as more insurers begin to cover the cost of in-home care. Home care is also less expensive than nursing home care, and many patients prefer the convenience of receiving treatment at home.

Skilled nursing services available at home include postsurgical wound care, IV therapy, injections, and monitoring for vital health stats (blood pressure, oxygen saturation level, etc.). Types of specialty care provided at home include physical and respiratory therapy; social services, such as psychosocial assessment and counseling; resource referral and advocacy; and discharge planning. Durable medical equipment (DME), such as hospital beds, wheelchairs, oxygen concentrators, and blood pressure monitoring/transmission equipment, can also be provided to patients at home.

Long-Term Care

Long-term care (LTC) is a general term that describes supportive care provided to individuals who are no longer able to live independently at home. In LTC, the patient is typically referred to as a *resident* since the LTC facility becomes the patient's residence. Many LTC residents are not sick but are unable to care for themselves.

Long-term care facilities provide medical services such as medication administration, vital signs monitoring, physical and respiratory therapies, and nonmedical support—assisting residents with activities of daily living. **Activities of daily living (ADLs)** include eating, bathing, dressing, toileting, transferring (walking), and continence (the ability to control bladder and bowel functions), the kinds of things that an individual could normally do in the course of daily living. The extent to which the resident can perform ADLs determines the level of care provided.

A LTC facility may provide more than one service. A **skilled care facility** provides nursing or rehabilitation care for patients in need of speech, physical, respiratory, psychological, or other therapy.

An **intermediate care facility** provides care to disabled and elderly individuals with nonacute chronic illness. This facility type offers less intensive care than a hospital or a skilled long-term care facility.

Residential care/assisted living facilities provide support services to adults who cannot live alone but do not require skilled or intermediate care. Residents in these facilities live independently in their own apartments but may share meals in a communal dining room. On-site nursing staff are available for vital signs monitoring, routine wellness checks, and medication administration. These facilities often provide transportation to doctors, shopping centers, and other planned activity sites as well.

Adult day care is an organized program of services provided in a community group setting during the daytime hours only. Adult day care provides older and disabled individuals with social, physical, and emotional support and provides respite for the primary in-home caregiver.

Hospice

The philosophy of **hospice** care is to provide symptom and pain control to patients in the terminal phase of an illness, commonly defined as someone with a life expectancy of less than six months. Hospice is provided in a variety of settings, including in the home, in a long-term care facility or acute care hospital, and in a facility specifically for hospice patients. The terminally ill patient, family, and close friends are all considered hospice clients. The type of services provided varies depending on the individual hospice program. Typical hospice services include physician services, nursing care, social services, homemaker services, trained volunteer support, **respite care** (temporary institutional care of a dependent elderly, ill, or handicapped person to provide relief for his or her usual caregivers), and **bereavement** (grief) support for the patient's caregivers and family members.

Behavioral Health Care

Behavioral health care is the preferred term for mental health care and substance abuse treatment. Care is provided in inpatient, residential, and outpatient facilities and through community-sponsored programs.

Accreditation for Alternative Care Facilities

The Joint Commission is the primary accrediting body for healthcare facilities; however, there are a number of other accrediting organizations for alternative care facilities. Table 2.2 lists the accrediting bodies for each facility type.

Table 2.2 Accreditation for Alternative Care Facilities

Type of Facility	Primary Accrediting Bodies
Long-Term Acute Care	Joint Commission
Rehabilitation Care	Joint Commission
	Commission on Accreditation of Rehabilitation Facilities
	Comprehensive Outpatient Rehabilitation Facility (CORF)
Ambulatory Care	Joint Commission
	Accreditation Association for Ambulatory Health Care (AAAHC)
Home Health	Joint Commission
	Community Health Accreditation Program (CHAP)
Long-Term Care	Joint Commission
Hospice	Joint Commission
Behavioral Health Care	Joint Commission
	Commission on Accreditation of Rehabilitation Facilities
	National Committee for Quality Assurance (NCQA)

Healthcare Organizations and Associations

The **American Hospital Association (AHA)** is the national professional organization that represents hospitals and healthcare networks. The AHA advocates for its members on issues of healthcare policy and regulation. It also conducts research and provides education and training.

The **American College of Surgeons (ACS)** was founded in 1913 to improve the quality of care for surgical patients through improved education and training. Surgeons can earn the designation FACS (Fellow, American College of Surgeons). This designation is awarded after an extensive evaluation of the surgeon's education and training, qualifications, surgical competence, and ethical conduct. The ACS conducted its first review of health records more than 100 years ago using documentation to learn more about how care was provided. These early reviews were instrumental in the creation of the Joint Commission and served as a catalyst for initiatives to improve the quality of care.

The **World Health Organization (WHO)** provides leadership on global public health issues and initiatives and works within the United Nations to coordinate and direct public health programs. WHO is neither a regulatory agency nor a direct provider of health care.

Chapter Summary

Health care is provided in a number of different settings, from routine ambulatory care provided in physician offices to in-home services provided to dying patients. It is important for anyone working in health care to be knowledgeable about the setting and the type of care provided in each setting.

Since Blue Cross's first offerings in the 1920s, health insurance has evolved as the primary way individuals pay for health care. Many people purchase health insurance in the private market from for-profit and nonprofit companies. Federal and state government offer public insurance programs for the elderly, children, and other groups that meet specific criteria.

The insurance marketplace is highly competitive, but the market is also changing. The passage of the federal Patient Protection and Affordable Care Act has resulted in the creation of federal and state health insurance exchanges in which people can comparison shop for policies.

Healthcare facilities are highly regulated by governmental agencies and by professional organizations such as the Joint Commission that provide voluntary accreditation and certification. Each licensing, certification, and accreditation entity has its specific requirements, including many important standards and guidelines that govern the maintenance and the use of patient health information.

HIM Review

Check Your Understanding

Test your understanding of the material covered in this chapter by completing the following multiple-choice questions. For each question, select the best answer from the choices provided.

1. _____ is the preferred term for mental health care and substance abuse treatment.

    a. Rehabilitation care

    b. Behavioral health care

    c. Substance abuse care

    d. Social work intervention

2. _____ is an insurance plan with contracts in place for physicians, providers, and hospitals to provide medical care at a reduced cost for members of the plan.

   a. Indemnity insurance
   b. Medicare Part B
   c. Original Medicare Plan
   d. Managed care

3. _____ is a first-line physician who directs preventive and sick care.

   a. A physician extender
   b. A case manager
   c. A primary care physician
   d. A medical staff member

4. Utilization of home health care is growing because _____

   a. of advances in technology.
   b. insurers are covering more of this type of care.
   c. it is more convenient for patients.
   d. All of the choices are correct.

5. _____ describes a payment arrangement in which the insured pays a share, usually a percentage, of the claim.

   a. Coinsurance
   b. A copay
   c. A deductible
   d. Health insurance

6. The goal of hospice care is to _____

   a. relieve pain and control symptoms.
   b. provide supportive services to the family.
   c. provide supportive care to friends.
   d. All of the choices are correct.

7. LTAC is the appropriate treatment facility for _____
   a. a patient who needs care at a level between an acute care hospital and a nursing home.
   b. a patient under observation to determine if hospital admission is appropriate.
   c. rehabilitation treatment regardless of the patient's medical condition.
   d. a condition requiring skilled nursing care.

8. Things an individual normally does to take care of himself or herself are referred to as _____
   a. care plans.
   b. activities of daily living.
   c. maintenance activities.
   d. self-care.

9. _____ is used to help a patient develop to his or her fullest potential.
   a. Occupational therapy
   b. Behavioral health care
   c. Physical therapy
   d. Rehabilitation

10. A chronic illness is defined as _____
    a. a complication of another illness.
    b. a condition in which the patient is constantly experiencing symptoms.
    c. a long-developing, persistent illness.
    d. an illness with rapid onset that is severe in nature but short in duration.

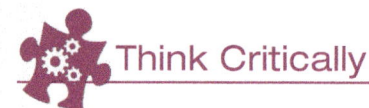

Think Critically

Consider the following real-world scenario and draft a response.

The acute care hospital where you work is due to undergo a Joint Commission accreditation survey within the next six months. You have been asked to prepare a short presentation for the noncredentialed HIM staff to help them understand Joint Commission accreditation. Access the document *Facts about Hospital Accreditation* at http://IntroHIM.ParadigmCollege.net/HospitalAccreditation. Use this document to draft an outline for your presentation. You may also use other resources to create your outline.

Sharpen Your Comprehension

Complete the following matching exercise by selecting, from the list provided, the answer that best matches each of the numbered statements. For each statement, only one answer is correct.

a. accreditation
b. acute illness
c. bereavement
d. Conditions of Participation
e. gatekeeper
f. medical staff
g. Medigap policy
h. Patient Protection and Affordable Care Act
i. point of service
j. provider

1. _____ State of sorrow following a death or a loss

2. _____ Physicians who have admitting privileges at a hospital

3. _____ The primary care physician whose role is to authorize access to medical care

4. _____ Recognition given to an organization that has met a set of standards

5. _____ Health insurance plan that includes elements of both HMO and PPO plans

6. _____ Guidelines developed by the Centers for Medicare & Medicaid Services

7. _____ Law intended to improve the quality and the cost of care, improve consumer protections, and expand access to health care

8. _____ Has a rapid onset that is severe in nature but of short duration

9. _____ An individual or an institution that provides direct patient care

10. _____ Covers out-of-pocket expenses that are not covered under Medicare

Chapter 2   Healthcare Organizations

Connect Theory to Practice

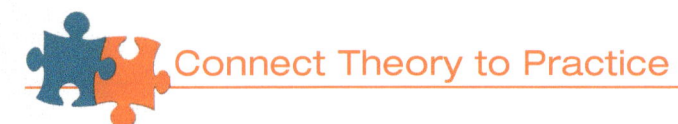

To help translate the concepts presented in this chapter to the workplace, complete the following exercise.

Choose five of the different types of healthcare facilities discussed in this chapter and compare and contrast the patient care provided by each type of facility. Explain why you think these different levels of care are necessary.

Student eResources

*To enhance your comprehension of the chapter material, go to **Navigator+** and complete the additional practice items as advised by your instructor.*

Chapter Terms

accountable care organization (ACO)
accreditation
activities of daily living (ADLs)
acute care hospital
acute illness
adult day care
ambulatory care
American College of Surgeons (ACS)
American Hospital Association (AHA)
American Medical Association (AMA)
behavioral health care
bereavement
Blue Cross (BC)
Blue Shield (BS)
Centers for Medicare & Medicaid Services (CMS)
certification
Children's Health Insurance Program (CHIP)
chronic illness
coinsurance
Commission on Accreditation of Rehabilitation Facilities (CARF)
community hospital
comprehensive outpatient rehabilitation facility (CORF)
Conditions for Coverage (CfCs)
Conditions of Participation (CoPs)
copay
critical access hospital (CAH)
deductible
emergency department (ED)
fee-for-service
for-profit/investor-owned hospital
formulary
gatekeeper
governing body
health insurance
health insurance exchange
health maintenance organization (HMO)
home health care
hospice

indemnity plan
intermediate care facility
Joint Commission
level one trauma center
license
long-term acute care hospital (LTAC)
long-term care (LTC)
managed care
Medicaid
Medicare
Medicare Part A
Medicare Part B
Medicare Part C/Medicare Advantage Plan
Medicare Part D
Medigap policy
military hospital
nonprofit hospital
Original Medicare Plan
osteopathic hospital

outpatient surgery
Patient Protection and Affordable Care Act/Affordable Care Act (ACA)
point of service (POS) plan
preferred provider organization (PPO)
premium
primary care physician (PCP)
private health insurance
provider
public health insurance
rehabilitation
residential care/assisted living facility
respite care
rural hospital
skilled care facility
teaching hospital
urban hospital
workers' compensation
World Health Organization (WHO)

Hospital History

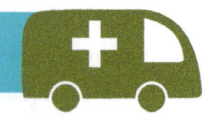

Johns Hopkins Hospital in Baltimore, Maryland, is considered the birthplace of modern surgery in the United States. The hospital's founding professors (William Osler, professor of medicine; William Stewart Halsted, professor of surgery; Howard A. Kelly, professor of gynecology; and William H. Welch, professor of pathology), known as the "Big Four," developed many groundbreaking medical practices and procedures. Read more about the contributions of the Big Four at http://IntroHIM.ParadigmCollege.net/BigFour.

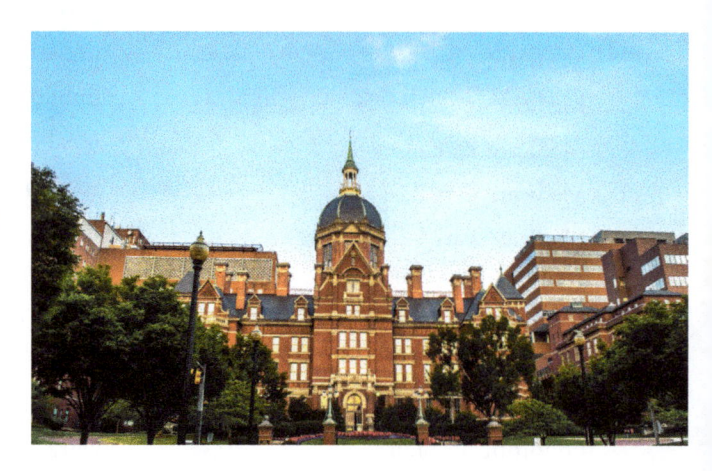

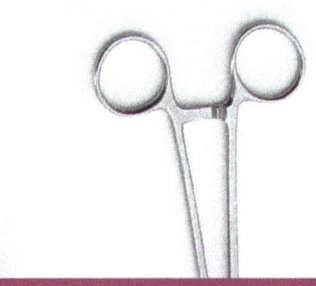

Hospitals' Must-Do Strategies for Success

- Align hospitals, physicians, and other providers across the care continuum
- Utilize evidence-based practices to improve quality and patient safety
- Improve efficiency through productivity and financial management
- Develop integrated information systems
- Join and grow integrated provider networks and care systems
- Educate and engage employees and physicians to create leaders
- Strengthen finances to facilitate reinvestment and innovation
- Partner with payers
- Advance through scenario-based strategic, financial, and operational planning
- Seek population health improvement through pursuit of the "triple aim"

Source: American Hospital Association, *Hospitals and Care Systems of the Future*, 2011

Chapter 3

Hospital Organization and the Medical Staff

The Law of Least Action

Deepak Chopra, MD, believes that the law of least action, one of the classic laws of physics, can be applied to improve human productivity. In simplified form, the law of least action says that nature takes the shortest, most efficient route to accomplish things.

Says Chopra, "If the Law of Least Action was applied to the human brain, productivity would increase tenfold, because making a decision would be an automatic, effortless computation of all the variables involved."

To improve productivity, follow Chopra's *Tips for Promoting Least Action*:
- Get enough sleep.
- Promote an open environment for the exchange of ideas.
- Allow free communication at every level of work and management.
- Support the whole group emotionally.
- Ask for honest feedback.
- Make every worker feel valued.

Source: Excerpted from Deepak Chopra, "Productivity Hacks: The Law of Least Action," LinkedIn.com, January 21, 2014.

Fast Facts

The largest US hospitals based on the number of beds:
1. New York Presbyterian Hospital — 2,236 beds
2. Florida Hospital Orlando — 1,972 beds
3. Jackson Memorial Hospital (Miami) — 1,756 beds
4. University of Pittsburgh Medical Center Presbyterian — 1,590 beds
5. Methodist Hospital (San Antonio) — 1,536 beds

Source: *Becker's Hospital Review*, 2013

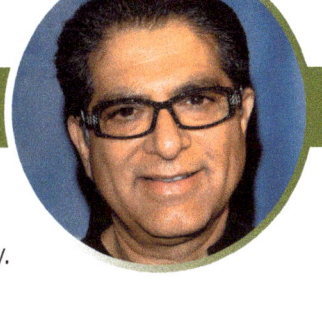

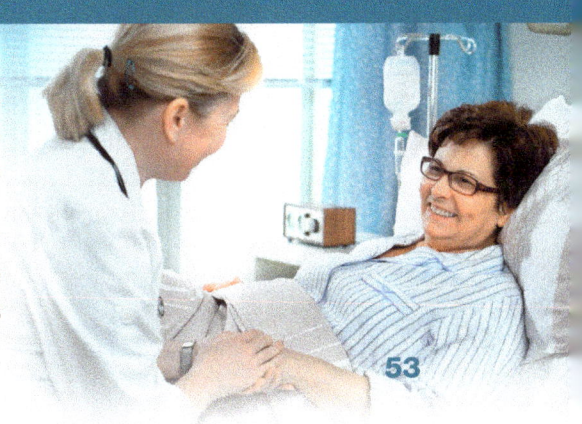

Learning Objectives

- Know what departments and services are found in a healthcare setting.
- Be familiar with occupations available in health care.
- Describe specialty healthcare units and clinics.
- Be familiar with medical specialties.
- Know the basic structure and privileges of the medical staff.
- Understand the differences between hospital and medical staff leadership and reporting structures.

Hospital Organization

Every hospital type—whether for-profit, nonprofit, or public—has a similar organizational structure. At the top of the structure, the **board of directors** (also called the *board of governors*) oversees hospital management and appoints the hospital's chief executive officer (CEO). The board is responsible for ensuring that the organization meets overall financial and quality performance measures. The board of directors is made up of business and community leaders and members of the medical staff. Board members are elected; board service is voluntary and unpaid.

The **chief executive officer (CEO)**, also referred to as the *hospital president*, is responsible for the overall success of the organization. The CEO provides the strategic vision for ongoing and future hospital operations and reports directly to the board of directors. The CEO heads the organization's executive leadership team, which typically includes the **chief operating officer (COO)**, who is responsible for all hospital operations, the **chief financial officer (CFO)**, who is responsible for the organization's financial stability and integrity, and the **chief nursing officer (CNO)**, also referred to as the *vice president of nursing* or *patient care*. The CNO is a registered nurse and is responsible for all patient care initiatives. This position is required by regulation in most states and by the Joint Commission.

The director of the health information management (HIM) department generally reports to the CFO. In some cases, the HIM director reports to another member of the executive leadership team, such as the COO, or, as has become more common in recent years, to the **chief information officer (CIO)**. The CIO is responsible for overseeing the hospital's information technology and network infrastructure.

Large hospitals (hospitals with more than 600 licensed beds) and teaching hospitals often include other executive leadership positions, such as the **chief human resources officer (CHRO)** and the **chief medical officer (CMO)**. The CHRO, also referred to as the *vice president of human resources*, oversees recruitment, benefits, compensation, employee relations, and workers' compensation. The CMO position is found in organizations that employ a large number of physicians and/or residents and medical students. The CMO is a licensed practicing physician who is responsible for the medical-staff services department, medical staff education, quality management, and all of the medical directors employed by the organization.

An **organizational flowchart** diagrams the departments, personnel, and lines of authority in a business or an organization. Example 3.1 shows the structure and the organization of a typical small- to medium-sized hospital.

Example 3.1 Organizational Flowchart for a Small- to Medium-Sized Hospital

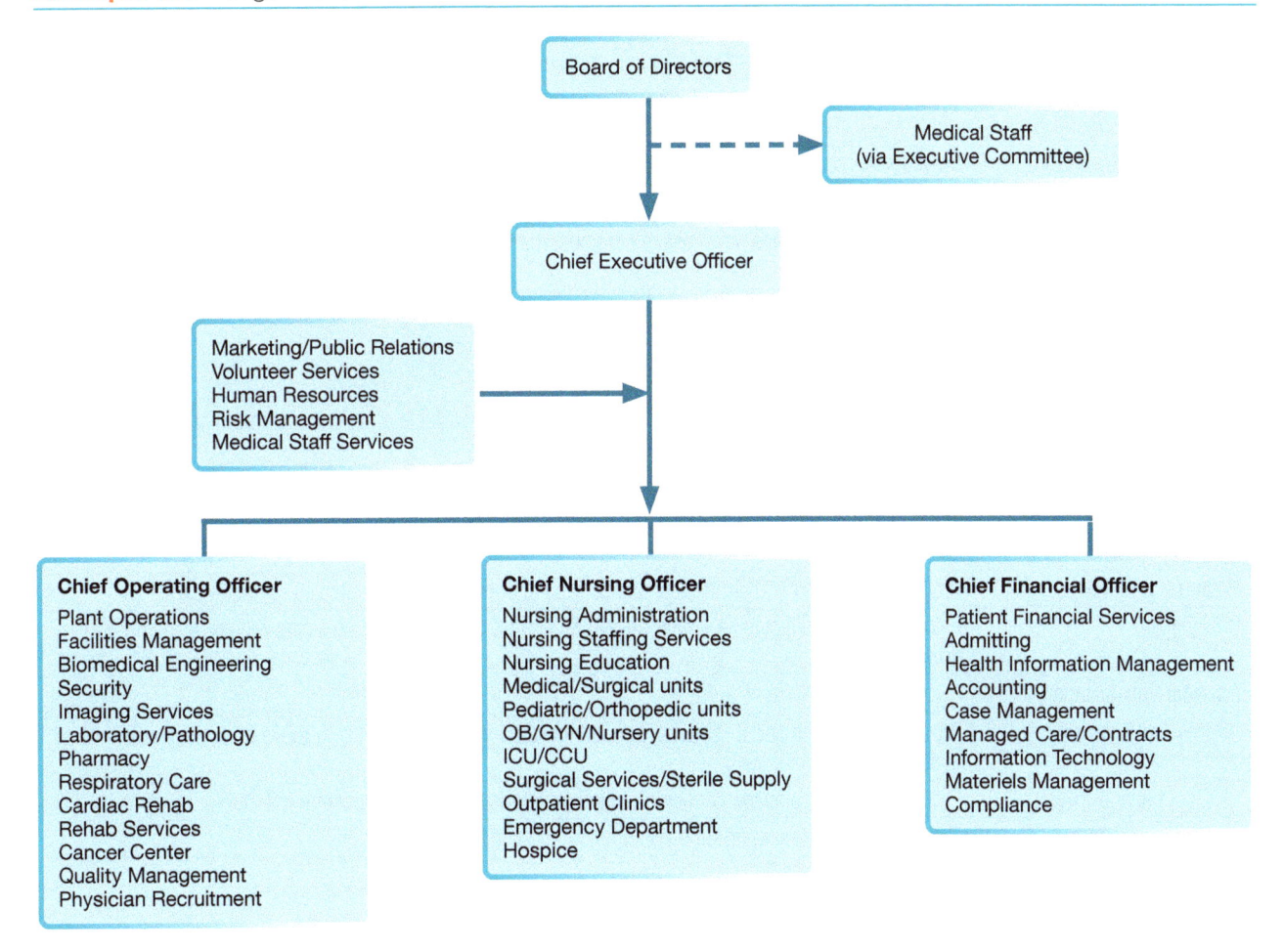

```
                          Board of Directors
                                 |
                                 | - - - - - -> Medical Staff
                                 |              (via Executive Committee)
                                 v
                         Chief Executive Officer
                                 ^
    Marketing/Public Relations   |
    Volunteer Services           |
    Human Resources  ----------->
    Risk Management              |
    Medical Staff Services       |
                                 v
        _____|_____
       |                        |                        |
Chief Operating Officer   Chief Nursing Officer    Chief Financial Officer
Plant Operations          Nursing Administration   Patient Financial Services
Facilities Management     Nursing Staffing Services Admitting
Biomedical Engineering    Nursing Education        Health Information Management
Security                  Medical/Surgical units   Accounting
Imaging Services          Pediatric/Orthopedic units Case Management
Laboratory/Pathology      OB/GYN/Nursery units     Managed Care/Contracts
Pharmacy                  ICU/CCU                  Information Technology
Respiratory Care          Surgical Services/Sterile Supply  Materiels Management
Cardiac Rehab             Outpatient Clinics       Compliance
Rehab Services            Emergency Department
Cancer Center             Hospice
Quality Management
Physician Recruitment
```

Hospital Departments

Hospitals typically include a large number of departments, more than many other businesses, because of the number and the diversity of services provided. The largest department in a hospital is **patient care services**, also referred to as the *department of nursing*. Patient care services includes nurses, technicians, therapists, and other employees who provide direct patient care. Patient care services may also include departments that provide **clinical services**. These departments (e.g., laboratory, radiology, and pharmacy) have direct patient contact and impact patient health.

Chapter 3   Hospital Organization and the Medical Staff

Table 3.1 Hospital Departments

Hospital Department	Department Services
Admitting	Registers each patient visit, ensuring all patient demographic information is complete and accurate, and assigns medical record number
Business Office	Prepares bill for each patient visit and responds to insurance questions, verifies insurance information, and completes collection process
Cardiology	Conducts all diagnostic heart procedures including EKGs, cardiac catheterizations, stress tests, and carotid doppler studies
Case Management	Provides assessment, planning, and coordination of a patient's health needs
Dietary	Provides nutritional counseling as well as food and supplements to all patients
Emergency Services	Provides urgent, emergent, and trauma services
Health Information Management	Manages and protects health information to ensure quality documentation, which supports patient care
Human Resources	Provides all recruitment, employment, benefit, and employee advocacy services for the organization
Laboratory	
Diagnostics	Collects body fluids and other tissue samples, runs tests, and provides results; also includes culture and sensitivity
Blood bank	Stores, processes, and distributes all blood products, maintaining strict controls to ensure patient saftey
Pathology	Reviews all specimens removed during diagnostic and operative procedures
Genetic testing	Provides testing for possible genetic disease
Marketing	Provides information to consumers regarding services available and coordinates patient outreach activities
Materiels Management	Provides all supplies and equipment for the organization
Nursing (Patient Care Services)	The largest department in hospital organizations; provides patient care and education in a variety of settings
Patient Advocates	Provides mediation and arbitration services to patients to remove obstacles to health care
Pharmacy	Provides drug and biological treatments and ensures patient safety regarding proper dosaging and drug interactions
Physical Rehabilitation	
Physical Therapy	Provides diagnoses and treatment for patients who have limited ability to move and perform functional activities in their daily lives
Occupational Therapy	Promotes health by enabling people to perform meaningful and purposeful activities
Speech Therapy	Provides diagnoses and treatment of speech and swallowing conditions
Radiology	
Diagnostic Imaging	X-rays of all body parts
CT Scan	Provides a three-dimensional computer model that allows in-depth slicing of the area being reviewed
Tomography-PET	Used for cancer, heart disease, brain, and nervous system disease; reveals cellular level metabolic changes occuring in an organ tissue
Fluoroscopy	Real-time moving images; includes upper and lower gastrointestinal (GI) procedures
MRI	Magnetic Resonance Imaging uses magnetic field and radio frequency for good contrast review of soft tissues
NM	Nuclear Medicine; radiopharmaceuticals are administered to the patient to allow an image of the extent of a disease/process based on cellular function
Ultrasound/sonography	Uses real-time tomographic images without harmful radiation
Special Procedures	Radiologic guided biopsies, insertion of cancer treatment devices, and other invasive procedures
Utilization Review	Analysis of the necessity, appropriateness, and efficiency of medical services and procedures
Volunteer/Auxillary Services	Provide nonpaid services under the nonprofit direction and training of the Auxillary

Departments that do not provide direct patient care, sometimes referred to as *behind-the-scenes departments*, include HIM, business, marketing, administration, materiel management, and volunteer services. Table 3.1 outlines the departments found in a typical hospital setting and lists the core services provided by each department.

Nursing

According to the American Association of Colleges of Nursing (AACN), nurses make up the largest workforce in health care. There are more than 3.1 million registered nurses nationwide, making them one of the largest segments of the US workforce. Nurses are the primary providers of inpatient hospital care and deliver most of the nation's long-term care. HIM professionals interact and work with nurses on teams and committees and consult with nurses on medical documentation.

Nurses are licensed by the state in which they work. There are many types of nursing credentials, and the type of credential defines the level of care and treatment a nurse is qualified to provide. Table 3.2 lists nursing credentials, acronyms, educational requirements, and the level of care a nurse with that credential is qualified to provide.

In addition to the nursing staff, the HIM staff often works closely with physician assistants. A **physician assistant (PA)** performs duties similar to a nurse practitioner. A physician assistant is licensed by the state and works under the direction of a licensed physician. A PA may gather patient health history and conduct physical exams, order and interpret tests, counsel patients on preventive health measures, assist in surgery, give medical orders, and write prescriptions.

Table 3.2 Nursing Credentials

Acronym	Title	Education	Qualified to Perform
RN	Registered nurse	Two- to four-year college degree	Fully licensed. Permitted to perform all nursing duties.
LVN LPN	Licensed vocational nurse (LVN)/licensed practical nurse (LPN)	12–14 months of vocational training	Works under the direction of a RN. Performs basic duties and drug administration and procedures (with limitations).
CNS	Clinical nurse specialist	Graduate degree plus certification in a specialty area	A clinical expert, consultant, educator, or researcher in a specialty area, such as diabetes, wound care, colostomy care, women's health, or oncology.
CRNA	Certified registered nurse anesthetist	Graduate degree plus additional training	Works under the direction of a licensed anesthesiologist. Administers anesthesia, monitors patients during operative procedures, and conducts postoperative assessments. Can order certain pharmaceuticals (limited by license).
NP	Nurse practitioner	Graduate degree plus additional training	Provides general patient care. Gathers patient health history and conducts physical exams. Orders tests and writes prescriptions.

Specialty Units

Some hospitals and health systems operate **specialty units**, which are inpatient units, such as psychiatry or neonatology, designated for the treatment of specific illnesses or conditions. These units are staffed by physicians, nurses, therapists, and counselors who have specialized training. Some units require specialized equipment.

IT REALLY HAPPENS

A medical center was constructing a specialty unit in its psychiatric service division. While processing invoices for the new unit, the facility's accounting manager was surprised to see an invoice for a child's sandbox. The unit was built to treat patients with dissociative identity disorder (multiple personality disorder). The sandbox was intended for patients' child personalities to use during therapy.

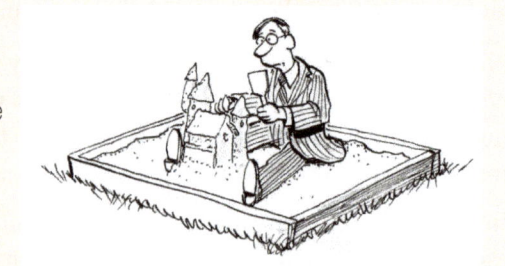

Some specialty units are referred to as *exempt units* (the exemption refers to billing and reimbursement procedures). Exempt units provide unique services and are subject to special licensing requirements (state licensing, for example). Physical rehabilitation and drug and substance abuse rehabilitation are examples of exempt units. Table 3.3 lists some common hospital specialty units and the types of treatment provided.

Table 3.3 Specialty Units

Specialty Unit	Treatment Provided
Alcohol and chemical dependency	Medically managed detoxification and rehabilitation for individuals addicted to alcohol and other chemicals.
Alzheimer's care	Provides care for patients with memory loss, dementia, and Alzheimer's disease.
Behavioral health/psychiatric care	Care, education, and recovery services for patients with behavioral health conditions.
Neonatal intensive care	Specializes in the care of ill or premature newborn infants.
Transplant unit	Specializes in the care of organ, bone marrow, and reconstructive transplant patients.
Ventilator unit	Provides short-term weaning and long-term care for patients on a ventilator.
Burn care	Treats burn injuries. Treatment includes emergency care, intensive care, recovery care, and rehabilitation care.

Specialty Clinics

Specialty clinics provide outpatient treatment of specific diseases and conditions. Table 3.4 lists some common specialty clinics and the types of treatment provided.

Table 3.4 Specialty Clinics

Specialty Clinic	Treatment Provided
Arthritis	Diagnosis and treats rheumatoid arthritis, lupus, Sjögren's disease, and similar conditions.
Fertility	Fertility assessment, egg harvesting, and in vitro fertilization.
Hemodialysis	Dialysis treatment and monitoring of patients with chronic renal failure.
Pain	Multidisciplinary care of individuals with acute, chronic, and cancer-related pain.
Radiation therapy	Treatment for patients with cancer and hyperthyroidism.
Sleep lab	For the diagnosis and the treatment of sleep disorders.
Wound care	For the treatment of nonhealing wounds, pressure ulcers, and diabetic foot ulcers. Treatments include compression, debridement, vacuum-assisted closure, biosurgery (sterile maggots), and hyperbaric oxygen treatments.

The Medical Staff

In years past, the family physician treated illnesses and injuries, delivered babies, and even performed surgery. Over the years, however, physicians have become more specialized. While some still provide general care, many doctors have chosen to specialize, providing care to a specific patient population (gynecology or gerontology, for example) or focusing on a particular type of treatment (such as oncology or fertility).

The **primary care physician (PCP)** is often the first point of contact for patient care. The PCP is usually licensed in family practice, internal medicine, or pediatrics. Primary care physicians diagnose and treat minor illnesses and injuries and perform some diagnostic testing and treatment for more serious conditions. If a patient requires tests or treatment beyond the scope of primary care, the PCP provides the patient with a **medical referral** to a physician **specialist** who has advanced education and clinical training in a particular area of medicine. Table 3.5 lists medical specialties and the area(s) of concentration for each specialty.

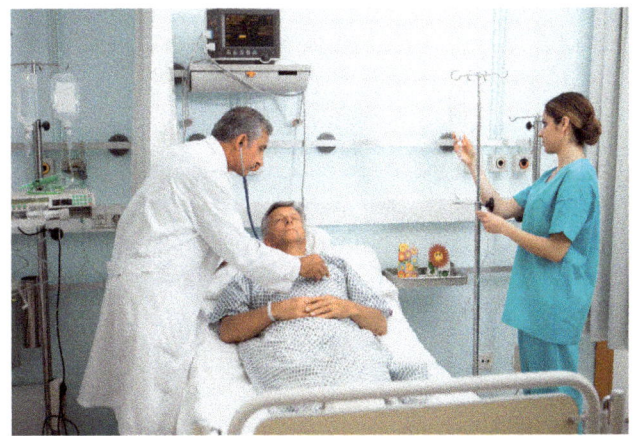

Physicians are permitted to provide specific types of care based on their education, training, licensure, and experience.

> **! BE AWARE**
>
> A cardiologist is different from a cardiac or cardiovascular surgeon. A *cardiologist* performs diagnostic tests, such as EKGs and Doppler studies, cardiac catheterizations, and minimally invasive procedures, such as stent and balloon insertions. A *cardiac* or *cardiovascular surgeon* performs major, high-risk procedures, including bypass surgery, cardiac valve replacement, and heart transplantation.

Table 3.5 Medical Specialties

Specialty	Area(s) of Concentration
Anesthesiology	Pain management and anesthetics administration for surgical procedures
Cardiology	Heart and blood vessels
Dentistry	Mouth and teeth
Dermatology	Diseases of the skin
Endocrinology	Diseases of the glands, such as diabetes and thyroid disorders
Family practice	General care of all family members, which includes basic diagnostics, testing, and treatment
Geriatrics	Diseases and disabilities of older adults
Gynecology	Female reproductive system
Hematology	Diseases of the blood and the blood-forming tissue
Immunology	Immune system function and diseases
Internal medicine	Adult general care and nonsurgical problems
Neurology	Nerves, brain, and spinal cord injuries and diseases
Neonatology	Newborn infants
Nephrology	Diseases of the kidneys, including chronic renal failure
Obstetrics	Infertility, pregnancy, childbirth, and postpartum care
Oncology	Cancer and tumors
Ophthalmology	Diseases and conditions of the eyes
Orthopedics	Diseases and injuries of the bones, the joints, the muscles, and the tendons
Otorhinolaryngology	Conditions and diseases of the ears, the nose, and the throat
Plastic and reconstructive	Repairs or reforms the structure and the appearance of the body
Pediatrics	Children under the age of 18
Physical medicine and rehabilitation/physiatry	Provides diagnostics, evaluation, and management for patients with physical and/or cognitive impairment and disability (e.g., stroke, sports injuries, and post–hip replacement)
Radiology	Medical imaging of all body parts as well as special studies utilizing imaging equipment
Urology	Urinary organs in females (such as the bladder and the urethra) and urinary and genital organs in males

One fairly new type of specialized physician is a hospitalist. The term **hospitalist** was first used in the *New England Journal of Medicine* in 1996. The Society of Hospital Medicine defines a hospitalist as a physician who provides general medical care to patients in the hospital. Hospitalists do not provide follow-up care after the patient has been discharged from the hospital.

Physician Designations

Many medical professionals have the designation of "doctor." Table 3.6 lists the most common types of doctors and describes their areas of authority.

Table 3.6 Physician Designations

Physician Type	Physician Authority
Doctor of medicine (MD)	Performs procedures, prescribes drugs, orders tests, and recommends treatment according to license specifics
Doctor of osteopathic medicine (DO)	Able to perform the same tasks as an MD, but has additional training in osteopathic manipulative medicine
Doctor of dental surgery (DDS)	License limited to treatment of the oral cavity, the maxillofacial area, and the adjacent structures. Must partner with an MD or a DO to admit a patient to a hospital
Doctor of podiatric medicine (DPM)	License limited to the treatment of the foot, ankle, and lower leg. Must partner with an MD or a DO to admit a patient to a hospital
Doctor of chiropractic (DC)	Treats neuromusculoskeletal system disorders; cannot prescribe medications and rarely works in hospital settings
Resident	Licensed physician-in-training who works under the direction of an attending physician

> **BE AWARE**
> A psychiatrist is different than a psychologist. A *psychiatrist* is a licensed medical doctor (MD or DO) who can prescribe medications and perform procedures. A *psychologist* is a doctor of philosophy (PhD) who provides counseling and suggests therapies. Psychologists are not licensed to prescribe medication or perform procedures.

Hospital Privileges

In an acute care hospital, the medical staff are typically not hospital employees; they are physicians with hospital privileges. **Hospital privileges**, also referred to as *medical staff privileges*, permit the physician (or the dentist) to provide patient care in that hospital (see Table 3.7). The hospital governing board grants privileges based on a physician's professional license, experience, and competence. A physician may have privileges at more than one hospital. A physician with privileges is referred to as a *member* of the medical staff. A physician may request privileges in one of five categories.

> **BE AWARE**
> The medical staff includes all physicians who have been granted admitting privileges at a hospital. In most cases, physicians are not hospital employees, although this is changing in some larger hospitals and health systems.

Table 3.7 Hospital Privileges

Privilege	Status
Active	Physicians with active privileges are the only physicians who can admit patients to the hospital (based on specialty/licensure). To maintain active status, active members must admit a minimum number of patients to the hospital annually, actively serve on medical staff committees, and participate in medical department meetings. Active members have voting privileges and may hold office.
Associate/provisional	Physicians with associate or provisional privileges are being considered for advancement to the active medical staff. Associate members may not vote or hold office.
Consulting	Physicians with consulting privileges are recognized specialists who consult on patient care. Consulting members must be active members at another hospital. They may not admit patients, vote, or hold office, and they have no assigned responsibilities.
Courtesy	Courtesy privileges allow a nonmember physician to occasionally admit a patient to the hospital. Courtesy staff members may not vote or hold office.
Honorary	Honorary privileges may be given to retired physicians. Honorary members have no voting rights but may attend medical staff educational activities and other functions.

The Joint Commission requires hospitals to limit physician privileges to terms of two years or less, after which time the physician must reapply. The hospital's medical staff credentialing committee reviews all new applications and those up for renewal to ensure that the physician has the appropriate licensure, training, and experience. In addition, physicians seeking to renew privileges must meet additional requirements. For example, a physician must perform a minimum number of a specific procedure—e.g., appendectomies—annually to be allowed to perform the specific procedure for which credentials are requested during the next two-year period. The hospital's board of directors must approve medical staff credentialing committee recommendations.

Medical Staff Organization

The medical staff is a distinct organization, separate from the hospital staff organization. It has its own leadership structure that reports to the hospital board of directors. The medical staff is governed by **medical staff bylaws** that dictate medical staff governance and structure and by **medical staff rules and regulations** that outline policies and procedures. These policies and procedures address, among other issues, health information management practices such as record completion, patient privacy requirements, and the legal ownership of health information.

The medical staff leadership includes a president or a chief of staff, a vice president or a vice chief of staff, a past president, a treasurer, and a secretary. Voting members elect the officers. If the facility is very small, the treasurer and the secretary positions may be combined. The chief of staff appoints active medical staff members to chair committees and serve as medical department chiefs.

The medical staff meets annually or biannually, depending on the requirements set forth in the bylaws, to elect leadership and consider proposed changes to the bylaws. A *quorum* (a set minimum number of members) must be present to vote on recommended changes. Because the medical staff bylaws can only be revised every six to 12 months, it is important for the HIM professional to be aware of changes to federal and state regulations that may impact medical staff practices—for example, new federal privacy regulations or Joint Commission changes to documentation requirements. Medical staff meetings are closed to nonmembers, so it is important for an HIM professional to work with physicians who can sponsor and advocate for any necessary bylaw changes.

All medical staff committees and medical departments report to the medical staff executive committee, chaired by the chief of staff. The Joint Commission and the state department of health regulations require some committees while others are optional. Table 3.8 provides examples of medical staff committees.

Table 3.8   Examples of Medical Staff Committees

Infection Control

Reviews statistical findings of *nosocomial* (hospital-acquired) infections, develops policies and procedures to reduce the incidence of infections, and educates hospital staff.

Quality/Performance Improvement

Develops policies and procedures related to and provides oversight of quality improvement measures, identifying safety issues and areas in need of improvement and monitoring and reporting to regulatory agencies.

Utilization Review/Documentation Improvement/HIM

Includes medical staff members and is attended by HIM, utilization review, nursing, and administrative personnel. This committee reviews delinquent records reports, identifies opportunities for documentation improvement, reviews hospital utilization reports, and evaluates requests for continuing patient stays.

Pharmacy and Therapeutics

Maintains the hospital's *drug formulary* (a list of medications available from the hospital pharmacy) to ensure the safety and the proper use of medications and biological treatments, investigates reported drug interactions and errors, and educates providers on the proper use of pharmaceuticals.

Blood Transfusion

Reviews blood transfusion interactions to ensure safe and appropriate transfused-blood delivery, blood storage procedures, and blood transfusions provided without meeting indication of need.

Cancer

Evaluates care provided to cancer patients to ensure all patients receive the most appropriate care; reviews the statistical data gathered on cancer cases (such as survival rates and comparison data with national averages of the top 10 cancer types). American College of Surgeons (ACS) requires accredited facilities to have this committee.

Tissue Review

Reviews normal tissue that has been removed (e.g., a normal appendix that was thought to be the cause of pain), confirms the accuracy of specimen review (sent out at random for external review), and assesses the turnaround times for preliminary specimen findings when the patient is in surgery.

Medical Staff Departments

Active members of the medical staff are organized within specific medical departments, according to each physician's specialty and training. Medical departments in small- to medium-sized hospitals typically include medicine, surgery, emergency medicine, pediatrics, obstetrics and gynecology, laboratory, pathology, and radiology. In larger hospitals, these departments are often broken down into smaller subspecialties. For example, surgery subspecialties would include general surgery, urology, orthopedics, cardiovascular, and neurology.

> **BE AWARE**
>
> Hospital departments and medical departments often have similar names, so it is important to pay attention to the order of the words. The *cardiology department* is a physical hospital department where cardiac treatment is provided. The *department of cardiology* is an organized group of medical staff members. It is not a place.

To remain active members, physicians must attend and participate in department committee meetings as specified under the medical staff bylaws. The department's committee chair reviews new medical staff applications and applications from members up for renewal (these applications are then forwarded to the credentials committee), establishes *medical protocols* (guidelines for medical treatment), establishes medical policies and procedures, and assesses the quality of patient care.

Physician Employment

Traditionally, physicians have not been hospital employees, but this is changing. Faced with physician shortages, particularly a shortage of primary care physicians, hospitals are increasingly recruiting physicians to work on staff. This trend is driven in part by provisions in the Patient Protection and Affordable Care Act (ACA) and efforts to reform healthcare delivery models through the creation of accountable care organizations. The definition of an **accountable care organization (ACO)** is evolving, but, in general terms, an ACO is a group of healthcare providers (primary care physicians, specialists, hospitals, and other healthcare facilities) working together to coordinate patient care across care settings for individual Medicare patients. ACOs are intended to improve patient care and reduce the cost of care. Hospitals and physicians with participating ACOs will be eligible to participate in Medicare's Share Savings Program, which financially rewards providers who meet quality and cost standards.

> **EXPAND YOUR KNOWLEDGE**
>
> The cost of hiring a physician is very high. On average, a hospital can expect to lose $150,000–$250,000 per year during the first three years of a physician's employment. Read the full *New England Journal of Medicine* article to find out why at http://IntroHIM.ParadigmCollege.net/HiringPhysicians.

Chief Executive Officer versus Medical Chief of Staff

The hospital and the medical staff are separate organizations with separate leadership. The CEO is responsible for all the day-to-day operations of the hospital. The medical chief of staff oversees the medical staff. Both report to the hospital's board of governors. The CEO and the medical chief of staff work collaboratively to ensure high-quality patient care, but each has different areas of influence and responsibility. Table 3.9 compares the responsibilities of the CEO to the medical chief of staff.

Table 3.9 CEO versus Medical Chief of Staff

CEO	Medical Chief of Staff
• is appointed by the governing board	• is elected by his or her peers
• is an employee of the hospital	• is not employed by the hospital
• can hire, fire, and direct hospital employees	• cannot hire, fire, or direct hospital employees
• cannot hire, fire, or direct individuals with privileges granted by the medical staff	• has direct responsibility for granting or removing clinician privileges

TAKE THE CHALLENGE

Read the two scenarios below and write a short paragraph for each case explaining who is responsible for decision making (the CEO or the medical chief of staff) and why.

1. The hospital has not met its financial goals because a member of the medical staff stopped scheduling surgeries at the hospital. In turn, the hospital has decided to lay off staff. Who is responsible for the employee layoffs?

2. The hospital's operating room is losing money because physicians in a group practice are scheduling surgery under another physician's name. This practice occurs when a physician's hospital privileges are suspended due to delinquent records (which makes him or her ineligible to schedule patients) and this same physician schedules procedures under a partner's name. The operating-room staff prepares the surgical suite by opening a sterile packet of surgical supplies for the physician listed on the schedule. When the suspended physician shows up to perform the procedure, the sterile package opened for the physician listed on the schedule must be thrown away and a new package opened (sterile packets are very expensive). Who is responsible for fixing this problem?

Chapter 3   Hospital Organization and the Medical Staff

Chapter Summary

Every department in a hospital plays an important role in ensuring that patients receive the highest quality care. And every department contributes to the hospital's financial success.

Hospital operations are overseen by the hospital's board of governors, also referred to as the *board of directors*. The CEO is responsible for hospital operations. The medical chief of staff is responsible for the medical staff—all physicians with privileges at that hospital. The medical staff has its own governance and bylaws.

The largest department in a hospital is the patient care services department. This department includes the nursing and hospital departments (e.g., laboratory, radiology, and pharmacy) that provide direct patient-care services. Some hospitals operate specialty inpatient units (neonatal intensive care, burn care, substance abuse and chemical dependency, for example) that provide care and treatment for specific diseases or conditions requiring unique services and doctors with specialized training.

Physician designations are based on education and expertise. Physician designations include doctor of medicine (MD), doctor of osteopathic medicine (DO), doctor of dental surgery (DDS), doctor of chiropractic (DC), doctor of podiatric medicine (DPM), and resident.

Doctors are classified as primary care physicians and specialists. The PCP is usually the patient's first point of contact in the health system. A specialist is a physician who has advanced education and clinical training in a specific area of medicine. In a hospital, active members of the medical staff practice within specific departments, according to their specialty and training. Typical departments include medicine, surgery, emergency medicine, pediatrics, obstetrics and gynecology, laboratory, pathology, and radiology. In larger hospitals, departments are often broken down into subspecialties.

Typically, physicians are not employed by a hospital but work independently or in a group practice. Physicians must apply for and be granted hospital privileges to treat patients at a specific hospital. Only physicians with active privileges may admit patients to a hospital. Some physicians have privileges at more than one hospital.

HIM Review

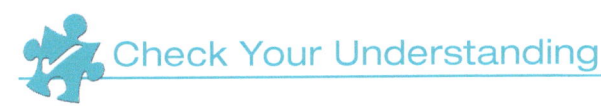

Check Your Understanding

Test your understanding of the material covered in this chapter by completing the following multiple-choice questions. For each question, select the best answer from the choices provided.

1. The type of privilege granted to a physician who may occasionally admit a patient to the hospital is the _____ privilege.

    a. associate

    b. consulting

    c. courtesy

    d. active

2. _____ is the hospital department that bills patients for services provided.

    a. Patient advocacy

    b. Health information

    c. Utilization management

    d. The business office

3. A(n) _____ is not performed in a radiology department.

    a. stress test

    b. MRI

    c. CT scan

    d. special procedure

4. The medical chief of staff is_____

    a. employed by the hospital.

    b. allowed to hire, fire, and direct hospital employees.

    c. elected by his or her peers.

    d. not responsible for granting or removing clinicians' privileges.

5. The _____ reviews all new physician applications and those up for renewal.

    a. credentialing committee

    b. utilization review committee

    c. cancer committee

    d. quality/performance improvement committee

Chapter 3 Hospital Organization and the Medical Staff

6. Physical therapy, occupational therapy, and speech therapy are all part of which department?

    a. nursing
    b. physical rehabilitation
    c. emergency services
    d. radiology

7. _____ is not a physician specialty.

    a. Internal medicine
    b. Transplantation
    c. Immunology
    d. Otorhinolaryngology

8. Which correctly describes the activities permitted by the credential?

    a. An RN can administer drugs with limitations.
    b. An LVN can perform all nursing procedures.
    c. An RN can perform all nursing duties.
    d. An LVN can perform all nursing duties.

9. ACO stands for_____

    a. acute coronary operation.
    b. access, controls, and optimization.
    c. the American College of Osteopathics.
    d. accountable care organization.

10. Which of the following dictates how the medical staff operates?

    a. medical staff rules and regulations
    b. medical staff bylaws
    c. medical staff privileges
    d. medical staff committees

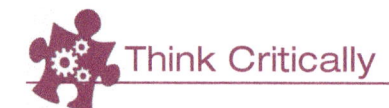

Think Critically

Consider the following real-world scenario and draft a response.

As the director of health information management, you have reviewed the medical staff rules and regulations and noted that the regulations do not require the completion of all medical record documentation within 30 days—the standard set by the Joint Commission and required by Medicare. What steps would you take to ensure this requirement becomes part of the medical staff rules and regulations?

Sharpen Your Comprehension

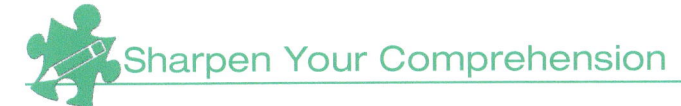

Complete the following matching exercise by selecting, from the list provided, the answer that best matches each of the numbered statements. For each statement, only one answer is correct.

a. board of directors
b. specialty clinic
c. licensed vocational nurse
d. accountable care organization
e. pharmacy and therapeutics
f. fluoroscopy
g. patient advocate
h. admitting
i. clinical nurse specialist
j. geriatrics

1. _____ Creates incentives for healthcare providers to work together to treat an individual patient across care settings

2. _____ Has overall responsibility for the financial and quality outcomes of the organization

3. _____ Assigns the patient's medical record number

4. _____ Works under the direction of a RN and performs basic nursing duties

5. _____ Specialty involving care for the medical conditions of the elderly

6. _____ Subdepartment that creates real-time moving images, including upper and lower GI procedures

7. _____ Committee that ensures the safety and the proper use of medications and biological treatments

8. _____ Provides mediation and arbitration services to patients to remove obstacles to health care

9. _____ Is a clinical expert, consultant, educator, and researcher for a specialty area

10. _____ A place that patients go to receive treatment for a particular disease or condition on an outpatient basis

Connect Theory to Practice

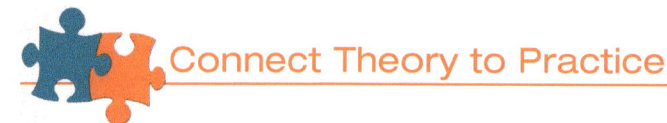

To help translate the concepts presented in this chapter to the workplace, complete the following exercise.

Do an Internet search for a copy of your local hospital's medical staff bylaws that includes the rules and regulations section. If your local hospital does not publish its bylaws, select another hospital. For this assignment, you will need to provide your instructor with the hospital name and the URL for the hospital's bylaws.

Review the bylaws you selected and complete the following exercises:

1. List the titles of the medical staff departments.

2. List the names of the medical staff committees. (Note: Your answer should include committee titles such as Infection Control Committee or Pharmacy and Therapeutics Committee.)

3. Locate the section of the bylaws that lists possible penalties for physicians who fail to complete medical record documentation in a timely way and then provide the following information:

   - The title of the section (including the section number and section title) where the information is located.

   - The timeframe listed for records completion.

   - Any penalties or restrictions listed for failing to complete documentation within the stated timeframe.

Student eResources

*To enhance your comprehension of the chapter material, go to **Navigator+** and complete the additional practice items as advised by your instructor.*

Chapter Terms

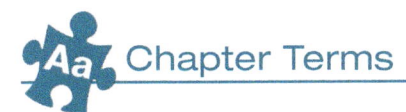

accountable care organization (ACO)
board of directors
chief executive officer (CEO)
chief financial officer (CFO)
chief human resources officer (CHRO)
chief information officer (CIO)
chief medical officer (CMO)
chief nursing officer (CNO)
chief operating officer (COO)
clinical services
hospital privileges
hospitalist
medical referral
medical staff bylaws
medical staff rules and regulations
organizational flowchart
patient care services
physician assistant (PA)
primary care physician (PCP)
specialist
specialty clinic
specialty unit

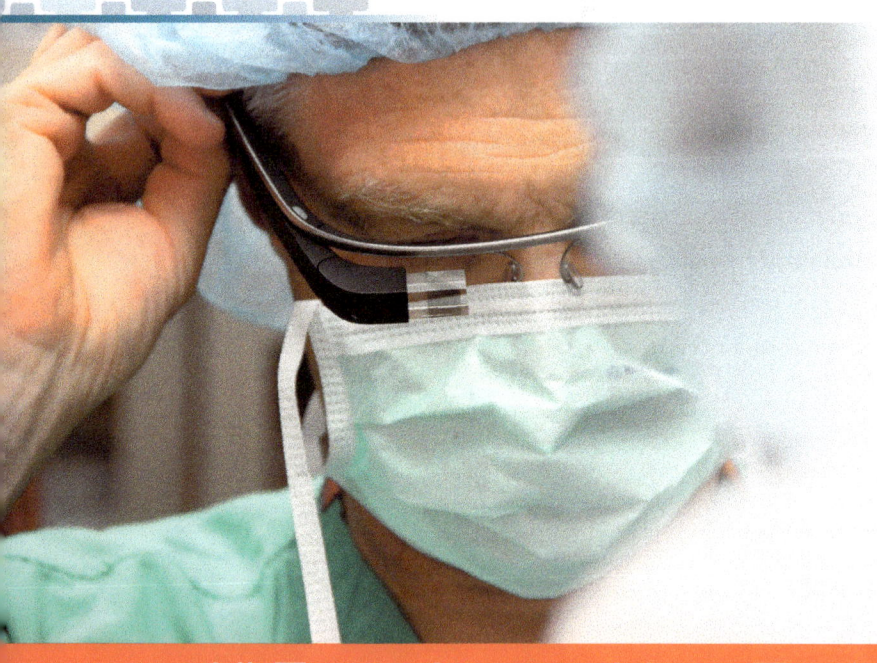

All Eyes Are on New Technology

Some physicians now use hands-free, wearable Google Glass technology to view patient charts, take photos or video consultations during surgery, and assist in treating patients en route to the emergency room by ambulance.

Future Trends

Computers can't and won't replace the interaction between the patient and the physician. However, they are capable of crunching vast amounts of data and identifying patterns that humans can't. *Artificial intelligence* (the use of computers to perform activities normally thought to require intelligence) allows physicians to take full advantage of electronic medical records, transforming them from mere e-filing cabinets into full-fledged doctors' aides that can deliver clinically relevant, high-quality data in real time.

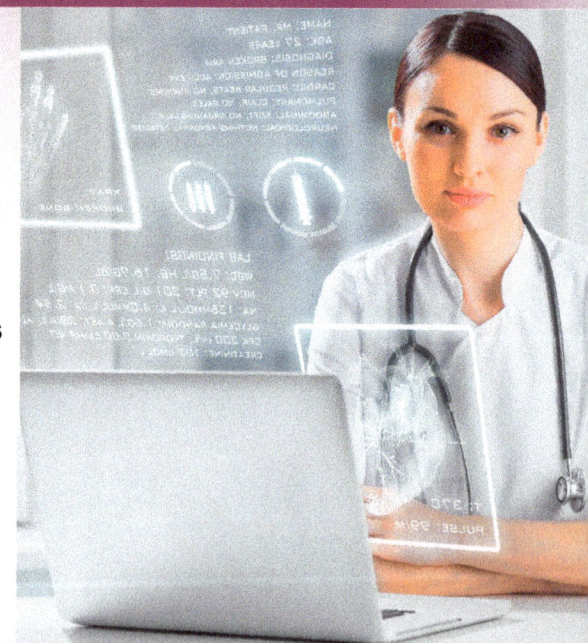

Chapter 4

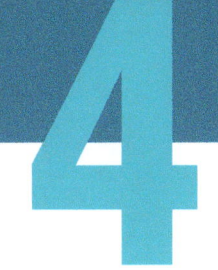

Health Record Purpose and Components

Medicare and other healthcare providers are using the Blue Button Connector app to allow patients to easily and securely download and share personal health information. The US Department of Veterans Affairs created Blue Button in 2010 to allow veterans to download parts of their medical records. Since then, HealthIT.gov has made Blue Button technology available to millions of Americans. For more on the Blue Button, go to http://IntroHIM.ParadigmCollege.net/BlueButton.

Fast Facts

Access to quality health care is far from equal. Commonly underserved populations, such as racial and ethnic minority populations; people with limited English proficiency; people with disabilities; and members of the lesbian, gay, bisexual, and transgender communities often have reduced access to health care and health insurance. These healthcare disparities result in poorer health outcomes.

The Institute of Medicine reports that lack of data on patient race, ethnicity, and language is contributing to the disparity in health care. In an effort to remedy that lack of data, the Affordable Care Act requires that all health surveys sponsored by the US Department of Health and Human Services include standardized information on race, ethnicity, sex, primary language, and disability status.

Learning Objectives

- Explain the purpose of the patient health record.
- Describe the content of the patient record.
- Understand the difference between paper, electronic, and hybrid patient health record formats.
- Describe the role of the forms/screen committee.
- Apply selected requirements governing the patient health record.
- Discuss the importance of and emerging issues related to information governance.
- Describe clinical documentation improvement and its advantages.

The Patient Record

The **patient record**, also referred to as the *medical record* and the *health record*, documents a patient's medical history and all care and services provided to the patient during episodes of care. An *episode of care* may involve a visit to a physician, a lab or X-ray procedure performed at a stand-alone or hospital outpatient clinic, or an inpatient stay in a hospital or other type of healthcare facility.

"If it's not written down, it didn't happen. If it did, prove it."

—Association of Clinical Documentation Improvement Specialists (ACDIS)

Patient records may be maintained in paper or electronic formats or as a *hybrid record* (a combination of both formats). Health information is entered into the patient health record every time a service is provided and in every healthcare setting, although different information may be recorded in different types of care settings.

The Joint Commission requires that the medical record contain these components:

- information unique to the patient, which is used for patient identification
- information needed to support the patient's diagnosis and condition
- information needed to justify the patient's care, treatment, and services
- information that documents the course and the result of the patient's care, treatment, and services
- standardized formats to document the care, treatment, and services it provides to patients

In an ambulatory care facility, such as a physician's clinic, the patient record is a record of care provided during every encounter between a patient and a provider of care. An *encounter* may take many forms including a physician, physician assistant, or nurse practitioner giving an exam; a technician drawing blood; or a nurse giving an injection or educating a patient about a procedure. Some entries in the record are related to illnesses or injuries while others document preventive care services, such as an annual physical examination or immunization. Phone calls and emails between a patient and a care provider are not considered an encounter and are not formally entered into the record, although notation may be added to the record.

In general, the ambulatory record includes:

- patient identification information
- the patient's health history; the onset of current illness, which includes the reason for the visit
- a problem list of the dates and the reasons for all visits
- the results of the physical examination

The ambulatory record may also include test results, a list of medications prescribed, a record of educational materials provided to the patient, and instructions for follow-up care.

In an inpatient hospital setting, the patient record documents all care provided from the time of admission to the time of discharge. The record includes forms documenting admission and consent for treatment, physician orders, diagnostic test results, and documentation of all medications and treatment provided to the patient. The hospital record also includes various log forms, such as **vital signs** (temperature, pulse, respiration, and blood pressure), information on procedures performed, nurses notes, provider notes, and a discharge summary. If a patient is hospitalized for an extended period or undergoes multiple or certain types of complex procedures, the hospital patient record may become quite large.

Purpose of the Patient Record

The primary purpose of the patient record is to support direct patient care. The record documents patient care management and the progress of the patient's condition, and it serves as a communication tool between all of the providers involved in the patient's treatment.

The patient record also serves a number of secondary uses, including as a legal document and a business record for the provider and the facility. Data contained in patient records and data compiled from those records is a valuable resource. These secondary uses of the record are unrelated to direct patient care.

Primary Uses

First and foremost, the patient record is used to support patient care. The information available in an appropriately documented record:

- helps to determine the appropriate course of treatment during an outpatient visit or an inpatient stay. The record contains information from the physical examination and diagnostic results, which are used to determine the appropriate treatment.
- provides patient-specific context for treatment based on the patient's condition, health status, age, medical history, and other factors. Patient-specific data is combined with established *treatment protocols* (guidelines for the standard of care) to develop a treatment plan.

- provides continuity of care over time and between the clinicians and the care providers. Providers refer to the patient record for past medical information when a patient returns for follow-up care or when a patient seeks care from a different physician or care provider.

- supports communication with referring and consulting colleagues. During a *consultative evaluation* (usually a one-time examination to provide a secondary or expert opinion), the record provides the consulting physicians with the information necessary to examine the patient. The record is also used to communicate the consulting or referred physician's opinion on the diagnosis and the treatment.

Secondary Uses

In addition to the primary purpose of supporting direct patient care, the patient record contains valuable information that is used for other internal and external activities, such as demonstrating the facility's compliance with reporting requirements established by external entities.

Within the healthcare organization, secondary uses of the patient record include:

- serving as a legal document for the protection of the patient, providers of care, and facility
- substantiating claims for insurance payment
- supporting quality improvement activities
- monitoring facility operations
- monitoring public health and other external reporting
- strategic planning
- planning activities for facility evaluation

External users of secondary data include:

- governmental agencies
- accrediting organizations
- educational institutions for the approval of clinical internships and other educational programs
- insurance companies
- specific disease-related organizations (e.g., American Lung Association, American Cancer Society)

Patient health information is also used both internally and externally in research, education, and for statistical analysis after the record has been de-identified. **De-identified** means that all patient identifying information has been removed from an individual patient record or from a group of patient records. Data abstracted from a group of patient records for statistical reporting purposes is called **aggregate data**. Aggregate data is used to track variables over time, across groups, or across patient populations, for example.

Uses for de-identified information and/or aggregate data include:

- clinical research
- educational programs for healthcare professionals
- statistical reports for external reporting to governmental agencies, accreditation organizations, payers, and others
- statistical reports for strategic planning (internal use)

As more providers adopt the use of electronic health records, new uses for patient data are emerging. More patient information is readily available in the electronic record, and it is easier and faster to aggregate and analyze patient information stored in digital form.

It is important for health information management (HIM) professionals to understand and be able to recognize what information must be maintained in the patient record to support primary and secondary uses of the information, and to be familiar with the rules and the guidelines governing documentation in the record. These include licensing requirements, accreditation guidelines, Medicare and other payer requirements, and the medical staff bylaws.

The HIM professional needs to know record-keeping requirements and understand how the information is collected and organized in paper or electronic format to form the patient record. To comprehend the complexity of the patient record, one must know:

- who is responsible for the creation, authentication (the establishment of authorship), and procedure for incorporating information into the patient record
- what information must be included in each individual report or document included in the record
- where the information comes from (for example, admission information and consent forms are obtained during the admissions process; a report dictated by a physician must be **transcribed** in typewritten form to become a part of the record; lab reports generated from lab equipment are sent to the record electronically; and log sheets and notes are completed by the nursing staff)
- when the reports are considered complete and the timeframe in which they are required to be available for use for patient care
- why the information is necessary for the provision of medical care and why timeliness is important in many instances (For example, the history and physical examination must be in the patient record and accessible before surgery is performed.)

Many of the individuals who provide patient care and work with the patient record understand most of these issues, but they do not have the overall picture. The HIM department can provide guidance on documentation and completion requirements.

In an inpatient setting, after the patient is discharged, the record must be complete. A **complete record** is one in which all required reports, signatures, and dates have been entered. The completed record is then filed in a permanent filing area, or if it is an electronic record, it is designated as complete in the electronic health record (EHR) system.

Internal Uses

After the patient has been discharged, the patient record may still be accessed for a variety of internal and external uses.

- A physician may review information in the record on the previous diagnosis and treatment if the patient returns to the hospital for follow-up or additional care.

- The billing department may need to make copies of the record to substantiate payment of the claim.

- An infection-control committee may review the chart of a patient who developed a nosocomial infection. A **nosocomial infection** is an infection that is acquired in a hospital.

- A committee may review the charts of a physician under review for medical staff membership.

- The Joint Commission or state department of health may review patient charts while conducting a survey.

- An HIM staff member may abstract data from patient charts for a statistical report.

- Student interns may need the record to complete a case study of a patient they have encountered. (Special permission, Health Insurance Portability and Accountability Act of 1996 [HIPAA] training, and de-identifying any notes and reports are all required in most facilities for this kind of access.)

External Uses

Copies of the patient record are also needed by other care providers and for payment, research, and regulatory activities.

- A patient may request a copy of the record or specific reports from the record.

- The patient may authorize the release of information to third-party payers, other healthcare providers, attorneys, or other entities.

- Data from patient records may be submitted in a statistical report for submission to the Joint Commission, a state licensing board or other governmental agency, payers, and/or educational institutions.

- The record may be released in response to a subpoena or court order to provide the record as evidence in court.

- External auditors, such as the federal **Recovery Audit Contractor (RAC)**, may use patient information to identify and recover improper Medicare payments. The role of the RAC is to detect and correct past improper payments and to implement actions to prevent future improper payments.

Forms/Information Included in the Patient Record

To get a true sense of the amount of data gathered in the patient record, it is useful to review the individual forms and the types of information obtained during a patient encounter. The forms discussed below are typically a part of a paper record. This same information is captured in an electronic record but entered in data fields, and may be accessed in a variety of formats.

The Hospital Record

To understand the standard (general) hospital record, the forms and screen views that make up the record, and the specialty records that vary from this standard, it is important to understand how patients are classified or grouped. Hospital inpatients are typically classified into groups based on service assignment. The *service assignment* identifies the type of service the patient will receive. A service assignment may be made by location in the hospital, diagnostic category, or another defining attribute. The basic assignment of a patient to a service utilizes the following four diagnostic categories:

- **Medical** The patient is admitted for the diagnosis and the treatment of a medical condition; no surgery is planned, and the patient is not an obstetric or newborn patient. Myocardial infarction and pneumonia are examples of a medical service assignment.

- **Surgical** The patient is admitted for a surgical procedure, such as an appendectomy, tumor removal, a hip-fracture repair, or a coronary bypass procedure.

- **Obstetrical** The patient is admitted for an obstetrical condition, such as delivery, false labor, or uterine hemorrhage postdelivery.

- **Newborn** The patient was born in the facility.

In large hospitals that provide many types of services, service categories may also include cardiac medicine, cardiac surgery, psychiatry, gastrointestinal medicine, obstetrics (OB) delivery, OB surgery, OB medicine, and other categories. Grouping patients by service category allows healthcare facilities to better track the number and the types of patient conditions treated.

There probably is no "standard" patient record, but some forms and screen views are common to all types of patient records. The following items are included in the standard chart for medical service patients.

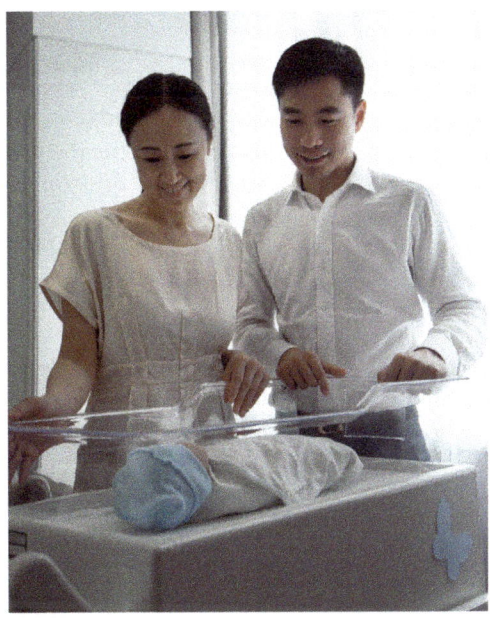

"Newborn" is a common service assignment category for infants born in a hospital.

Chapter 4   Health Record Purpose and Components

Acute Care Documentation

Acute care hospital records are the most comprehensive and the most complex because of the level of care provided. Common types of forms found in the acute care patient record include admission, patient history and physical exam, assessment plan, physician orders, diagnostic findings, patient care documentation, log and flow sheets, and discharge summaries.

Patient records maintained by other types of facilities (e.g., long-term care, ambulatory care, home health, or rehabilitation) may include some of the same forms, depending on the type of care provided, as well as forms specific to that setting and type of care.

In an acute care setting, medical-service patient records are the most general and include the most commonly used forms, which are described here.

Admission

Admission forms include the following:

- registration information and documents to initiate the treatment
- preadmission/admission
- demographic, emergency contact, and insurance information (also called the *Face Sheet*)
- emergency department (ED) documentation if the patient was transferred from the ED
- consent for treatment and payment
- **advance directive** (a written statement detailing the patient's wishes for medical treatment should he or she be unable to communicate with the care provider)

Medical History and Physical Examination

The medical history includes a history of the present illness, a past medical history, current medications, allergies, social history, family history, and a review of body systems. The physical exam reflects the physical assessment by the physician and includes vital signs, general appearance, physical findings, provisional diagnosis, and care plan.

These two reports are almost always documented together and referred to as the H&P (history and physical). The Joint Commission requires that the H&P and any updates be in the record 24 hours after registration or inpatient admission and before surgery or any procedure requiring anesthesia services.

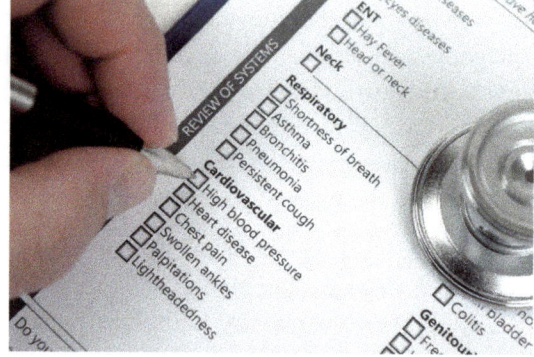

The review of systems form is a screening tool used to identify dysfunction and disease. The form lists symptoms organized by body system (e.g., respiratory, cardiovascular, digestive, etc.).

HEART: Sounds are normal

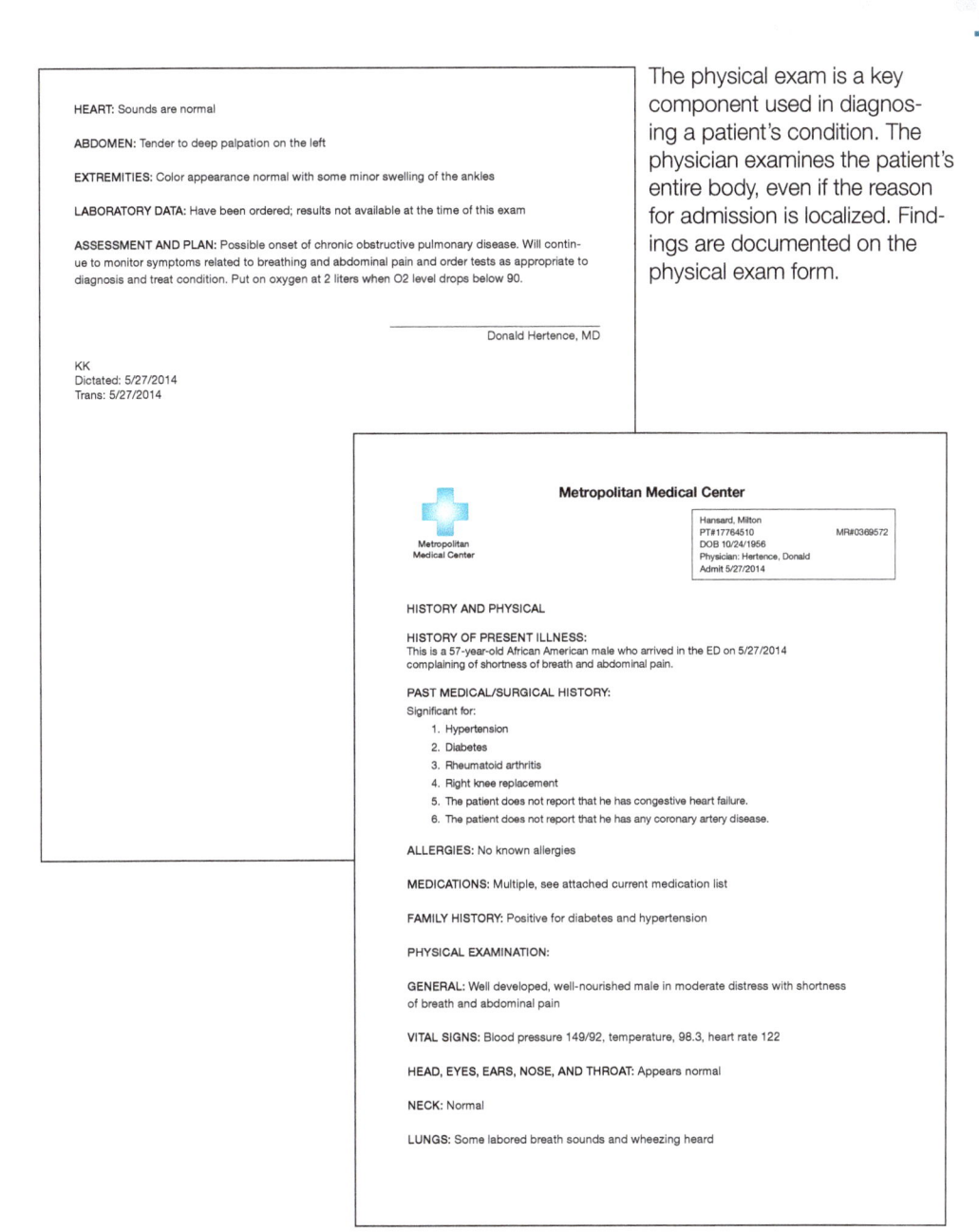

ABDOMEN: Tender to deep palpation on the left

EXTREMITIES: Color appearance normal with some minor swelling of the ankles

LABORATORY DATA: Have been ordered; results not available at the time of this exam

ASSESSMENT AND PLAN: Possible onset of chronic obstructive pulmonary disease. Will continue to monitor symptoms related to breathing and abdominal pain and order tests as appropriate to diagnosis and treat condition. Put on oxygen at 2 liters when O2 level drops below 90.

_____
Donald Hertence, MD

KK
Dictated: 5/27/2014
Trans: 5/27/2014

The physical exam is a key component used in diagnosing a patient's condition. The physician examines the patient's entire body, even if the reason for admission is localized. Findings are documented on the physical exam form.

Metropolitan Medical Center

Hansard, Milton
PT#17764510   MR#0369572
DOB 10/24/1956
Physician: Hertence, Donald
Admit 5/27/2014

HISTORY AND PHYSICAL

HISTORY OF PRESENT ILLNESS:
This is a 57-year-old African American male who arrived in the ED on 5/27/2014 complaining of shortness of breath and abdominal pain.

PAST MEDICAL/SURGICAL HISTORY:
Significant for:
1. Hypertension
2. Diabetes
3. Rheumatoid arthritis
4. Right knee replacement
5. The patient does not report that he has congestive heart failure.
6. The patient does not report that he has any coronary artery disease.

ALLERGIES: No known allergies

MEDICATIONS: Multiple, see attached current medication list

FAMILY HISTORY: Positive for diabetes and hypertension

PHYSICAL EXAMINATION:

GENERAL: Well developed, well-nourished male in moderate distress with shortness of breath and abdominal pain

VITAL SIGNS: Blood pressure 149/92, temperature, 98.3, heart rate 122

HEAD, EYES, EARS, NOSE, AND THROAT: Appears normal

NECK: Normal

LUNGS: Some labored breath sounds and wheezing heard

Assessment, Plan, and Provisional Diagnosis

This information may be included as a part of the history and physical exam or as a separate document. It includes:

- an assessment of the patient's condition to guide treatment
- a plan listing treatment goals and procedures; this plan may include referrals, additional testing, and services
- a provisional diagnosis, or the initial diagnosis made before testing and evaluation

Physician Orders

Physician orders are written orders that communicate the physician's instructions for the patient's care to others (nurses, lab, radiology, pharmacy, dietary, etc.).

Diagnostic Findings

Diagnostic findings are the results of testing conducted to aid in diagnosis and treatment. Testing may involve:

- labs
- imaging (e.g., X-rays and computerized tomography [CT] or other scans)
- pathology
- cardiology (electrocardiograms [EKGs or ECGs])

Patient Care Documentation

A lot of patient information is captured via log sheets and flow sheets (see Example 4.1). **Log sheets and flow sheets** provide a graphic summary of changes in the patient's vital signs, health status, or treatment, such as changes in weight, blood pressure, treatment, and medications administered. Commonly used log and flow sheets are identified in the following sections.

Example 4.1 Vital Signs Flow Sheet

Vital Signs Flow Sheet

Patient:
DOB:
M/F:
Physician:

Notes:

Date	Weight	Temp.	BP	Pulse	Respiration	Pain	Initials

Intake and Output

Used to monitor fluid balance, *intake* measures all fluids, by mouth or intravenously, taken in by the patient, and *output* measures the patient's urine and emesis (vomit).

Medication Records

A **medication record** documents the administration of each drug each time it is given to the patient, including the date and the time of administration and the initials of the nurse who administered the medication (see Example 4.2). If the patient refuses or is unable to take the medication, that is also documented.

Example 4.2 Medication Record

Ward/Unit:			Weight (kg)		Name and Check Label Correct:										
Date	Medicine (Print Generic Name)				Date										
1/2	Oral Sucrose					1/2	1/2	2/2	2/2	2/2					
Route	Dose	~~Hourly Frequency~~ **PRN**		Max Does 24 hrs	Time	08 30	16 15	08 20	16 30	10 30					
PO	0-2-1ML			5ML											
Pharmacy Additional Information					DOSE	0.5ML	1ML	0.5ML	0.8ML	0.5ML					
Initialed by CNS															
Indication		Dose Calculation (e.g. mg/kg per DOSE)			Route	po	po	po	po	po					
Procedural Only															
Prescriber Signature		Print Name		Contact Pager	Sign	JL	JL	JL	JL	JL					
J. Lowell															

Restraint Logs

Restraints may sometimes be needed to secure a patient to a bed or a chair. **Restraint logs** are maintained to document justification for the use of restraints and to record monitoring of the patient by the staff. When restraints are used, the Joint Commission requires that the staff assess and document the patient's status every 15 minutes. In addition, the Joint Commission requires facilities to document:

- orders for the use of restraints (in a timely manner)
- the results of patient monitoring
- reassessment of the patient's condition
- any unanticipated changes in the patient's condition

Patient Care Notes

Progress notes are brief notes written by the providers throughout a patient's stay to document changes in the patient's condition.

Nursing notes are notes made by the nursing staff regarding the patient's general condition. Nursing notes might record how much or often the patient is sleeping and eating, whether the patient is able to get out of bed, the patient's reports of pain, and whether the patient is able to urinate. These notes are documented throughout each nursing shift as events occur or the patient's condition changes.

Transfer Record

A **transfer record** captures basic patient care information to ensure continuity of care when a patient is transferred to another location within in the facility (e.g., from the ICU to a standard room) or when patient is transferred to or from another healthcare facility (e.g., from a long-term care facility to an acute care hospital).

Consultation Report

A **consultation report** is used by a consulting provider to record diagnoses, notes, care plans, and other information. Consultants may be other physicians or representatives of other patient care areas, such as dietary, respiratory care, physical or occupational therapy, social work, palliative (pain relief) care, or wound care.

Discharge Summary

A **discharge summary** is completed at the conclusion of the hospital stay to provide information to other providers and to facilitate the continuity of care for the patient. The discharge summary should include:

- the reason for hospitalization
- the procedures performed
- the care, treatment, and services provided
- the patient's condition and disposition at discharge
- a summary of the information provided to the patient and his or her family
- the provisions for follow-up care

A discharge summary is not required when the patient is seen for a minor problem or intervention and the patient's stay is short, as defined by the medical staff bylaws. In that instance, a final progress note may be substituted for the discharge summary, but the note must document the outcome of care, disposition of the patient, and provisions for follow-up care.

Additional Forms for Surgical Service Patients

Additional forms are required for patients undergoing a surgical procedure. Forms listed in this section may be included in the surgical patient record.

Consent for Surgery

Laws in all 50 states require providers to obtain a patient's written consent prior to treatment. It is the surgeon's responsibility to ensure that the patient understands the procedure and associated risks and that the patient signs a consent form before a surgical procedure. As shown in Example 4.3, the **consent for surgery** outlines the specifics of the procedure, options, and associated risks. The patient must express an understanding of the information provided. A witness must also sign the form, attesting that the patient has verbally confirmed that he or she understands the procedure.

Example 4.3 Sample Consent for Surgery

Metropolitan Medical Center

INFORMED CONSENT TO SURGICAL PROCEDURE

The purpose of this form is to verify that you have received and have given your consent to the surgery or special procedure recommended to you. You should be involved in any and all decisions involving your medical care. Read this form carefully and be sure to ask your doctors any questions that you many have about the operation or procedure, the risks, and any potential alternative treatments before you give your consent. Your signature below indicates that you have read and understand this paragraph and indicates your consent to the procedure.

_____   _____

Name of Patient or Authorized Representative   **Date**

I, _____, hereby authorize Dr. _____ and any associates or assistants the doctor deems appropriate, to perform (**circle one:** LEFT, RIGHT, BOTH, UNILATERAL) _____.
I consent to have _____ (name and title) perform the following tasks (list): _____.

The risks and benefits associated with the procedure have been explained to me. I understand there is no certainty that I will achieve the described benefits of this treatment and no guarantee has been made to me regarding the outcome of the procedure(s). I also authorize the administration of sedation and/or anesthesia as may be deemed advisable or necessary for my comfort, well being, and safety.

The risks and possible undesirable consequences associated with the procedure not limited to blood loss, transfusion reactions, infection, heart complications, blood clots, loss of or loss of use of body part or other neurological injury or death. Other risks may include: _____ _____. I understand that blood or blood products that may be used during this procedure carry a risk of HIV/AIDS, Hepatitis, or reactions such as the symptoms of fever, chills, hives, or in more severe reactions, the destruction of the transfused red cells (Hemolytic Transfusion Reaction), antibody stimulation, bacterial infections, or, in rare situations, death.

Reprinted with permission from the American Health Information Management Association. Copyright © 2014 by the American Health Information Management Association. All rights reserved. No part of this may be reproduced, reprinted, stored in a retrieval system, or transmitted, in any form or by any means, electronic, photocopying, recording, or otherwise, without the prior written permission of the association.

Anesthesia Report

The anesthesiologist who administers anesthesia to the patient during surgery must submit a report. The report includes:

- a preoperative evaluation by the anesthesiologist
- anesthesia notes recorded during the procedure
- a graph showing vital signs and tracking the amount of anesthesia administered
- a postoperative anesthesia evaluation by the anesthesiologist

Recovery Room Report

The **recovery room report** records the patient's condition during recovery from anesthesia until the patient is returned to his or her hospital room or discharged.

Operative Report

An **operative report** is a narrative description of the surgical procedure, beginning with the type of and the location of the incision made and including an exact description of the procedure (what was removed or repaired), observations of the operative site, and an explanation of how the surgical wound was closed (type of suture material, kind of sutures, dressing applied, etc.).

The Joint Commission requires that operative reports contain:

- a provisional diagnosis
- a write up at the completion of the surgical procedure that includes:
    - the name of the licensed practitioner who performed the procedure plus the name of the participating assistants
    - the name of the procedure
    - a narrative description of the procedure
    - the procedure's findings
    - an estimate of blood loss
    - any specimens removed
    - a postoperative diagnosis

Pathology Report

A **pathology report** is a detailed report of the findings from the analysis of specimens removed during surgery.

Postoperative Evaluation and Follow-Up

The postoperative evaluation and follow-up is the surgeon's final report. It documents the condition of the patient, provides a summary of the surgical procedure, and includes instructions for patient care after the surgery.

Additional Forms for Obstetric Patients

Specific forms are required for OB patients who are admitted for delivery or for other OB conditions before or after delivery (e.g., false labor or postdelivery hemorrhage). These forms include:

- an OB/prenatal report from a physician's office, which provides the history of the pregnancy
- labor and delivery monitoring charts and logs

- labor and delivery notes
- OB anesthesia notes

Additional Forms for Newborn Patients

A baby delivered alive in the hospital is admitted as a patient. The newborn (NB) is assigned a patient number, and a new record is started. The NB patient record includes:

- portions of the mother's OB record, including the prenatal record
- observations after birth
- delivery room care
- a physical exam
- log and flow sheets recording temperature, weight, urination, and stool
- feeding information
- a phenylketonuria (PKU) report documenting the results of metabolic-disease screening tests
- the name of the person to whom the NB is released

The birth certificate issued to a newborn patient utilizes information from both the mother and the NB patient records; however, the official birth certificate is not incorporated into either patient record. Many hospitals do keep a copy of the birth certificate worksheet with the patient record for future reference. States vary on what information is collected on the birth certificate when the mother and the father are not married. Some states require that the father sign a form acknowledging paternity before adding his name to the birth certificate. This form is submitted with the birth certificate to the required agency.

Organization of the Patient Record

There are no regulations stipulating how healthcare facilities should organize the patient record. Licensing and accrediting entities require that the record be complete and the information in the record be accessible in a timely fashion. It is up to the individual healthcare facility to decide how to organize documents in the patient record to best meet the facility's needs and support patient care. Two commonly used organizational strategies are the problem-oriented medical record (POMR) and the source-oriented medical record.

Problem-Oriented Medical Record

In a **problem-oriented medical record**, documentation is organized by the patient's medical problems as identified in the medical history and physical examination. Problems may be *active*, a condition(s) that requires medical management or further diagnostic workup, or *inactive*, a previous and resolved condition(s) that may continue to impact the patient's health. Rehabilitation and behavioral health facilities often use the POMR. Teaching facilities also use the POMR because different practitioners address different aspects of patient care.

A POMR includes several components:

- a database that includes the medical history and physical examination and laboratory data
- a complete **problem list** (a list of conditions or problems for which the patient is seeking treatment or for which treatment should be considered)
- a diagnostic plan, a therapeutic plan, and a patient education plan to address the items identified on the problem list; a SOAP (subjective, objective, assessment, and plan) note (discussed below) recorded for each of the identified problems:
    - the diagnostic plan
        - includes the type of diagnostic testing to be done
        - may change as conditions are ruled out, as symptoms and/or conditions change, and as additional tests are needed
    - the therapeutic plan
        - details the treatment to be started
    - the educational plan
        - outlines the need for education about the condition
        - identifies the needs for care and patient compliance
- daily progress notes written by the physician and other direct care providers
- final progress note or discharge summary that documents the final status of each problem on the list

Table 4.1 illustrates how a physician office would organize a problem list. Each dated entry corresponds to a separate patient visit and includes all supporting documentation. The inclusion of information from previous visits allows the physician to follow up on issues or problems identified during previous visits, if warranted.

Documentation is entered into the POMR by problem. The information for Problem #1, urinary tract infection, maintained together would be the diagnostic plan, the lab report culture and sensitivity (C&S), medications and educational information, practitioner progress notes, and any other related documentation.

If a patient is treated for two problems during the same visit, information for each problem is maintained separately.

Table 4.1 Physician Office POMR

Date	Problem	Problem #	Plan	Phys.	Date Resolved	Date Recurred
1/10/15	Urinary tract infection (UTI)	#1	**DP** Urinalysis C&S **RX** Meds. based on C&S **CE** UTI info. sheet	Garcia	1/17/15	
6/8/14	Hypertension	#2	**DP** None at this time **RX** Clonidine 0.1 mg and lifestyle changes **CE** Hypertension info. and salt-free diet plan	White	7/8/14 Under control with meds.	
9/30/14	Epigastric pain, recurring	#3	**DP** Esophagoscopy **RX** Prilosec OTC **CE** Acid reflux info. **FUP** Return in two weeks if symptoms persist. Dr. will call with results of esophagoscopy.	Garcia		

DP diagnostic procedure; RX prescription; C&S culture and sensitivity (lab test); CE clinical education; FUP follow-up

Source-Oriented Medical Record

The **source-oriented medical record** is one of the most common methods of organizing documentation in the patient record. It is used by hospitals, large specialty clinics, and rehabilitation facilities. Information is organized by source (where the information came from) or by category. Categories include:

- practitioner documentation (history and physical, consultation reports, orders)
- discharge summary
- progress notes
- diagnostics (labs, X-rays, EKGs, and other diagnostic tests)
- monitoring sheets (vital signs, medical log sheet, intake/output logs, etc.)
- operative block of documentation (anesthesia notes and log sheet, pre- and post-surgery notes, operative report, recovery record, pathology report)
- therapist documentation (evaluations and treatment records) and nursing notes

The advantage of having the information maintained by documentation source or category is that all similar information is kept together, making it easier to review and compare information over time. For example, if a physician just wants to see all of a patient's lab work to monitor changes, all of the labs are filed in chronological order. The physicians won't have to sift through progress notes, log sheets, and other documentation. Having all of the physician orders in one place makes it easier for the nursing staff to follow up and verify that all physician orders have been acted upon. The major disadvantage of this arrangement of information is that care providers need to access different sections of the record to see all of the most recent information.

SOAP Notes

Both the POMR and source-oriented medical record are ways of organizing information in the patient record. A **SOAP note** is a format for organizing information documented in the record. SOAP stands for subjective, objective, assessment, and plan.

SOAP notes have been used for a number of years to improve the organization and increase the level of detail in medical documentation. As shown in Table 4.2, a SOAP note is divided into four parts: the patient's subjective description of the condition or the complaint; the physician's objective assessment based on preliminary testing; the physician's preliminary diagnosis; and the treatment plan.

SOAP notes provide a means of organizing information in the patient record. The same information may be provided in other documentation formats but will not be identified by the subjective, objective, assessment, and plan designations. The SOAP note format is used with both paper and electronic health records.

Table 4.2 Components of a SOAP Note

Components	Definition	Examples
1. Subjective	A description of the condition in the patient's own words (onset, symptoms, and the reason for seeking care)	"I have had a throbbing headache for four days, and nothing I take makes it any better." "I just don't feel well—sort of weak and shaky, not hungry, and not sleeping very well." "I feel like my blood pressure is high."
2. Objective	Factual, straightforward, and repeatable facts	Vital signs (temp, pulse, blood pressure, and respiration) Physical examination Results of lab and other studies Measurements (height, weight, and age)
3. Assessment	The preliminary diagnosis based on the physician's assessment of the subjective and objective information	"A 53-yr.-old male experiencing headaches with noted elevated blood pressure and recent, rapid 10 lb. weight gain" "A 76-year-old woman with vague symptoms; vital signs are within normal range, but tests indicate abnormalities of the blood chemical profile" "42 y.o. woman presents with elevated blood pressure, but no other symptoms present; cause unknown at this time"
4. Plan	A plan for treatment based on the physician's assessment; the plan may recommend more testing, monitoring of the condition, medication, surgical intervention, or a referral to another practitioner	"Treatment will begin for hypertension and fluid retention." "Additional blood tests ordered to monitor the chem profile and rule out possible conditions. A review of symptoms and past history will be done in an attempt to determine the cause of the abnormalities." "Start patient on a different blood pressure (BP) medication, and monitor. Will continue to evaluate the patient systemically. Order urinalysis, blood, urea, nitrogen (BUN), glomerular filtration rate (GFR), and creatinine blood work to evaluate kidney function and an ECG to check for heart arrhythmias to determine if there is an underlying cause for the elevation in BP."

Electronic Health Record Organization

An electronic health record is more than just a digital version of a paper record. All of the information stored digitally in a patient's EHR is available whenever and wherever it is needed. Patient information can be accessed and organized in many different ways. A simple query to the EHR can produce a report showing the results of diagnostic tests for the previous year or highlighting the patient's medication history for a specific condition during a set period of time. The EHR is covered in greater detail in Chapter 7.

Required Documentation in the Patient Record

The patient record is a legal document, and documentation in the record must conform to legal and regulatory standards. These include state licensing guidelines, Joint Commission standards, and Centers for Medicare & Medicaid Services (CMS) Conditions of Participation (CoPs). Healthcare facilities should have written policies based on these standards and regulations to ensure the uniformity of the patient record's content and format.

Documentation formatting must also take into account payer policies and professional practice standards. Whether the records are maintained in paper or electronic format, documentation must support the care of the patient and facilitate other required uses.

The acute care inpatient record includes the greatest variety of documentation, so requirements for the acute care record are discussed here. Other types of healthcare facilities may require other forms and documentation that are specific to the care provided. For example, the patient record at a long-term care facility may contain very little diagnostic information and a lot of nursing notes and assessment documentation.

Table 4.3 lists some of the Joint Commission and CMS documentation requirements for the acute care patient record. Note that some of the requirements have similar wording, but there are some important variations. It is also interesting to note that the Medicare CoPs are much more prescriptive in terms of what must be documented.

Good documentation is fundamental to quality patient care. The **National Committee for Quality Assurance (NCQA)**, an independent nonprofit organization focused on improving the quality of patient care, developed guidelines for documentation in the patient health record. These guidelines are commonly accepted standards of practice and are used by organizations to develop their own documentation standards. According to the guidelines, the patient record must be legible and should include:

- the patient's name
- the patient's identification number (could be a medical record number)
- the date the report was generated
- the printed name and signature of the report author

> **EXPAND YOUR KNOWLEDGE**
> To view a complete list of NCQA documentation guidelines, go to http://IntroHIM.ParadigmCollege.net/NCQAGuidelines.

Table 4.3 Sample Joint Commission and CMS Documentation Standards for the Acute Care Record

Documentation Requirements	Joint Commission	Conditions of Participation
The hospital initiates and maintains a medical record for every individual assessed or treated.	IM.7.1	
A medical record must be maintained for every individual evaluated or treated in the hospital.		482.24
Only authorized individuals make entries in medical records.	IM.7.1.1	
Every medical record entry is dated, its author identified and, when necessary, authenticated.	IM.7.8	
All entries must be legible and complete and must be authenticated and dated promptly by the person (identified by name and discipline) who is responsible for ordering, providing, or evaluating the service furnished.		482.24 (c) (1)
The author of each entry must be identified and must authenticate his or her entry.		482.24 (c) (1) (i)
Authentication may include signatures, written initials, or computer entry.		482.24 (c) (1) (ii)
The medical record contains sufficient information to identify the patient, support the diagnosis, justify the treatment, document the course and results, and promote continuity of care among healthcare providers.	IM.7.2	482.24 (c)
All records must document the following as appropriate: • admitting diagnosis results of all consultative evaluations of the patient • results of all consultative evaluations of the patient and appropriate findings by clinical and other staff involved in the care of the patient • documentation of complications, hospital-acquired infections, and unfavorable reactions to drugs and anesthesia • properly executed informed consent forms for procedures and treatments specified by the medical staff, or by federal or state law if applicable, to require written patient consent • all practitioner's orders, nursing notes, reports of treatment, medication records, radiology, and laboratory reports, vital signs, and other information necessary to monitor the patient's condition		482.24 (c) (2) (iii) 482.24 (c) (2) (iii) 482.24 (c) (2) (iv) 482.24 (c) (2) (v) 482.24 (c) (2) (vi)

Source: Excerpted from *Documentation Requirements for the Acute Care Inpatient Record (AHIMA Practice Brief)*; Joint Commission and Medicare Conditions of Participation updates added

TAKE THE CHALLENGE

Review the CT scan below and determine if it is **compliant** (conforms to the rules) with the NCQA guidelines listed in Table 4.3. Check the CT report for each of the NCQA requirements listed above, and indicate whether each of the required items is present in the report.

Patient Name:	Helen Small	Requesting DR:	Audrey Zinder, MD
MR#:	06975432	Attending DR:	Lee Her, MD
Account #:	113-222555	Family DR:	
Date of Birth:	10-24-1958	Transcribed Date:	10-11-2014
Order Location:		Transcriptionist:	Juanita Ramiro
Room #:			
Service Date:	10-09-2014		
Report Date:	10-12-2014		

STUDY: CT PELVIS WITH CONTRAST
REASON FOR PROCEDURE(S): LIVER MASS BY ECHO

CT PELVIS WITH CONTRAST

Spiral scanning during bolus infusion of contrast was performed.

No adenopathy is seen. There are no masses demonstrated. No fluid collections are noted. The GI tract was unremarkable. Note is made of small areas of increased density along the subcutaneous fat in the anterior abdominal wall and small collections of air consistent with injection sites.

IMPRESSION: Normal Exam

Transcriptionist: Juanita Ramiro
Reading Radiologist: Sheera Osborn MD
This report has been reviewed and released by: Audrey Zinder, MD

Printed on 10-12-2014   ORIGINAL REPORT   Page 1 of 1

Electronic Health Record Documentation Requirements

As noted, the healthcare industry is transitioning from paper patient records to the electronic health record. EHRs offer a number of advantages, including improved and real-time access to patient information, enhanced decision support, enhanced coding and billing functions, and increased opportunities for patient engagement. EHRs will be discussed in depth in Chapter 7.

HIM professionals are often involved in the planning and the development of EHR systems to ensure that all required information is captured in the EHR, the privacy and the security of patient information is maintained, and the system is interoperable (compatible) with other systems in the facility (lab, pharmacy, etc.) and with providers outside the facility.

Like paper record documentation, documentation in the EHR must comply with Joint Commission standards, CMS Conditions of Participation, and other regulatory and payer documentation guidelines.

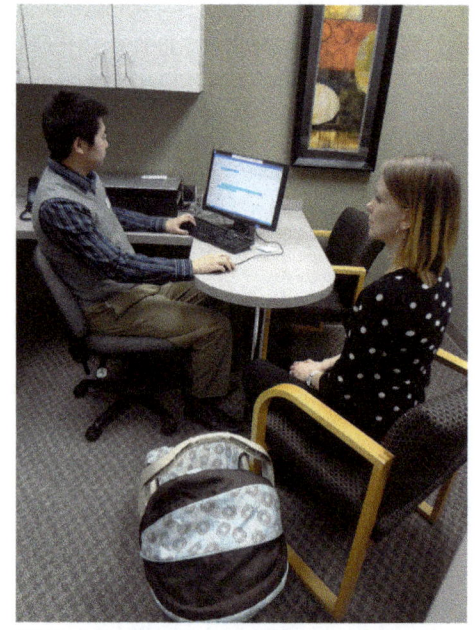

Bedside terminals, computer workstations, laptops and other types of portable devices are now commonly used to record information that will become part of the patient health record.

EHR documentation guidelines require the following:

- The record should include sufficient information to identify the patient, justify the diagnosis and treatment, document the results of care, describe the condition of the patient upon discharge, and document the instructions given to the patient upon discharge.
- All entries in the record should be accurate, relevant, timely, and complete.
- All entries in the record must be concise, without irrelevant text.
- The title of a note should match the content of the note and the author's credentials (physician notes written by the physician, nurses notes written by a nurse, etc.).
- All notes should be reviewed and signed by the author of the note in a timely manner. (In many systems, unsigned notes are not available for review by others except for the pharmacy.)
- Prompts from the EHR system for additional information or authentication should be responded to in a timely manner.
- Authentication should include the identity and the credentials of the author, and the date and the time signed.

- The electronic **copy and paste function** should be used sparingly, if at all, and with caution. (The copy and paste function allows providers to copy information from one section of a patient record to another, much like copy and paste in a word processing document.)

- A complete record (all documentation incorporated, signatures and dates obtained) should not be edited or altered without the approval of the physician or the medical record committee as per the facility bylaws. Only the original author of an entry in the record can initiate the retraction of information.

- Addendum notes can be added to clarify or add additional information to the original document. Addendums are linked to the original document and must be authenticated as required for original documents. Addendums cannot be backdated.

Forms Committee

Just think of the number of different forms that could be created if every hospital unit or provider could design a form to meet its specific needs and preferences. For example, what if nurses in the intensive care unit, the newborn nursery, and the obstetric delivery area all developed separate forms for recording vital signs and medication administration? It would be chaos. There would be no consistency, and many forms would likely not provide the necessary information or meet regulatory standards. To support patient care and meet clinical documentation requirements, healthcare facilities must have standardized, well-designed forms.

To ensure the uniformity of documentation in the patient record, most healthcare facilities have a forms committee. The committee typically meets monthly, and membership may vary. The committee is likely to include members of the medical staff and the departments of nursing, health information management, purchasing, and administration. The committee is charged with reviewing existing forms, approving new forms, and monitoring the use of paper forms and electronic data capture (EDC) screens to ensure that required information is collected and produces useable documentation when retrieved.

The forms committee is responsible for ensuring that:

- forms (paper charts) and formats (electronic records) that become a part of the permanent, legal health record support patient care, quality improvement, risk management, financial activities, teaching, and research

- approved forms meet all federal, state, and Joint Commission documentation requirements

- the consolidation and the design of forms reduce duplicate and redundant information in the legal health record

Document Design

The forms committee reviews form drafts and provides guidance for users in developing new forms. Design considerations may include such things as:

- standards for form layout and identification
- required information for patient identification
- signature and date lines/fields for providers and patients
- ease of the entry of required documentation
- compliance with the approved list of abbreviations (Words not included on the approved list should be spelled out.)
- how the form will be used and where it will be placed in the patient record

Authority/Responsibility for Documenting

As outlined in Table 4.3, the Joint Commission and the CMS Conditions of Participation have established standards for documenting in the medical record. To earn or maintain accreditation and to ensure high-quality patient care, facilities must comply with the documentation standards listed here.

A physician's authority and responsibility to document in the record is based on licensing and accreditation requirements, and facilities are required to demonstrate that they are in compliance with those documentation requirements.

In some facilities, the medical staff bylaws may permit a physician to delegate his or her authority to document in the record to someone else—for example, a physician assistant or a medical student. In this circumstance, the individual doing the documentation (the delegate) must be identified in the record and authenticate (sign) the report. The physician must review the documentation, document any needed changes, cosign the entry, and accept responsibility for the information entered. Authority/responsibility also applies to nursing, respiratory and all other providers responsible for documenting care provided. Policies should be in place indicating those who have the authority to document and the requirements for documenting.

Timelines

The Joint Commission and Medicare CoPs require that documentation in the inpatient record be completed within a specific timeframe. As shown in Table 4.4, the amount of time allowed to complete documentation in the record varies depending on the type of documentation. Individual facilities may choose to set more stringent requirements.

Records not completed within the timeframe specified by the medical staff bylaws are considered delinquent. Physicians who fail to complete records within the time specified may be sanctioned. Disciplinary actions may include the loss of hospital admission privileges for a specified time or until records are complete, temporary suspension from the medical staff, or probation (if the provider has continued or repeated delinquent records).

> **BE AWARE**
>
> When correcting an error in a paper medical record, erasing or covering the error with correction fluid is not permitted. To correct an error, strike through the text with a straight line, making certain it remains legible. Write the word "error," the author's initials, and the date and the time of the correction above the error. Editing an error in an EHR entry requires that the original, erroneous entry be noted and maintained and a correction added.

Table 4.4 Standards/Guidelines for Documenting in the Inpatient Record

The H&P, nursing assessment, and other screening assessments must be completed within 24 hours of admission.
If the H&P was performed within 30 days of admission, a durable and legible copy may be used in the record, indicating any changes since the H&P was completed.
An H&P update must be written before a surgical procedure.
Before surgery, the H&P, diagnostic test results, and a preoperative diagnosis must be completed and in the patient record.
There must be a complete H&P in the patient chart before surgery (except in the case of emergency surgery). The H&P must be completed no more than 30 days before or 24 hours after admission. (Oromaxillofacial surgeons have a 48-hour timeframe to complete the H&P since a medical doctor will do the complete H&P (except the portion related to what the oromaxillary surgeon will do.)
A care plan, usually developed by a nursing professional, must be developed and documented in the record before an operative procedure is performed.
A preoperative diagnosis must be recorded before surgery.
Operative reports must be dictated or written immediately after surgery.
If the report is not placed in the record immediately after surgery, a progress note is entered immediately after surgery and before the patient is transferred to the next level of care. The surgeon is required to make sure the patient has signed an informed consent form before surgery.
The surgeon must authenticate the completed operative report within the timeframe specified in the hospital bylaws, and the report should be filed in the record as soon as possible after surgery.
Documentation of a presedation or preanesthesia assessment is required before sedation and anesthesia.
Documentation that a preanesthesia evaluation was performed is required within 48 hours before surgery. For inpatients, a postanesthesia follow-up report must be completed within 48 hours after surgery.
Verbal and telephone orders—though infrequently used—should be signed as soon as possible or per medical staff bylaws.
Discharge summary/clinical summary or death summary is typically completed within 30 days unless individual state guidelines specify a shorter time.

Signature Requirements (Authentication)

The Joint Commission requirements specify that every patient record entry must be dated, the author of the entry identified, and, when required, the record or the entry be **authenticated**. When a practitioner signs, or authenticates, a report, he or she is attesting to the validity of that report. A handwritten signature is required to authenticate a paper record. An **electronic signature** is used to authenticate an electronic record. The electronic signature may consist of a digital facsimile of the provider's handwritten signature or a code consisting of letters, numbers, characters, and/or symbols that is executed as the individual's signature.

Incomplete versus Complete Records

Ensuring that the documentation in the patient record is complete, accurate, and up-to-date is important for optimal patient care. Information contained in the record provides the basis for diagnostic and treatment plans. Supported by medical staff bylaws, continuous efforts are made to reduce the number of incomplete and delinquent patient records to improve patient care. The patient record is not complete until all required documentation and signatures have been entered into the record. Until that point, it is considered an **incomplete record**. The record is rarely complete before a patient is discharged because the discharge summary is not dictated until after the patient is discharged. Final lab results and other reports may also not be available or incorporated into the record yet. Once completed, a record is ready for permanent storage/filing.

Joint Commission guidelines specify that facilities set a reasonable timeframe for completing patient records. Joint Commission standards also set limits on the number of delinquent records a facility may have at a given time, based on the number of patients discharged. The number of incomplete records should not exceed the facility's monthly average discharge rate. For example, if Good Health Hospital discharges an average of 1,250 inpatients per month, the hospital should have no more than 1,250 incomplete records at any given time. Some records may be incomplete for more than a month, but the total number of incomplete inpatient records should not exceed 1,250.

Medicare CoPs specify that if a record is incomplete after 30 days, it is considered a **delinquent record**. Medical staff bylaws at an individual facility may specify a shorter period of time. The Joint Commission standard requires that no more than half of the average discharge records from the previous 30 days be delinquent. Facilities must file the required form for reporting incomplete and delinquent records (Example 4.4) quarterly. A facility with a history of incomplete and delinquent records may be put on a probationary status for noncompliance and given a specific timeframe—six months, for example—to achieve compliance.

IT REALLY HAPPENS

California regulations require that all inpatient medical records be completed within 14 days from the date of discharge. (CA Code of Regulations, Title 22, Section 70751). To be in compliance, California providers should not have any delinquent records.

Example 4.4   Delinquent Records Reporting Form

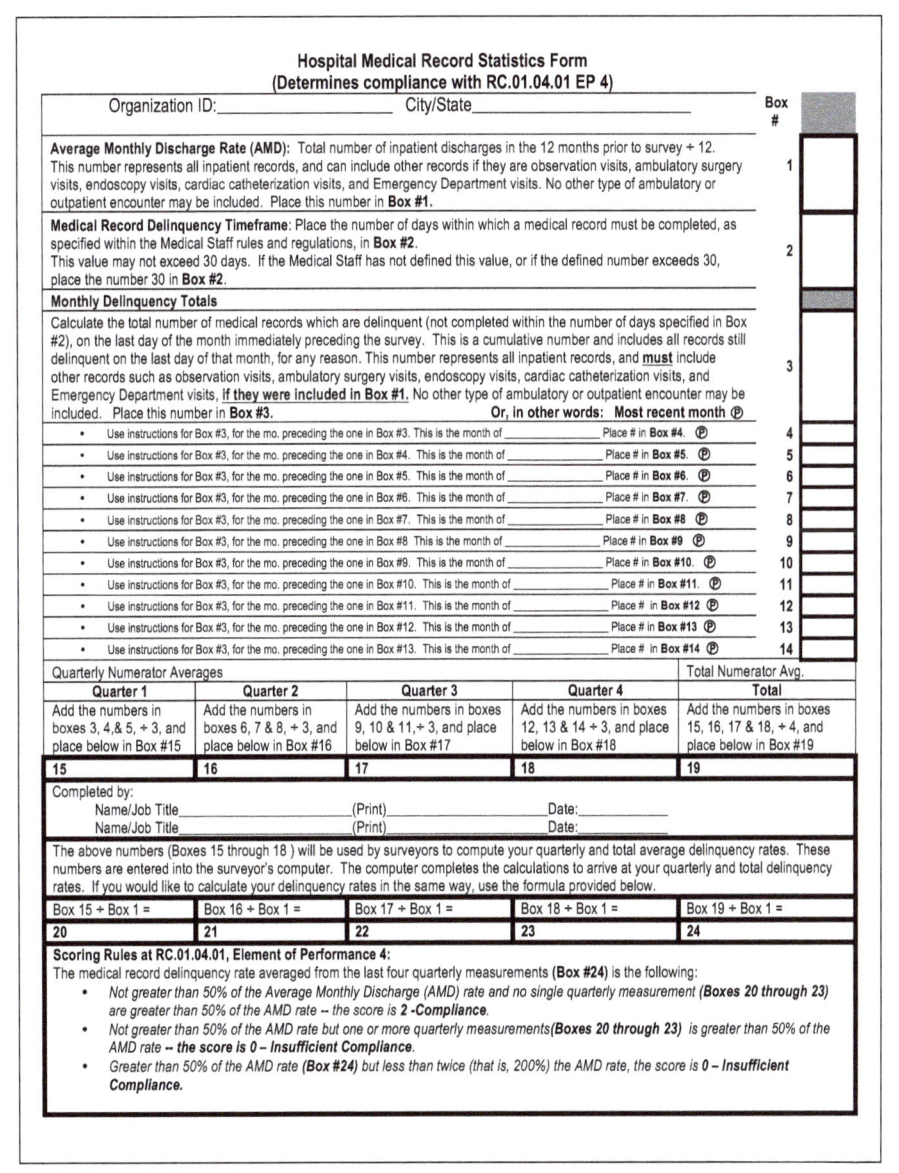

Hospital Medical Record Statistics Form (Determines compliance with RC.01.04.01 EP 4). Form reproduced from The Joint Commission.

© The Joint Commission, 2014. Reprinted with permission.

Information Governance

Healthcare organizations are becoming increasingly concerned with the issue of *information governance*. **Information governance (IG)** refers to the structures, principles, and practices needed to standardize, manage, protect, access, and communicate data in a business environment.

The amount and the type of data created in the healthcare environment are increasing steadily as are the demands to share and process that data for clinical, financial, and patient-related needs. With the widespread adoption of the EHR, there is a growing need to protect the integrity of patient health information and to ensure that information is accurate, timely, relevant, valid, and complete.

EXPAND YOUR KNOWLEDGE

Interested in learning more about information governance? Read the article "IG 101: The Role of HIM Professionals," published in the *Journal of AHIMA*, at http://IntroHIM.ParadigmCollege.net/IG.

> " ... the hoped-for efficiency and quality gains from electronic records and related applications will evaporate if hospitals and medical practices don't support them with organizational changes."
>
> —Julia Adler-Milstein; assistant professor of information, School of Information, and assistant professor of health management and policy, School of Public Health; University of Michigan; *Harvard Business Review*; April 2009

Improving the quality of care while reducing costs is one of the challenges facing the healthcare system. Patient information can be a major asset to a facility as a resource for evaluating the cost and the quality of care. For example, a facility may want to know the average cost for a Medicare patient who has undergone a total hip replacement. By breaking down the data further, the data may show that a brand of prosthetic hips commonly used at the hospital has a higher postoperative infection rate than other brands, which increases the patient's length of stay and the overall cost of the procedure. An effective IG program can provide opportunities like this to improve decision making and reduce costs.

Clinical Documentation

Clinical documentation is the capture and the recording of clinical information. It is a vital component of every patient encounter. **Clinical information** used in making patient care decisions includes the patient's medical history and physical exam, labs, and X-rays along with evaluations by the practitioner(s). Clinical documentation must be completed in a timely manner, be accurate, and reflect the range of services provided to the patient.

Clinical documentation includes data from:

- assessments, including lab tests, lab results, and assessments by a physical therapist or another provider
- consultations, including a secondary opinion from another physician or another type of care provider
- imaging exams, such as X-rays, CT scans, and magnetic resonance imaging (MRI) scans
- treatment, which includes all medications given, therapy reports (e.g., respiratory or physical therapy), and nurses notes
- the patient's past and current medical status
- clinical diagnostics and evaluations performed
- events where communication was exchanged, such as family meetings
- transfer information

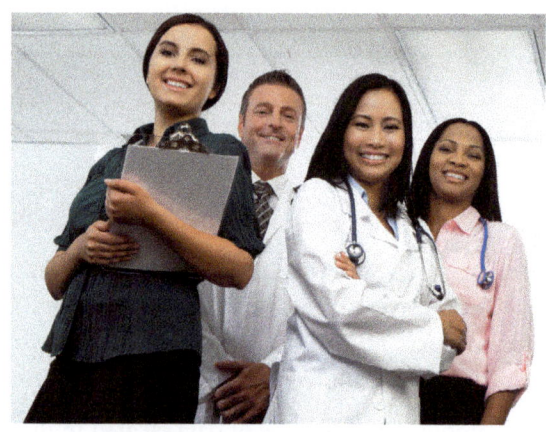

Clinical documentation provides the basis for patient care. It is also used in billing, research, and education. It is reported to external agencies used in other statistics to evaluate care quality.

- the patient's response to clinical interventions
- clinical care plans
- future goals for patient health

Clinical Documentation Improvement

Most healthcare facilities have a work group or a committee assigned to **clinical documentation improvement (CDI)**, a program to improve the quality of documentation to ensure that it is complete, legible, timely, concise, clear, patient-centered, and accurate. The quality of documentation is important to patient care, and it also affects the facility's financial reimbursement. Healthcare providers must be able to accurately document all of the care and the services provided to the patient. Clinical documentation that is complete and accurate can be more easily and accurately translated into the medical and procedural codes used to bill insurers and other third-party payers for reimbursement. By improving the quality and the accuracy of clinical documentation, healthcare facilities can improve the quality of patient care, insure proper revenue, reduce the number of denied claims, and help to reduce coding errors that can lead to fraudulent billing.

CDI program goals generally include:

- identifying and clarifying missing, conflicting, or nonspecific physician documentation related to diagnoses and procedures
- supporting accurate diagnostic and procedural coding, severity of illness, and expected risk of mortality, leading to appropriate reimbursement
- promoting health record completion during the patient's course of care
- improving communication between physicians and other members of the healthcare team
- educating providers on appropriate documentation
- addressing negative findings stemming from quality reviews
- improving coders' understanding of the disease process, so they can identify the appropriate information necessary to code as specifically and accurately as possible

As shown in Table 4.5, CDI programs encourage providers to use well-defined, objective statements to convey the most complete information.

Table 4.5 Clinical Documentation Improvement

Vague	Well Defined
Breathing improving	Breathing improved, oxygen saturation rate 95%, and patient can walk without getting short of breath
Pneumonia	Aspiration pneumonia, status poststroke patient with dysphagia
Patient ambulated	Patient ambulated 50 ft. at 9:00 a.m. and 3:00 p.m. with the aid of a walker

Chapter Summary

To truly understand the health record, one must understand the individual pieces of information and the forms that comprise the record and the specific data that is recorded on those forms. Documentation in the medical record is governed by a variety of regulations with the primary focus on supporting patient care. A great deal of information is available in the patient record, however, and that information is used to support many activities other than direct patient care, including billing and reimbursement, statistical reporting, research, and education.

The acquisition of data and its maintenance, usage, and storage are also key to understanding the patient record. While patient records have traditionally been maintained as paper documents, healthcare facilities are now in the process of transitioning to the electronic health record. Documentation requirements are the same for paper and electronic records; however, these requirements may be met in different ways. For example, requirements for record storage and access are implemented very differently depending on the format of the record.

Clinical documentation improvement programs have grown out of the transition to electronic health records and the increased access to patient data that EHRs afford. The patient record is considered to be a resource for the facility and should be treated as such from a management perspective. The patient health record is at the core of what HIM professionals do but is also a crucial component of what others do in the healthcare setting—from the physicians, the nurses, and other direct care providers; to admissions and billing; and to administrative support functions.

HIM Review

Check Your Understanding

Test your understanding of the material covered in this chapter by completing the following multiple-choice questions. For each question, select the best answer from the choices provided.

1. _____ is a method of organizing a patient record by the medical condition(s) for which the patient is being treated.

    a. A SOAP note

    b. Clinical documentation

    c. A POMR

    d. A source-oriented record

2. A discharge summary is _____
    a. a series of summary notes made by the providers of care.
    b. a set of educational materials provided to the patient upon discharge.
    c. part of the patient's bill, used to substantiate care provided.
    d. a summary of the patient's stay from admission to discharge.

3. The goal of clinical documentation improvement is _____
    a. to ensure all patient information is created and maintained electronically.
    b. to have patient information that is complete, legible, timely, concise, clear, patient-centered, and accurate.
    c. to decrease the number of incomplete and delinquent patient records.
    d. All of the choices are correct.

4. _____ is a tool for managing patient information as a resource.
    a. Information governance
    b. Clinical documentation improvement
    c. POMR
    d. The National Committee for Quality Assurance

5. Records that are not completed within the timeframe established by the medical staff bylaws are _____
    a. considered incomplete.
    b. filed away as they are.
    c. delinquent.
    d. abstract.

6. An electronic signature is _____
    a. a code of letters, numbers, and characters, similar to a PIN (personal identification number).
    b. a computer-generated signature code.
    c. an electronic image of a handwritten image.
    d. All of the choices are correct.

7. _____ is/are a means of documenting that provides structure and thoroughness by recording findings from an objective and subjective manner, providing assessment comments and plans for care.

   a. The POMR
   b. The source-oriented medical record
   c. SOAP notes
   d. The electronic health record

8. A problem list is _____

   a. a document providing dates and conditions for all visits.
   b. a POMR.
   c. a tool to manage information.
   d. clinical documentation.

9. Data that is tracked by variables such as over time, across groups, or across patient populations is _____

   a. abstracted data.
   b. aggregate data.
   c. the Minimum Data Set (MDS).
   d. a problem list.

10. The goals of a clinical documentation improvement program include _____

    a. identifying missing or conflicting physician documentation of diagnoses and procedures.
    b. supporting accurate coding.
    c. improving communication between the healthcare team.
    d. All of the choices are correct.

Think Critically

Consider the following real-world scenario and draft a response.

Access the medical record forms in Appendix D or on Navigator+ website. Find the copy of the physical examination paper record and one other paper-based form of your choosing. Design a template for an electronic health record that would capture this same information at a computer workstation. Research resources for suggested screen/template design for data capture.

Sharpen Your Comprehension

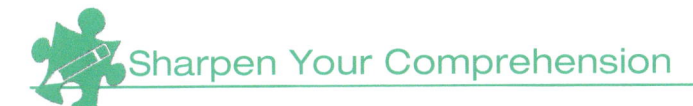

Complete the following matching exercise by selecting, from the list provided, the answer that best matches each of the numbered statements. For each statement, only one answer is correct.

- a. abstract
- b. authenticate
- c. de-identifying
- d. incomplete record
- e. nosocomial
- f. protocol
- g. public health
- h. source-oriented medical record
- i. transcribe
- j. vital signs

1. _____ Organized activities to prevent disease, promote health, and prolong life among the general population

2. _____ Missing any of the required components and signatures

3. _____ To create a written copy

4. _____ Information is organized by where the information came from

5. _____ Establish authorship

6. _____ To extract or find information

7. _____ Includes measurements of temperature, pulse, and blood pressure

8. _____ Removing information that could potentially identify the patient

9. _____ Infection acquired by the patient while already in the hospital

10. _____ Guidelines based on data and to be followed in the treatment of specific diseases

Connect Theory to Practice

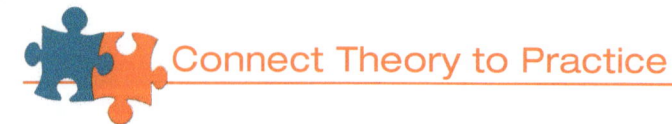

To help translate the concepts presented in this chapter to the workplace, complete the following exercise.

Refer to the Delinquent Records Reporting Form, Example 4.4 on page 99. Using the data below, calculate the statistics required to complete the form.

# of discharges for the year	10,583 patients
Medical Record Deficiency Timeframe	20 days

# of delinquent records for the year by month, most recent first:

December	320
November	295
October	290
September	1101
August	1125
July	1134
June	498
May	593
April	1102
March	684
February	589
January	576

Student eResources

*To enhance your comprehension of the chapter material, go to **Navigator+** and complete the additional practice items as advised by your instructor.*

Chapter Terms

- advance directive
- aggregate data
- authenticated
- clinical documentation
- clinical documentation improvement (CDI)
- clinical information
- complete record
- compliant
- consent for surgery
- consultation report
- copy and paste function
- de-identified
- delinquent record
- diagnostic findings
- discharge summary
- electronic signature
- incomplete record
- information governance (IG)
- log sheets and flow sheets
- medication record
- National Committee for Quality Assurance (NCQA)
- nosocomial infection
- operative report
- pathology report
- patient record
- physician orders
- problem list
- problem-oriented medical record
- Recovery Audit Contractor (RAC)
- recovery room report
- restraint log
- SOAP note
- source-oriented medical record
- transcribed
- transfer record
- vital signs

Fast Facts

Adoption of Electronic Health Record Systems Varies Widely Across States

- In 2013, the percentage of physicians using an electronic health record (EHR) system that meets the criteria for a basic system ranged from 21 percent in New Jersey to 83 percent in North Dakota.
- The national average was 48 percent.
- Eight states fell below the national average: Connecticut, Maryland, Nevada, New Jersey, Oklahoma, Vermont, West Virginia, and Wyoming.
- Nine states exceeded the national average: Iowa, Massachusetts, Minnesota, North Dakota, Oregon, South Dakota, Utah, Washington, and Wisconsin.
- The percentage of physicians using any type of EHR system (all or partially electronic) ranged from 66 percent in New Jersey to 94 percent in Minnesota.

Source: National Center for Health Statistics Data Brief No. 143 (January 2014)

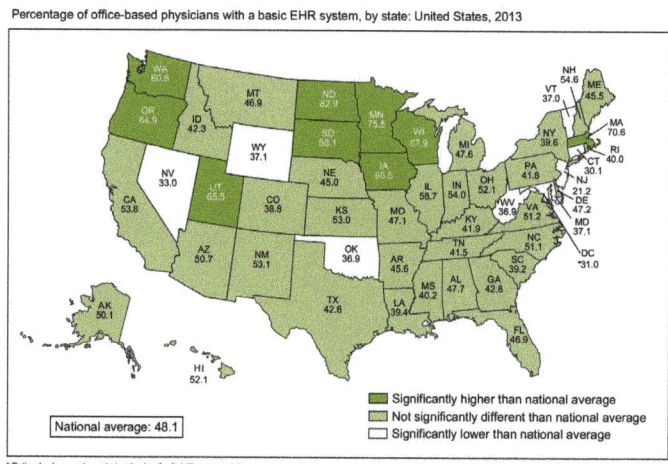

Percentage of office-based physicians with a basic EHR system, by state: United States, 2013

National average: 48.1

* Estimate does not meet standards of reliability or precision.
NOTES: EHR is electronic health record. Significance tested at $p < 0.05$.
SOURCE: CDC/NCHS, National Ambulatory Medical Care Survey, Electronic Health Records Survey.

Think Ethics!

EHRs are rapidly replacing paper records as the standard in health care. EHRs allow patients greater access to personal health information, but not all patients benefit equally. Elderly patients and patients with limited computer access or skills may find themselves on the wrong side of the digital divide. However, EHR technology may also help to reduce racial and ethnic disparities in health care. To learn more about the impact of EHRs on healthcare disparities, read the article "Bridging the Digital Divide in Health Care: The Role of Health Information Technology in Addressing Racial and Ethnic Disparities" at http://IntroHIM.ParadigmCollege.net/Disparities.

Chapter 5

Health Record Organization and Storage

> "There are uncountable hours lost each year in the workplace because of disorganization. But people mix up cleaning with organizing. Being clean is a visual thing, but being organized is being able to find things when you need them."
>
> —Julie Mahan, owner of Indianapolis-based company Simply Organizing

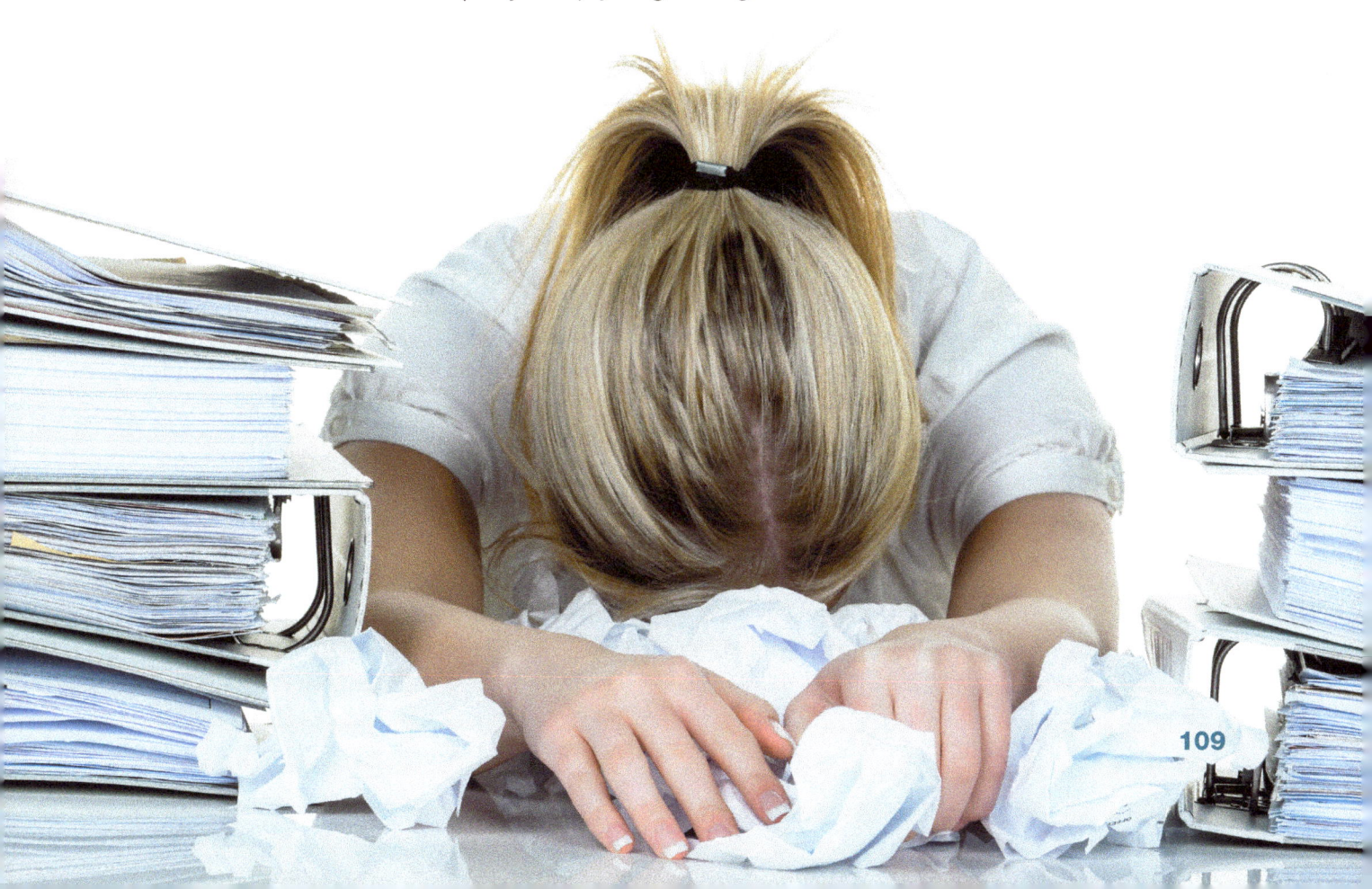

Learning Objectives

- Compare serial, serial unit, and unit numbering systems.
- Differentiate between the methods used for paper record filing.
- Explain the benefits and the drawbacks of different digital record storage mediums.
- Explain the retrieval process for patient health records.
- Describe advantages of electronic health record systems.
- Understand the stages of the health record life cycle.
- Understand the consequences of failing to file documentation in a timely manner.
- Summarize record retention and destruction practices.
- Describe the disaster-preparedness process.

The primary purpose of the patient health record is to document and facilitate all care provided to the patient. High-quality documentation and the proper organization and storage of the patient record are essential components of patient care. The health information management (HIM) department is responsible for ensuring that the content of the record is accurate and complete and that the record is available in a timely manner for patient care, billing, statistical reporting, and quality monitoring, whether the record is stored in paper, electronic, or hybrid form.

As healthcare facilities move from paper to electronic health records, the HIM department is playing an integral role in the transition, working with information systems, administration, medical staff, nursing, business, and other departmental stakeholders to assess the facility's needs and assist in the design and selection of the electronic health record (EHR) system. The HIM department also plays a key role in overseeing EHR implementation, and in monitoring and evaluating its performance.

Transitioning from paper to electronic records is a very long process. Because of the amount of planning required and the impact the switch will have on other facility systems, it may take two to three years from the time a facility decides to adopt an EHR system to the time the EHR system is fully functional. Even after the EHR system is fully functional, facilities will likely continue to retain some older and inactive patient records in paper format. HIM staff need to be familiar with storage and retrieval practices for both paper and electronic records.

Paper Record Storage

Patient health records in paper form are most often stored in file folders with some sort of fasteners to hold the individual pieces of paper together in the approved format. File folders are used extensively for both inpatient and outpatient records. Some facilities maintain their patient records in a three-ring binder. Patient records must be readily accessible but also secure to maintain the privacy and the security of patient information. The task of accessing or pulling a record from storage is referred to as **record retrieval**.

To reduce the amount of storage space required, paper records are often stored on moveable shelving systems set on tracks. Each unit slides forward and backward to create aisle space between units. In smaller facilities, patient files may be stored in standard filing shelves or cabinets.

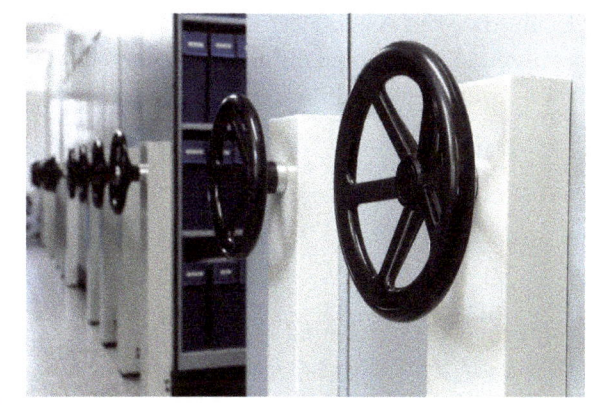

Moveable shelving units reduce the amount of floor space needed for the storage of paper files.

Maintaining a secure record-storage area is essential for the protection of patient privacy. The most current records—generally records of patients who have received care recently (within the previous six months to two years, depending on the type and the size of the facility)—may be filed in or near the HIM department. Paper records require a significant amount of storage space, however, so older or inactive records are often moved into permanent storage in a different location in the same facility or stored in a separate facility. Some records may be stored in a remote location. Regardless of where the records are stored, patient privacy and the security of the records must be maintained in accordance with legal and regulatory requirements.

After a patient record is completed and moved to permanent storage, the record may still be used within the facility, or it may be needed to respond to an external request. Internally, the record may be used for continued patient care, for administrative statistical reporting, or for review by committees such as blood usage, infection control, surgery, record review, or quality improvement. Externally, the record may be requested by an outside physician or treatment facility or for payment or legal purposes.

Health Record Numbering

In both inpatient and outpatient healthcare facilities, patients are given a patient or medical record number for identification purposes and to protect patient confidentiality. Patient identification numbers also help to distinguish between patients who share the same name. The type of numbering system used varies by facility. Patient identification numbers are assigned for both paper and electronic records.

Most healthcare facilities and individual providers use one of three numbering systems to identify patient records: serial numbering, serial unit numbering, or unit numbering.

In the **serial numbering** system, the patient is issued a new number at each visit. The record from each patient visit is filed with all of the other patient records in chronological order. Individual records for a single patient are shelved in many different locations in the facility's file room.

Chapter 5   Health Record Organization and Storage

To illustrate this system, let's use a hypothetical patient, Emma Stoddard, who was admitted to the hospital on three different occasions. At each visit, the clinic assigned her a new patient identification number:

Date	Patient/Record
4/15/1985	136250
7/22/1994	198824
2/15/2014	220417

Using the serial numbering system, Emma Stoddard's records would be filed in numerical order in three separate locations in the file room. When her records are needed for a subsequent visit or are requested by another care provider, the file clerk has to retrieve each record from a separate location in the file room. Very few facilities use this system anymore because it is time-consuming and may cause a delay in patient care.

In the **serial unit numbering** system, the patient is issued a new number at the time of each visit, but the patient's records from previous visits are brought forward and filed under the most recent number and in the same location. The benefit of serial unit numbering is that the records are all filed together in one place, facilitating the retrieval process. A file clerk must still locate the previous record to move it forward; however, unlike the serial numbering system, all of the records from previous admissions are already combined into a single file. The HIM department maintains a log showing all of the file numbers assigned to each patient in case a record is misfiled under a previous number.

The record log for patient Emma Stoddard would look like this:

Date	Patient/Record
4/15/1985	136250
7/22/1994	198824 (record #136250 moved forward and filed under this new number)
2/15/2014	220417 (record #198824, which includes record #136250, now filed under #220417)

Many facilities use this numbering system because it provides a sequential log of each patient's admissions over time. Compiling a patient's charts and moving the record forward at each visit also supports better quality care by simplifying and speeding up the retrieval process.

In the **unit numbering** system, the patient is assigned a patient/record number at the first visit, and all of the records related to that patient going forward are given the same number and maintained in a single file. Under this system, all of the records related to Emma Stoddard's hospitalizations would be filed under the same number:

Date	Patient/Record
4/15/1985	136250
7/22/1994	136250
2/15/2014	136250

The advantage of the serial unit numbering and the unit numbering systems is that all records for an individual patient are grouped together in a single folder, which makes it easy to locate information needed during subsequent visits. The unit numbering system has one additional advantage: staff do not have to move the record from a previous visit to a new location the next time the patient is seen.

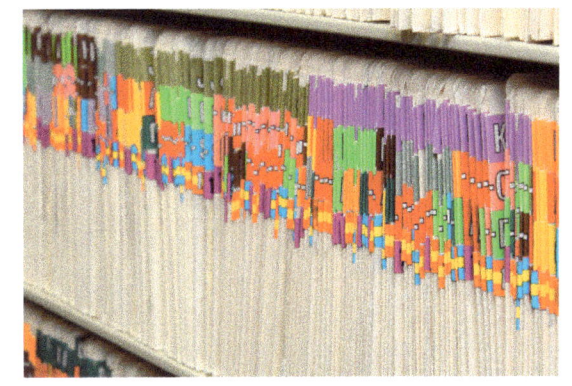

The color-coded file folders shown here make it easier to locate and refile patient records. Each color represents a number—for example, red for 1, blue for 2, etc.

Record Filing Systems

When patient records become inactive, the paper records are often moved to permanent storage. These records may be filed using one of several different methods. The most common filing methods used by hospitals include alphabetical filing, straight numeric filing, **terminal digit filing**, and **middle digit filing**. Two other filing systems, family numbering and subject category filing, are used to store records by patient group or type.

Physician offices and other outpatient settings commonly use alphabetical filing systems. With this method, patient records are stored using the letters of the patient's last name and then first name or a combination of letters and numbers. Straight numeric systems are as straightforward as the name sounds: records are filed in simple numerical order. These two filing schemes are easy to learn and use but do not offer the same level of patient privacy protection as other filing systems. The middle and terminal digit filing systems offer greater security because each pair of numbers in the file number represents a different part of the file's location (i.e., section or subsection) in the file room. A nontrained person would not know how to find a record filed using the middle or terminal digit methods.

The ease of retrieval and the availability of storage space are also determining factors in selecting a filing method. Inpatient hospital records tend to be much larger than outpatient records. Hospital stays often involve multiple and/or more complex procedures, and patients may be hospitalized for an extended period. In a hospital setting, more people need access to the patient record. Terminal digit and middle digit filing systems make it easier to distribute the records evenly throughout the storage area, which helps to maximize the use of storage space. Ambulatory records are smaller in size, and fewer employees have access to patient files. In ambulatory care settings, physical file storage is less of an issue, and simpler alphabetical or numerical filing systems provide easy access to records. Patients visit outpatient facilities more frequently; therefore, staff in these facilities need to access patient records more often. Table 5.1 provides more information on filing methods and the advantages and disadvantages of each.

Table 5.1 Paper-Record Filing Methods

System	Definition	Examples	Advantage(s)	Disadvantage(s)
Alphabetical	Organized by patient's last name, then first name.	Adams, Mary Adams, Samuel James, Cervenka James, Mary Nolan, Alexander Nolan, Alexandria	Easy to learn and retrieve.	Provides less privacy protection. Misfiles more difficult to identify. Filing space inefficiently used (as more files are added, the files need to be shifted to other shelves).
Straight numeric	Organized in chronological order.	054913 054914 054915 055915 060913	Easy to learn and retrieve. Color-coded numbers make misfiles easier to identify.	Provides less patient-privacy protection.
Terminal digit	The last two digits identify the primary location of the file (i.e., the section); the second two digits identify the subsection; and the first two digits identify the tertiary number.	05-43-13 06-43-13 05-49-14 05-49-15 05-59-15 The first file number (05-43-13), for example, would be shelved in section 13, subsection 43, and by the 05 (the tertiary number).	Greater privacy protection. Easy to incorporate color-coding to facilitate filing, retrieving, and finding misfiles. Best utilization of filing space because the 100 primary numbers are evenly divided on the shelves.	Complicated and difficult to learn.
Middle digit	The middle two numbers identify the primary location of the file; the first two digits identify the subsection; and the third two digits identify the tertiary number.	05-43-13 05-43-14 05-49-14 05-49-15 05-59-15 If the file number is 05-43-13, for example, 43 is the primary number, 05 the subsection, and 13 the tertiary. This file would be shelved in section 43, subsection 05, and by the 13 (the tertiary number).	Greater privacy protection. Easy to incorporate color-coding to facilitate filing, retrieving, and finding misfiles. Best utilization of filing space because the 100 primary numbers are evenly divided on the shelves.	Complicated and difficult to learn.
Family	Records for all family members are filed together. Used most often in family practice medicine.	Family #64313 01 = head of household 02 = spouse 03 = child 1st child, #1 03-1 2nd child, #2, 03-2, etc. 04 = other family members in the household 05 = household staff who live in the house	Family records stored together. Familial conditions easier to identify. Family history of disease known.	Difficult to organize. Changes in the family unit require the record to be reorganized. Care must be taken to release only those records authorized for release.

continues

Table 5.1 Paper-Record Filing Methods

System	Definition	Examples	Advantage(s)	Disadvantage(s)
Subject	Records organized by subject and then by name. Used most often in cancer registries in which separate patient records are typically maintained by the primary cancer site (e.g., lung). Also used in research facilities where records may be filed by the drug or the treatment under study.	Pancreatic cancer (subject) and then by Ali, Charma (name).	Like records are together and easily accessible.	Difficult to identify the subject if the patient is treated for more than one condition (e.g., the patient had pancreatic cancer and skin cancer). Within the subject area, records must still be organized using one of the existing filing systems (alphabetical, straight numeric, terminal digit, or middle digit).

In the future, as the electronic health record is fully deployed across all types of healthcare facilities, the use of paper records will be limited. As a facility transitions to an EHR, it is standard practice to establish a **go-live date**, the date the system becomes operational. After the go-live date, the majority of the patient record will be created electronically and miscellaneous paper documents will be scanned and stored electronically. Patient records created during a certain period before the go-live date (probably one to three years, depending on the number of records and the frequency of patient visits) are scanned into the electronic record. Older records continue to be stored in paper form. These records, however, must remain accessible to facility staff, the patient, and anyone authorized to view the record. Because access to medical records may be required for many years, HIM staff must know how to retrieve and refile paper records. Once a patient record meets the criteria for destruction established by the facility's record retention policy (e.g., the number of years since the patient's last visit, the state's **statute of limitations**—the time limit for bringing legal action), the record will be disposed of in an approved manner, which should reduce the need for paper file storage over time.

TAKE THE CHALLENGE

Use a spreadsheet or paper index cards to practice filing patient records using the names and the record numbers listed below. Arrange the list of patient records in the correct order using each of these filing systems: 1) alphabetical, 2) straight numeric, and 3) terminal digit.

John Garcia	379014
John Adams	496410
Alicia Contrero	602967
Elizabeth Schmidt	040829
Tom Adams	025002
Joseph Klein	108916
Alma O'Brian	052699
Bertha Newton	863102

Chapter 5   Health Record Organization and Storage

Off-Site Storage

Due to space limitations, some facilities choose to store older patient records at a remote location. Some healthcare facilities own these **off-site storage** facilities and others contract storage space from a vendor. The most recent records are kept at the facility where the records can be easily accessed for patient care and for other internal uses that usually occur during hospitalization or after discharge. Older, less-active records are sent to the off-site storage facility. Adequate procedures must be in place to ensure the security and the timely retrieval and delivery of records stored off site.

IT REALLY HAPPENS

Hutchinson, Kansas, boasts one of the most secure storage facilities in the world. Located in an abandoned salt mine, the storage facility sits 650 feet below ground in solid rock. Access to the mine is limited, and records stored there are protected from fires, floods, tornadoes, and other potential threats.

The constant temperature and humidity in the salt mine are perfect for storing medical records and other types of documents, as well as other items, including classic films, costumes, and museum artifacts.

Although the facility is remote, records can be retrieved via fax or digital transmission or they can be sent by courier or shipped overnight.

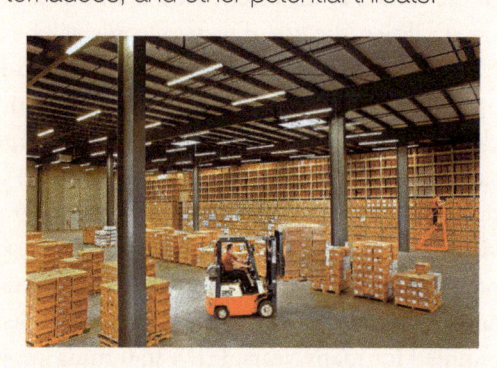

Microfilm and Digital Storage

For many years, facilities transferred patient files onto **microfilm** in order to reduce the amount of space needed for file storage. The paper image is copied in miniature form on microfilm strips. Most of the time, the facility or the provider kept the original paper record for two to five years, depending on the space available. Older records were transferred to microfilm, and then the paper records were then destroyed. Health records were most often stored on microfilm rolls or cassettes that hold approximately 2,400 images or pages each, or on **microfiche**, a flat film on which images were mounted in a matrix format. Documents on microfiche are stored in envelopes and filed in drawers or boxes. A microfilm reader/copier is required to view or make copies of records stored on microfilm or microfiche. Many healthcare institutions have now switched to scanning paper records to digital files and storing them on a computer. Digital images are easier to access and read, and they retain their integrity longer.

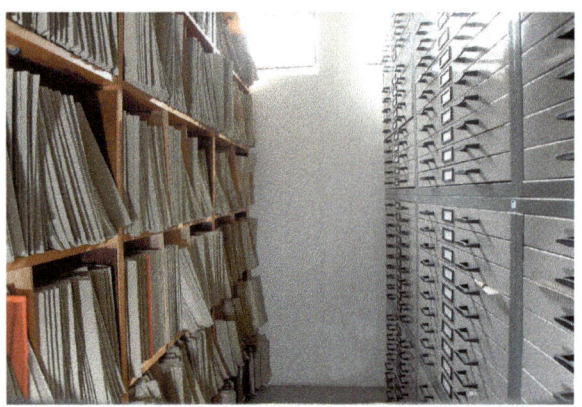

Microfilm storage (right) holds more records and takes up significantly less square footage than paper file storage (left).

Hybrid Records

Paper filing and microfilm storage have been used for many years, but as the healthcare industry transitions from paper to electronic records, many physician offices and hospitals have records that straddle both formats. These **hybrid health records** are stored in paper and electronic formats. The paper portion is stored in the file room, and the electronic record is accessible only through the EHR system.

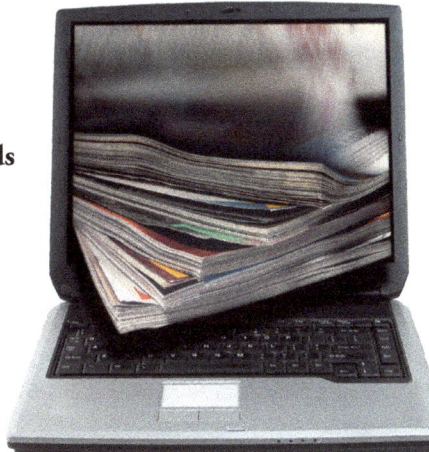

Healthcare organizations that are transitioning to electronic health records often end up using hybrid records for a period of time. Older parts of the patient record are stored on paper, and newer entries are in electronic format.

One important responsibility of the HIM department is to identify all of the data elements that make up the patient health record and the location in the record where each element is stored. Having this information is essential so that the full record may be assembled quickly when needed.

Digital Imaging

Digital imaging is the process of scanning paper health records into a computer system. Digital images offer several advantages over paper records. Digital imaging:

- allows multiple users to access the record simultaneously
- reduces labor costs related to the assembly, filing, retrieval, refiling, copying, purging, and destruction of paper records
- reduces filing errors
- reduces the need for physical storage
- facilitates data retrieval and auditing
- complies with regulatory requirements regarding quality documentation, accessibility, and use of information

Electronic Health Records

The electronic health record is a patient record in digital format. EHRs are created in real time during the patient encounter, and the information entered into the EHR is available instantly and securely to authorized users.

The EHR offers several advantages over paper records. Information in the EHR can be shared simultaneously with multiple providers in the same facility (one or more physicians, nurses, the pharmacy department, the X-ray department, etc.) and with providers in more than one organization or location (laboratories, pharmacies, emergency departments, specialists, medical-imaging facilities, etc.). All providers involved in the patient's care can document directly into the EHR. The storage space required for EHR equipment is a fraction of the storage space required for paper files. Computers located in exam rooms and patient rooms and in other areas of the facility allow fast, convenient access to patient records. Because EHRs are stored electronically, patient records do not need to be physically retrieved or refiled, which almost eliminates the problem of misfiled or missing records.

Misfiles are a common occurrence in facilities that use paper records because of the records' lengthy file numbers and the sheer volume of records that must be filed and refiled. Misfiles are eliminated in an EHR environment because records are never physically removed from the system.

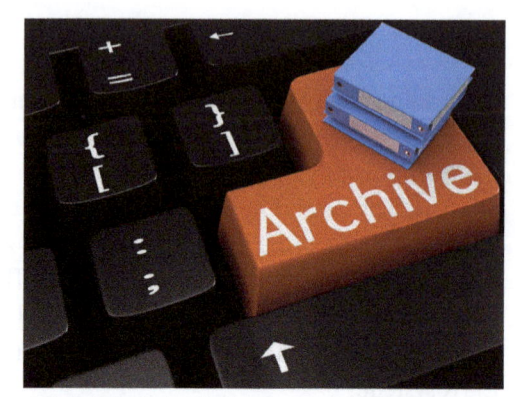

A 2013 study by the Pennsylvania Patient Safety Authority found that the use of hybrid medical records can increase potential for medical errors because clinicians need to look for information in more than one location.

Health Record Life Cycle

The health record life cycle begins at the time the patient checks in for an outpatient visit or is admitted to an inpatient facility and continues until the record is destroyed, as specified by the facility's record retention program. This health record life cycle is referred to as the **record retention cycle**. As illustrated in Figure 5.1, the record retention cycle includes four major stages: creation, utilization, maintenance, and destruction.

Figure 5.1 The Record Retention Cycle

The record retention cycle shows the ongoing life cycle of patient records. An individual patient may have a record at any or all stages at the same time.

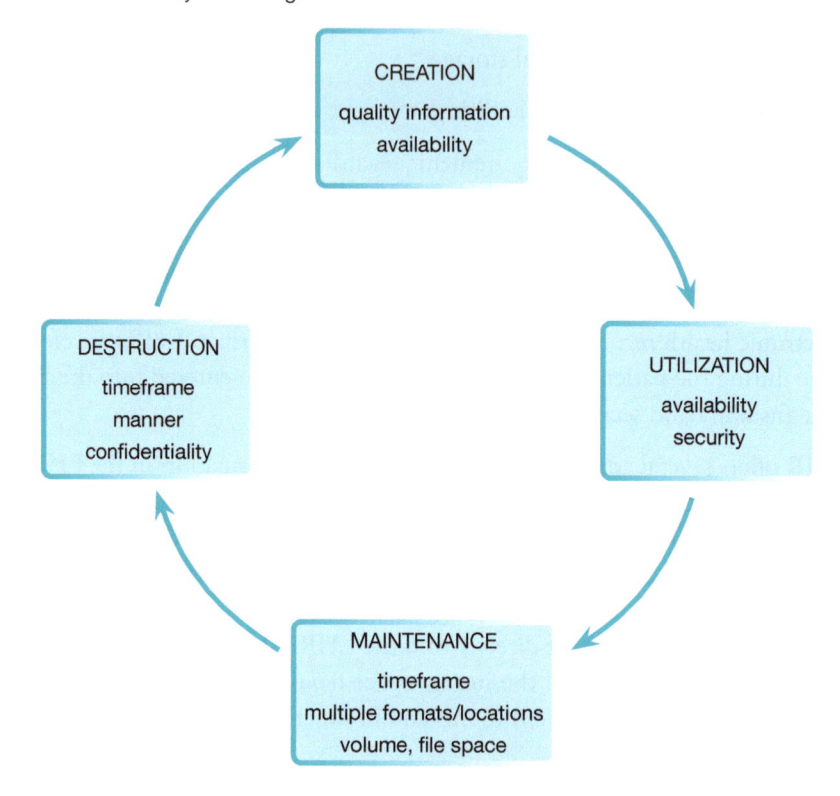

CREATION
quality information
availability

UTILIZATION
availability
security

MAINTENANCE
timeframe
multiple formats/locations
volume, file space

DESTRUCTION
timeframe
manner
confidentiality

The **creation** stage includes all documentation entered into the record during a single inpatient stay or outpatient visit, from the time of admission through the course of treatment. The information must meet regulations and quality guidelines. It is imperative that the record be available during this time to facilitate patient care.

During the **utilization** stage, the record is available to authorized personnel for internal and external uses during the patient stay or visit and afterward when access to the record is needed for insurance billing, committee review, and reporting to outside agencies. Protecting the privacy and the security of patient health information is essential during this time.

The **maintenance** stage refers to handling the record as it becomes inactive over time. The record may be moved to off-site storage or microfilmed or scanned for electronic storage, and it may be stored in multiple locations.

Destruction is the final phase. It occurs when the timeframe for keeping the record (the *record retention period*) has been met, and the information is no longer needed.

The disposal of patient records must be done in accordance with the facility's record retention policy and federal and state regulations protecting the privacy and the security of patient health information. The facility should have a destruction log, which is normally maintained by the HIM department, listing the file numbers of all records destroyed and the date and the method of destruction.

The retention cycle for electronic records is determined by the individual facility. EHRs have a longer life span and are potentially more useful than paper records because EHRs are easier to access, contain more data, and take up less filing space.

Late or Loose Documentation

Late or loose documentation and reports are documents that have not been incorporated into the patient record. During an inpatient stay, new documents (laboratory tests, X-rays, other diagnostic test results, etc.) are frequently added to the patient record. While the patient remains in the facility, these reports are usually taken to the nursing unit on the floor where the patient is located. In a paper record environment, the nursing staff files these documents in the patient file as soon as possible so that the record is up-to-date. However, some documentation, such as final lab and test results and the physician discharge summary, may not become available until after the patient has been discharged.

After the patient is discharged, the paper record is transferred to the HIM department for **chart analysis**. At this point, HIM staff review the record to identify any missing reports, signatures, or items needed to complete the record. The volume of loose documentation can be significant

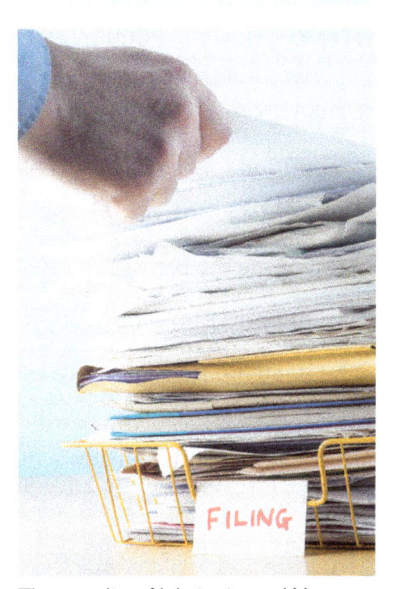

The results of lab tests and X-rays done just prior to discharge and the final summary notes from the physician and others involved in the patient's care are often unavailable until after the record has been moved to the HIM department.

and getting it all filed into the correct patient record can be a challenge for the HIM department. Late or loose documentation can easily become backlogged and can overwhelm the staff's ability to catch up. Late or loose documentation also poses problems for patient care if the complete patient record is not available for follow-up care.

Loose documentation is also quite common in outpatient care settings. Patient encounters are brief, and provider notes, lab results, and other test results are not available until after the patient visit. The process of filing loose documentation is the same in an outpatient setting as in an inpatient setting. Loose files are incorporated into the patient file as soon as possible to ensure they are available for subsequent visits.

Record Retrieval

Requests for paper records are often submitted to the HIM department by physicians and other direct care providers, by the billing department, and as part of an administrative review. Record requests for these types of internal uses do not require patient authorization. To respond to an internal record request, an HIM staff member retrieves the record from storage and then records the name of the individual who requested it and the delivery destination in the checkout log or electronic chart-tracking system before releasing the record. When the record is returned, the HIM staff member logs in the record and then returns it to permanent storage.

Regardless of the storage medium or filing system used, the timely retrieval of patient records is vital, especially when the record is needed for patient care. The federal Health Insurance Portability and Accountability Act of 1996 (HIPAA), Medicare Conditions of Participation (CoPs), and the Joint Commission all have regulations governing timely access to patient records.

The federal **Health Information Technology for Economic and Clinical Health (HITECH) Act** of 2009 requires healthcare providers to demonstrate meaningful use of patient information by 2015. **Meaningful use** is defined as the use of certified EHR technology to:

- improve quality, safety, and efficiency
- reduce health disparities
- engage the patient and the family
- improve care coordination and population and public health
- maintain the privacy and security of patient health information

Meaningful use regulations will be covered in greater depth in a later chapter. They are discussed here to illustrate the need for filing and storage systems to support the meaningful-use initiative related to timely patient access to health information.

Providers can give patients access to their personal health information through a **patient portal**, which is a secure website that allows patients to access their personal health information at any time from any computer. Many physician offices and other healthcare facilities are beginning to include access to patient portals on their websites. Patients do not have access to their full record, but they can access key documentation such as lab results, medications prescribed, lists of procedures, disease-specific educational materials, and other similar information.

Meaningful use criteria related to patient access to personal health information vary depending on whether the information is part of the record for a physician office, a hospital, an emergency room, or some other care setting. The examples shown in Table 5.2 are of criteria that require patient access within a specific timeframe.

Table 5.2 Meaningful Use Requirements and Timely Access Measures

Meaningful Use Criteria	Timeframe Requirements	To Be Compliant
Timely electronic access to changes in health information	More than 10 percent of all unique patients have timely electronic access to their health information (within four business days after the EHR is updated).	Provider must have a patient portal that provides real-time access to the EHR.
Electronic copies of health records	More than 50 percent of all patient requests for electronic copies of health information are completed within three business days.	A patient portal is helpful. Copies of health information can also be provided on a CD, a DVD, or a USB device.
Clinical summaries of office visits	Clinical summaries are provided to patients within three business days for more than 50 percent of all office visits.	Patient portal is not required. Information can be provided electronically, via a patient portal, or in print.
Patient-specific educational resources	More than 10 percent of all unique patients are provided with educational resources specific to the patient's condition.	Provide condition-specific educational information in print, on video, or through a patient portal with a built-in educational database.

Providing timely access to patient health information is essential, but access must be balanced with the need to protect the privacy and the security of protected health information. Facility policies and procedures must be consistent with HIPAA privacy laws and regulations.

The HIPAA Privacy Rule gives patients or their personal representatives the right to inspect, review, and receive a copy of the health record. When authorized by the patient, records may be provided to *covered entities*, defined under HIPAA as healthcare providers, health plans, and healthcare clearinghouses for the purpose of treatment, payment, or healthcare operations. *Treatment* refers to the provision, the coordination, or the management of health care and related services among healthcare providers. *Payment* includes those activities required to obtain payment or be reimbursed for services rendered. *Operations* refers to a covered entity's administrative, financial, legal, and quality improvement activities necessary to operate the business and to support the core functions of treatment and payment.

EXPAND YOUR KNOWLEDGE
To learn more about disclosures of patient information under the HIPAA Privacy Rule, visit http://IntroHIM.ParadigmCollege.net/PrivacyRule.

Release of Information

Patients have a legal right to access their personal health information. To do so, patients must submit a written request to review and/or copy records, and they may be required to pay for copying costs. Requests for copies may take several days to process.

Physicians and healthcare facility staff who need access to a patient record for treatment, payment, or operations reasons will be required to follow the procedures specified by the individual facility. Licensing and accreditation agency surveyors may access patient records to evaluate a compliance against standards.

In general, records cannot be released to external providers, third-party payers, or other entities without a signed authorization from the patient. Patient authorization is not required for release if the record is the subject of a subpoena.

Committee Requests for Records

In every healthcare facility there are committees that oversee various aspects of patient care. These committees make frequent requests for patient records. While patient authorization is not required for this type of internal facility review, patient-identifying information is generally removed and replaced by a number or other code in committee deliberations and documentation. As shown in the following examples, committees use patient information for a number of purposes, such as evaluating treatment provided to the patient, reviewing medication errors, and performing quality improvement activities.

- The blood usage or transfusion committee reviews the charts of all patients who receive blood or blood products to verify that the treatment was justified and documented appropriately. In cases in which a patient has a negative reaction to a transfusion, the committee reviews all aspects of patient care to determine if proper procedures were followed and documented appropriately, and it considers policy or procedural changes intended to reduce or eliminate potential future incidents.

- The pharmacy committee reviews patient charts when a medication error occurs or a patient has an adverse reaction to a medication to determine if the patient received the correct medication and dosage. Medication errors occur for a number of reasons: a misread medication order, incorrect dosage, a dispensing error in the pharmacy, or when medication is administered to the wrong patient. This committee also reviews trends and statistics related to medication errors and recommends changes in hospital policies and procedures to reduce errors.

- The quality improvement committee reviews the patient charts of most common diagnoses and procedures. The results of the review are used to identify treatments, procedures, and practices that may improve the quality of care.

Other committees that commonly request patient data include pathology, infection control, safety, credentials, HIM (for documentation issues), and ethics. Committee requests for patient health records are made in much the same way as other internal requests for patient records. Requests are submitted to the HIM department either by patient name or disease category. For example, a committee might request the records of 25 patients who had the most common operative procedure performed in that hospital in the last two months. Once the committee completes its review, the records are returned to the HIM department.

Purging Patient Records

Purging refers to the removal of individual documents or pages from a patient health record when those documents are no longer needed for the provision of immediate patient care. These unneeded documents might include a copy of a previous physical-exam report after a new one has been placed in a chart or physician order sheets that are several months old (physician orders must be redone and signed on a monthly basis). Often, the medical records for patients in long-term care, patients in mental health and rehabilitation facilities, and patients who are hospitalized for long periods of time can become very large and can be difficult to handle. To make it easier for care providers to find the most relevant and recent information, older and rarely accessed documents may be purged or removed from the active file. Purged documents are refiled in a separate location and remain easily accessible if needed.

Destruction of Patient Records

The length of time that a facility retains a patient record depends on a number of factors. These include the needs of the facility (teaching and research facilities may retain patient records for a long period of time); the method of storage; the amount of storage space available to the facility; and the legal requirements governing the retention of patient records.

Most facilities periodically destroy old and inactive patient records because of space limitations or financial (expenses incurred with storage) and legal considerations (to follow a business plan and/or the record retention plan). Destruction of patient records must be done in a manner consistent with the facility's retention policy and the statute of limitations set by the state where the facility is located. Any record related to an unresolved investigation, audit, or litigation cannot be destroyed. State requirements on the destruction of records vary, but records should always be destroyed in a way that ensures the record is unreadable and cannot be recreated.

Medicare CoPs, HIPAA, state law, and the Joint Commission all dictate specific requirements for the destruction of patient health records to ensure the protection of patient health information. Healthcare facilities use different methods to destroy records, depending on the type of record:

- paper records—burning, shredding, pulping, and pulverizing
- microfilm—recycling and pulverizing
- laser discs—pulverizing
- DVDs—shredding or cutting
- magnetic tape—demagnetizing
- computerized data—magnetic degaussing to erase data

Healthcare facilities are required to maintain a *destruction log* that lists the records destroyed, a description of each record, the method used to destroy the records, and a statement signed by the individuals supervising and witnessing the process, attesting that the records were destroyed in the normal course of business. The HIM department maintains the destruction log.

If the provider contracts with a business associate (BA) to handle the disposal of records, HIPAA requires the BA to document the time between the receipt of and the disposal of the records along with the safeguards in place to protect against any breach of privacy or security. The BA must also agree to take responsibility for any financial loss stemming from an information breach and to maintain a specified amount of liability insurance.

Disaster Recovery Planning

A **disaster** is defined as a catastrophic event that usually occurs suddenly and that may cause great loss of life, property damage, and hardship. Floods, tornadoes, hurricanes, and fires are examples of natural disasters that can disrupt access to patient records and damage or destroy records. Power outages and other types of system failure can also disrupt access to electronic health records.

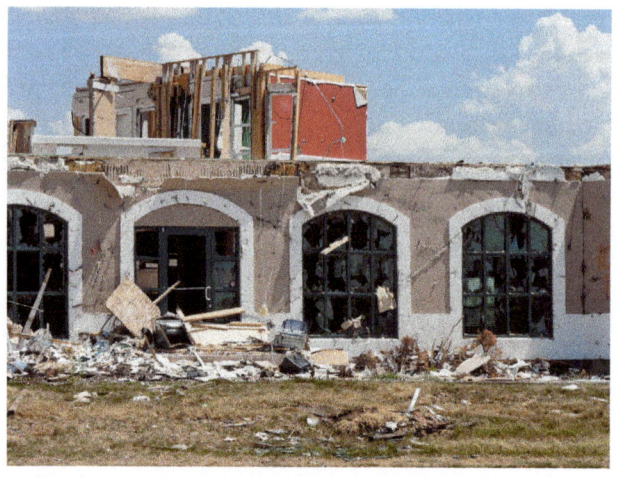

In 2011 and 2013, tornadoes caused widespread destruction to the communities of Joplin, Missouri, and Moore, Oklahoma. Healthcare facilities must have a plan for creating, accessing, and maintaining patient records if computer and communications systems are destroyed or inoperable.

HIPAA, state laws, and accreditation and licensing bodies all require healthcare entities to have a **disaster recovery plan**, also referred to as a *business continuity plan*, in place to protect and provide access to patient information during and after a natural disaster or other disruptive event. A disaster recovery plan identifies systems that may be impacted in a disaster and identifies solutions for restoring those systems.

"By failing to prepare, you are preparing to fail."
—Benjamin Franklin

Creating a disaster recovery plan involves a number of steps:

- Determine what precautions can be taken to reduce the risk or limit the impact during a disaster, including implementing policies and procedures, training employees, relocating equipment to a more secure location, and ensuring data is backed up frequently and stored in a secure location.

- Plan what actions will be taken during a disaster to safeguard patient records and EHR equipment and systems, address potential staff shortages, and create and maintain patient files if computers and other equipment are disabled.

- Identify steps to take once the major force of the disaster is over to return to normal operations as soon as possible.

Table 5.3 illustrates how a hurricane might impact access to patient information, coding, and release of information functions and how the hospital could respond both during and after the storm. A similar table may be created for other types of disasters (e.g., flood, fire, earthquake).

Table 5.3 HIM Departmental Disaster Planning

Potential Disaster: Hurricane			
HIM Activity	**Potential Issue for HIM**	**Solution**	**Alternative**
Access to patient information	Water damage to departmental records	Access backup system for electronic records. Contract with paper-recovery vendor in an attempt to salvage paper records.	Attempt to reconstruct parts of the patient record from physician office files; other facilities; and lab, X-ray, and pharmacy departments.
	Hospital patients and personnel evacuation	Move paper files and equipment to a more protected space if available. Secure area before evacuating. Access electronic-record backup system remotely.	In advance of the hurricane, ensure that the master patient index is backed up and/or stored in a secure location.
Coding	Billing may be delayed for a period of time.	Assure that late filing is complete and documentation in EHR is current. Access remotely if needed.	Reconstruct information needed to be able to code as soon as the facility is operational again. If needed, hire a coding vendor to help with the backlog after the disaster has subsided.
Release of information (ROI)	External release of information will be interrupted for a period of time. If the facility is still operational, providers will need access to records.	Establish procedures for notifying requesters that release of information will not be done for a period of time. If records are accessible and employees available, prioritize external release requests as time permits, especially requests related to continued patient care (if a patient is being treated by another provider).	If possible, reconstruct damaged records. Hire a ROI vendor to help eliminate the backlog after the disaster has subsided.

IT REALLY HAPPENS

After Hurricane Katrina struck the Gulf Coast in 2005, many hospital and long-term care patients were evacuated to inland hospitals that did not have access to their medical records or medical history. Healthcare providers had no way of knowing about patients' preexisting conditions, medications, or allergies, and some patients were too ill or incapacitated to provide reliable information. Since Katrina, disaster preparedness has received much more attention from regulators, patient advocates, and the medical community.

The HITECH Act and other initiatives promoting the adoption of electronic health records are intended to improve disaster preparedness. During Katrina, EHRs would have greatly increased providers' access to evacuated patients' health information. Now, most hospitals maintain computer backup systems and servers that are located far away from the facility. Along the Gulf Coast, hospitals' backup systems are located out of the reach of future hurricanes.

Chapter Summary

Electronic health records are the future of health care, but many hospitals, physician practices, and other types of care facilities continue to create, maintain, store, and use paper records. Even facilities that have transitioned to electronic health records may continue to store inactive and older files on paper. The HIM professional needs to be familiar with paper numbering and filing systems and record storage requirements for both paper and electronic health records.

The health record life cycle includes four stages: creation, utilization, maintenance, and destruction. It is the responsibility of the HIM department to manage the life cycle and ensure that patients and providers have timely access to patient health information while protecting patient privacy. The HIM department is required to have procedures for the release of information and the destruction of records, when warranted, and a disaster recovery plan. The disaster recovery plan should document the steps to take during and after a disaster to protect patient records and provide access to health information necessary for the continued care of patients.

HIM Review

Check Your Understanding

Test your understanding of the material covered in this chapter by completing the following multiple-choice questions. For each question, select the best answer from the choices provided.

1. _____ was enacted to stimulate the adoption of electronic health records and supporting technology.

    a. HIPAA

    b. HITECH

    c. Meaningful use

    d. The HIPAA Privacy Rule

2. _____ is an appropriate means of disposing of health records.

    a. Burning

    b. Shredding

    c. Pulping

    d. All of the choices are correct.

3. A disaster recovery plan requires _____

   a. conducting a risk assessment.

   b. developing contingency plans.

   c. taking a proactive approach to determining how to deal with potential disasters.

   d. All of the choices are correct.

4. _____ is the use of a certified electronic health record to improve patient care and access to health information.

   a. Meaningful use

   b. Providing a patient portal

   c. HITECH

   d. Quality improvement

5. Statute of limitations is _____

   a. a legal requirement for limiting access to patient information.

   b. the Privacy Rule.

   c. the maximum time period in which to bring legal action.

   d. the same in all states.

6. An off-site storage facility is typically used for _____

   a. a contractor who provides services to an HIM department.

   b. records filed away from the main facility.

   c. an outpatient clinic.

   d. the physician office.

7. This numbering system requires that patients receive a new number at every visit and records from previous visits be brought forward and filed with the current record.

   a. serial unit numbering system

   b. serial numbering system

   c. unit numbering system

   d. All of the choices are correct.

8. In a terminal digit filing system, which patient number would follow 05-43-13?

    a. 05-49-14

    b. 05-49-15

    c. 06-43-13

    d. 05-44-13

9. Purging patient records is _____

    a. done to destroy duplicate documents.

    b. done to destroy older records when updates are done.

    c. done to remove and store older information when the record becomes too large.

    d. not done so that there will always be a complete health record.

10. Advantages of EHRs include _____

    a. real-time access.

    b. access to multiple users at the same time.

    c. information that can be accessed in different formats.

    d. All of the choices are correct.

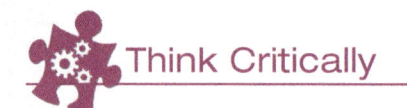

Think Critically

Consider the following real-world scenario and draft a response.

One of the employees in the HIM department is away on a six-week medical leave, and the staff is behind on filing loose reports. The loose sheets of paper are being put into boxes in the HIM department. As a supervisor in the file room, it is up to you to recommend what steps to take to reduce the backlog and to develop policies and procedures to make sure a backlog does not develop in the future. Write a two-page paper describing your recommendations for reducing the backlog of loose reports and for improving the process in the future. Be sure to prioritize your steps and offer specific examples, such as organizing documents as they come in to make it easier to file them later. There are no right or wrong answers. This is an opportunity for you to problem solve creatively.

Sharpen Your Comprehension

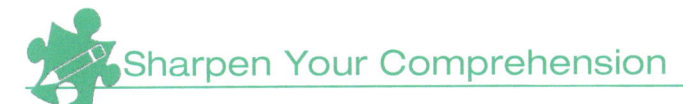

Complete the following matching exercise by selecting, from the list provided, the answer that best matches each of the numbered statements. For each statement, only one answer is correct.

- a. chart analysis
- b. disaster
- c. hybrid
- d. imaging
- e. loose reports
- f. patient portal
- g. purging
- h. record retention program
- i. retrieval
- j. internal

1. _____ Secure online website to provide patients with access to their health information

2. _____ Record requests for these uses do not require patient authorization

3. _____ Review of the chart for completeness

4. _____ When a health record is pulled from storage in response to a request

5. _____ Proactively manage timely maintenance and destruction of health records

6. _____ Reports that have not yet been incorporated into the patient record

7. _____ Event that occurs suddenly and that may cause great loss of life, damage, or hardship

8. _____ Capture (scanning) and digital storage of information from text

9. _____ Removal of pages that are no longer actively needed

10. _____ A record that is in multiple formats

Chapter 5 Health Record Organization and Storage

Connect Theory to Practice

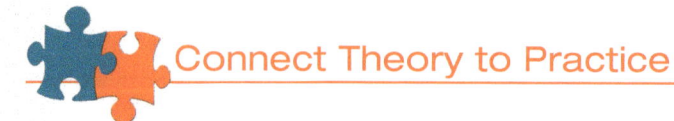

To help translate the concepts presented in this chapter to the workplace, complete the following exercise.

Select a hospital in your local area and conduct a disaster risk assessment using the table below. Interview the director of the health information management department and identify three to five major risks to the hospital's health records. Include both internal risks and external risks in your assessment, and write them in the table provided below. Rate the probability, impact, and category of risk using the scales indicated. Be sure to complete all of the columns for each risk you have identified.

Many online resources are available to provide additional information and examples of disaster risk assessments.

Hospital Name _____

Hospital Location _____

Risk Event and Consequence	Probability of Event Occurring: 1–5 (1 = low, 5 = high)	Impact on Records and/or Functioning of HIM Department: 1–5	Category of Risk: 1–10 (e.g., a lower-level risk would be a temporary loss to records; a high-level risk would be the complete destruction of records)	Preventive Activities
1.				
2.				
3.				
4.				
5.				

Student eResources

*To enhance your comprehension of the chapter material, go to **Navigator+** and complete the additional practice items as advised by your instructor.*

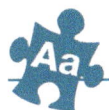

Chapter Terms

- chart analysis
- creation
- destruction
- digital imaging
- disaster
- disaster recovery plan
- go-live date
- Health Information Technology for Economic and Clinical Health (HITECH) Act
- hybrid health records
- late or loose documentation
- maintenance
- meaningful use
- microfiche
- microfilm
- middle digit filing
- off-site storage
- patient portal
- purging
- record retention cycle
- record retrieval
- serial numbering
- serial unit numbering
- statute of limitations
- terminal digit filing
- unit numbering
- utilization

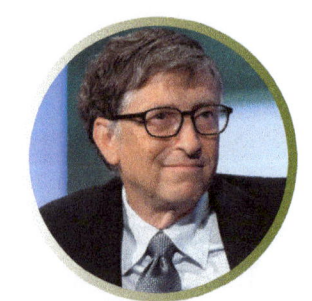

" I think it's fair to say that personal computers have become the most empowering tool we've ever created. They're tools of communication, they're tools of creativity, and they can be shaped by their user. "

—Microsoft founder Bill Gates

Fast Facts

Watson, the IBM supercomputer that beat two former champions to win the game show *Jeopardy!* in 2011, is now taking on the complexities of health care. Watson is harnessing the power of "cognitive computing" to improve health outcomes and to better analyze the massive amount of healthcare data generated each year.

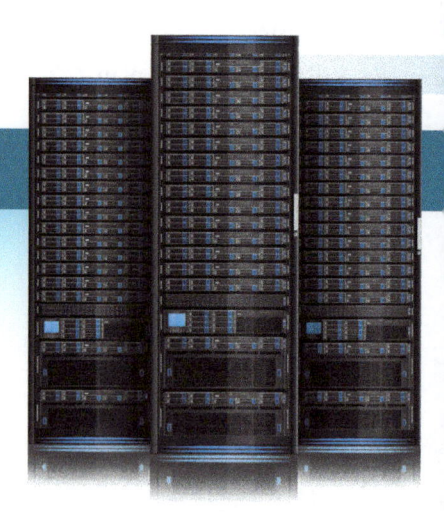

HIM and HIT Expertise: Three Areas of Convergence

- Maintaining the confidentiality and the security of patient information
- Using and maintaining data and information
- Terminology asset management (managing the use of clinical terminologies in electronic systems)

Source: "HIM and Health IT: Discovering Common Ground in an Electronic Healthcare Environment." *Journal of AHIMA* 79, no. 11 (2008): 69.

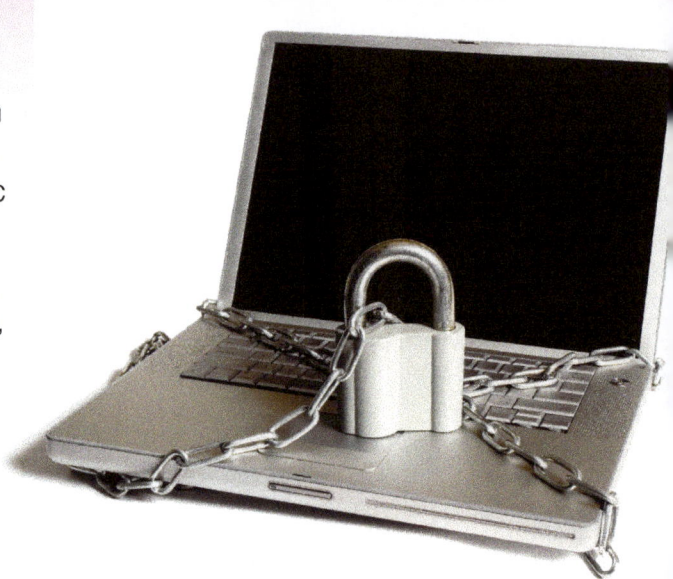

Chapter 6

Information Technology in Health Care

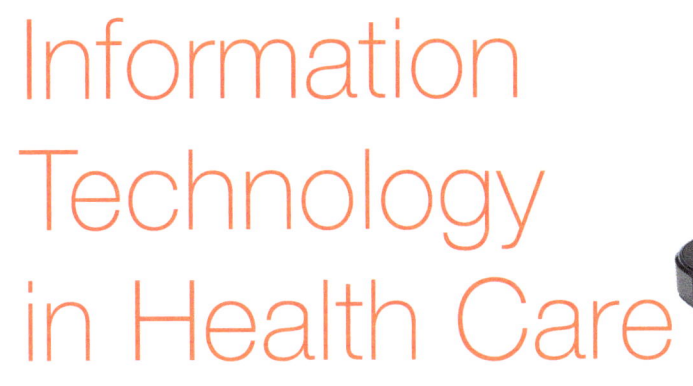

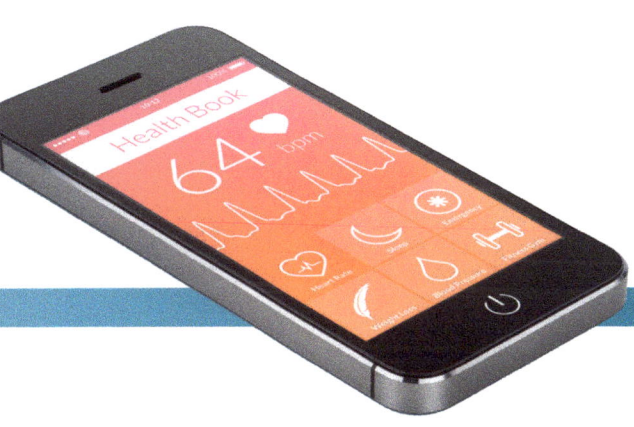

Heart Monitoring: There's an App for That

The first wireless electrocardiogram (ECG) heart-rate monitor was invented in 1977 as a training aid for the Finnish national cross-country ski team. Soon after, in the 1980s, personal heart monitors became popular among fitness enthusiasts to monitor their performance. Now, highly sensitive, smartphone-compatible ECGs are used routinely to diagnose and monitor arrhythmia, an irregular heart rhythm that can sometimes lead to a heart attack or a stroke.

Learning Objectives

- Define the terminology of information technology.
- Identify the difference between hardware and software.
- Understand how information is accessed and shared electronically.
- Understand data storage capabilities.
- Be familiar with the organization and the structure of the information technology department.
- Identify career opportunities in health information technology.

Computer technology drives our world. Cell phones allow us to video chat with friends and family around the globe, stream the latest movies, and monitor home security while we are away. In business, sophisticated robots are replacing humans on the assembly line, 3-D printers are creating custom products, and solar panels are converting the sun's rays into energy.

In the healthcare industry, bar-coded technology tracks pharmacy inventory and reduces medication errors; cardiac event devices allow healthcare providers to monitor a patient's vital statistics from miles or states away; robotic tools assist surgeons in the operating room; and medical records are recorded and stored in electronic formats.

Health information management (HIM) professionals must work closely with the information technology (IT) staff to implement and coordinate data sharing between specialized HIM computer systems. This close, working relationship is necessary to ensure the successful adoption and utilization of the electronic health record (EHR). To be able to communicate effectively with IT staff, HIM professionals need to be familiar with the terminology of information technology. Going forward, career and credential opportunities continue to grow in areas where the fields of healthcare IT and HIM meet.

Information Technology Basics

The Information Technology Association of America defines **information technology (IT)** as "the study, design, development, application, implementation, support, or management of computer-based information systems." Putting the emphasis on health care, the Office of the National Coordinator for Health Information Technology on its website, healthIT.gov, defines the term **health information technology (HIT)** as "a broad concept that encompasses an array of technologies to store, share, and analyze health information."

Discussions about IT usually include computers and their applications, which are referred to respectively as *hardware* and *software*.

Hardware

Within the context of information technology, the term **hardware** refers to the physical components of a computer system: the computer processor and all of its parts, input devices (e.g., mouse and keyboard), the monitor, the printer, and storage devices (e.g., hard disk drive and flash drive). Computer hardware comes in many shapes and sizes—from the desktop computers, laptops, tablets, and smartphones that we see all around us to the large **servers** (many computers connected together) that can take up an entire room or more.

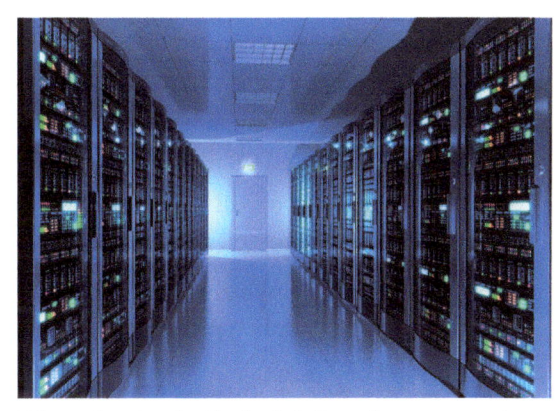

When planning for the installation of new computer systems, it is important to provide enough space for the equipment. Many hospitals are expanding data centers, such as the one shown here, to accommodate the increasing demand for technology.

The brain of any computer is the **central processing unit (CPU)**. This is where all calculations and processes take place. In small computers (**microcomputers**), the CPU is contained in one area called a **microprocessor**, which controls the logic of most digital devices. A **memory chip** stores data and information. Chips are plugged into the **motherboard**, the main circuit board of a microcomputer. To add memory to a computer, additional memory chips are added to the motherboard.

Software

The term **software** refers to the programs and the instructions that run the hardware, manage computer resources, process data, and communicate (network) with other computers. Software is divided into two main categories: **system software**, also known as the *operating system (OS)*, which controls the basic functions of a computer, and **application software**, which refers to a program or a group of programs designed to perform specific tasks. Most computers come with a preinstalled operating system, such as Microsoft Windows®, disk operating system (DOS) syntax, or Apple's Mac OS® system. Microsoft Office® is a well-known suite of application software programs that includes programs for word processing (Word®), spreadsheets (Excel®), databases (Access®), and email (Outlook®). In addition to these consumer-based products, the HIM department uses a number of specialized application programs, such as the chart analysis system, which identifies incomplete patient records.

Healthcare facilities utilize many different computer systems and software applications. The department that selects, deploys, maintains, updates, and determines access to each computer system is considered the owner of that system. The HIM department owns a number of specialty systems for coding, transcribing, and releasing information (to be discussed in greater detail in Chapter 7). In addition, the HIM department is a key stakeholder and user of the EHR.

The HIM staff is likely to have access to other departmental computer systems, including:

- **Human resources**   This system accepts applications for employment and tracks pre-employment checks (e.g., background, drug screens, and references), employee orientation, evaluation processes, departmental productivity (e.g., staffing numbers), and turnover.

- **Scheduling and payroll**   This system provides software for scheduling employees and verifying payroll submissions.

- **Materiel management/inventory control**   This system tracks departmental inventory and supplies, provides ordering service for supplies, and tracks supply expenditures.

- **Management information systems (MIS)**   This system provides reports and information to managers for day-to-day operations. The ownership of the MIS varies by organization.

Information Access

When a new disease, surgical procedure, or medication appears in a medical record, the HIM professional can access a variety of electronic resources to learn about these new discoveries. The most frequently used resource, the **Internet**, is an open-access, global network of networks or, in other words, the world's largest computer network. Most people access the Internet via the World Wide Web (WWW), more commonly referred to as *the web*. The web is made up of all of the documents and resources published on the Internet that are connected, or "linked," using Hypertext Markup Language (HTML), the publishing format used for web pages. HTML is a markup language used for website design only.

Users connect to the web via a **web browser**, or browser, a software application that is used to locate, retrieve, and display content on the web. Popular browsers include Internet Explorer, Google Chrome, Mozilla Firefox, and Apple Safari.

The web is a broad, global network of servers that contain all of the publically available texts, documents, and files (e.g., pictures, videos, and graphs) that are available as web pages. A **website** is a related collection of one or more web pages, usually starting with a home page. Each website is identified by a unique domain name. A **domain name** is much like an address on the Internet. Domain names often indicate the type of organization that purchased and owns the domain. For example, in the domain Harvard.edu, the *.edu* indicates that Harvard is an educational institution. Amazon.com is a commercial business. Medicare.gov is a federal government website. Many businesses, organizations, and even individuals own multiple domain names. ParadigmCollege.net, for example, is one of the domain names owned by the publisher of this textbook.

A **uniform resource locator (URL)** is like an "address" on the web, and each web page has a unique URL. Also called a *web address*, a URL has several parts, beginning with http:// or https://. The http portion stands for Hypertext Transfer Protocol; when the *s* is added, it indicates that the website uses a version of Hypertext Transfer Protocol

EXPAND YOUR KNOWLEDGE

Internet browsers are not all created equal. Some browsers offer greater security and privacy controls, and other browsers require more computer resources to operate. To learn more about browsers, read the article "Comparison on All Major Web Browsers: Internet Explorer, Safari, Firefox, and Google Chrome" at http://IntroHIM.ParadigmCollege.net/Browsers.

with additional security features. Websites that conduct e-commerce, such as those for banks and stores, often use https:// in their URLs.

Many companies and organizations use an **intranet**, a private communications network. Access to the intranet is password protected and accessible only to employees or other authorized users. The intranet is used to provide secure access to internal company information and data that are not intended for public use, such as organizational policy and procedures.

Cloud computing allows companies, institutions, and individuals to store, access, and back up data on a server that resides off-site (i.e., in the cloud—on remote servers owned by another company), rather than on a local computer's hard drive or a company's server. Cloud computing also allows multiple users in multiple locations to simultaneously access that data via the Internet. Cloud computing and storage allows companies to increase their data storage capacity without purchasing additional servers. Because many computers can access information stored on the cloud, including software programs, cloud storage can also reduce or eliminate the need for individual software licenses for each computer terminal. Cloud computing also has some disadvantages, however. Data stored in the cloud must be accessed via the Internet, so access can be impacted by heavy Internet traffic and connectivity issues. (For example, if the Internet connection is down, data stored on the cloud is unavailable.) Cloud-based storage may also be more vulnerable to external security threats.

Networking

The practice of linking two or more computing devices together in order to share data is called **networking**. The two most common network types in use are the **local area network (LAN)** and the **wide area network (WAN)**. A LAN connects computers located in a limited geographical area, such as in a home, an office building, or a hospital. A WAN uses telephone lines, fiber optic cables, and satellite links to connect computers and LANs located over a large geographical area, including across a country or around the world.

Computers can connect to a network or another device in two different ways—either with wires or wirelessly. An **Ethernet** is a system of wires and ports used to connect one computer to another or to a local network. Because it relies on cable connections, an Ethernet is described as a hardwired connection.

A computer can also connect to a network or a device wirelessly via a **wireless access point (WAP)**, router, and modem. The commonly used term **Wi-Fi** refers to any **wireless local area network (WLAN)** technology that connects computers and other electronic devices to each other or to the Internet. Wi-Fi networks can be used to connect a computer to a printer located in a separate room or your laptop computer or tablet to the Internet at a coffee shop or a local library. Although wireless networks offer convenience, wired networks can transmit data much faster and more securely.

Because they offer greater security, businesses often use a **virtual private network (VPN)** to share data between users in remote locations—between different branches of a bank, for example, or between different clinics in a health system—without leaving the security of the private network.

IT REALLY HAPPENS

As a registered health information technician, Lisa Hoffman reviews clinical documentation and coding for a physician office. Hoffman works from home and uses the physician office's secure VPN to access her client's EHR from her home office. She has real-time access to the EHR system without having to be on-site. Working from home, Hoffman doesn't have to spend time commuting to an office or dress in professional attire (she can work in her pajamas if she likes). However, she can still produce quality work in a secure environment.

Communicating over the Network

Not all computer programs "speak" the same language. Different software products store and share data in different ways, and this can cause problems when two systems are trying to communicate or share data. For example, a hospital's computer billing system may define the data field for insurance as a numeric value (Medicare equals "1"), and an insurance company's computer software may define the same data field alphabetically (Medicare equals "Med").

To share information, these two systems rely on an **interface**, a software program that facilitates the exchange of data between the two systems. When unrelated computer systems and software programs from multiple vendors work together and exchange data, they are said to be **interoperable**. In the United States, most software programs used in health care employ the information exchange protocol developed by a nonprofit organization called Health Level Seven International (HL7). HL7 provides a framework for different computer systems and software programs to exchange, integrate, share, and retrieve electronic health information.

Connecting to the Network

Computer ports provide communication links between other computers or peripheral devices; ports can be either physical or virtual connections. Physical ports provide access to cables that connect computers, routers, modems, and other peripheral devices (such as monitors, keyboards, mice, and printers).

Physical ports are usually located on the side or back of a computer and are used to connect the computer or the server via an Ethernet cable to another computer or peripheral device. Physical ports come in many different shapes and sizes.

Virtual ports use Transmission Control Protocol (TCP) and Internet Protocol (IP), commonly referred to as *TCP/IP*, to allow software applications

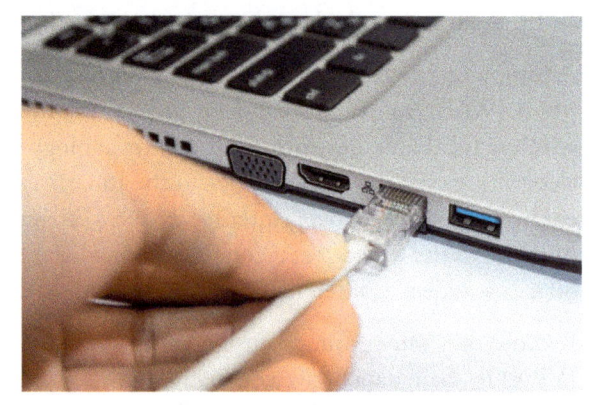

Computer ports are located on the side or back of a PC, laptop, or tablet. The user plugs the end of the device cord into the port in which it fits.

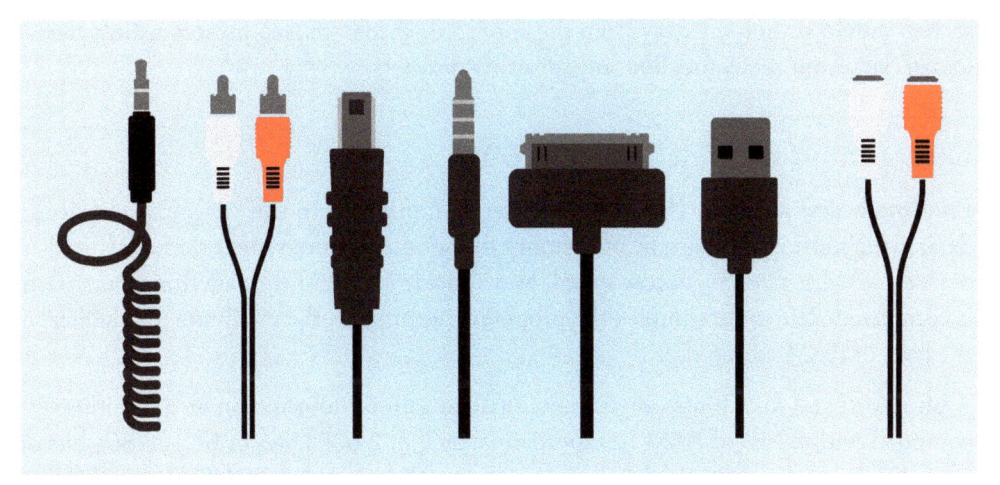

Each electronic device has a specific connection cord that is designed to fit into a specific port on a computer. Many cords are color-coded to match the computer ports.

to share hardware resources without interfering with each other. Web browsers, for example, use Hypertext Transfer Protocol (HTTP)— HTTP port 80 or HTTPS 443, in particular—to communicate securely with web servers.

Information Storage

Documents, files, reports, graphs, and illustrations must often be carefully saved for future access. Much of the time, this information is saved to a computer's **hard drive**, sometimes referred to as a *hard disk drive (HDD)*. The hard drive is an internal storage device, usually the C drive located on a desktop or a laptop computer. Data and information may also be stored on an external storage device, such as an external hard drive, a flash drive, or an optical disc.

An **external hard drive** is a large-capacity, portable storage device that can be used to store an exact copy of a computer's hard drive. External hard drives are often used to back up personal computers because the device can be stored securely in a separate location to protect data if the computer is lost or stolen, or if the internal drive fails.

A **flash drive**, also called a *thumb drive* or *jump drive*, is a small, rewritable, lightweight (1.1 oz.), and high-capacity device that can store up to one terabyte of data.

A compact disc (CD) or a CD-ROM (compact disc, read only memory) is a type of optical storage. CDs come in two formats: CD-R (compact disc, recordable) and CD-RW (compact disc, rewriteable). The CD-R format allows data to be recorded on the CD only once, but it can be read many times. After data is recorded on a CD-R, it cannot be altered or rewritten. Data stored on a CD-RW can be erased and replaced by new data multiple times. A typical CD-ROM holds about 737 MB of data.

Data (files, applications, and/or databases) stored on computer networks is often backed up on specialized in-house or remote servers.

To protect stored data, computer systems should be backed up at least once each day. Backup can be done automatically and can be scheduled to run at night or when system use is minimal. Critical information and systems used in healthcare settings, such as patient care information, are often backed up continuously in real time. Backup servers should be housed away from the core computer system to protect against the loss of data from theft, fire, flooding, or other disasters.

Calculating Data Storage Needs

Random access memory (RAM), computer memory used to run programs and store data, is the most common type of memory found in computers and other electronic devices. RAM is rated by **access speed**, how quickly a request for data from the system is completed. The more complex the programs running on the computer, the higher the level of RAM required.

A **bit**, shorthand for a binary digit, is the smallest unit of information on a machine. A computer with 8 MB of RAM has approximately 8,308,608 bytes or 67,108,864 bits of memory. Another way to think about it is that one byte is equal to eight bits, and eight bits is equal to one letter or number. A megabyte is roughly one million characters. Table 6.1 shows the different units of measurement used when discussing memory.

Table 6.1 Data Measurement

Data Measurement	Size
bit	single binary digit (1 or 0)
byte	8 bits
kilobyte (KB)	1024 bytes
megabyte (MB)	1024 kilobytes
gigabyte (GB)	1024 megabytes
terabyte (TB)	1024 gigabytes
petabyte (PB)	1024 terabytes

EXPAND YOUR KNOWLEDGE

Use a conversion calculator when comparing different computer-storage systems. If one vendor describes storage capacity in megahertz and another in terabytes, you can compare the amount of storage by converting the numbers into the same unit of measurement through the use of a conversion tool like this: http://IntroHIM.ParadigmCollege.net/ConversionTool.

Before installing a new software product, review the manufacturer's instructions. The instructions should describe the processing speed and the amount of memory required to run the program. For example, the standard system requirements for Microsoft Office Suites 2013 are one gigahertz or faster (computer and processor) and one gigabyte of RAM.

When considering electronic storage needs, say, for example, for a medical report, consider that a typical one-page typed document without graphics contains approximately 2 KB of data, and a 1 GB USB flash drive can store approximately 130,000 pages of text (although that number is a rough estimate and will vary, depending on the type of file and even the size of the type). Storing photographs, graphics, and other types of visual images requires significantly more memory than text documents.

Measuring Access Speed

When selecting computer hardware or before installing new software, it is important to consider the speed of the computer's CPU. CPU speed, the speed at which the computer processor can process data, is measured in **megahertz (MHz)** or

gigahertz (GHz). A megahertz is one million cycles per second, meaning data can be manipulated at least one million times per second; a gigahertz is at least one billion cycles per second. According to *PC Magazine*'s online encyclopedia, "a 1.6 GHz computer processes data internally (calculates, compares, copies) twice as fast as an 800 MHz machine."

Data Management

The word data is used frequently in IT settings. **Data**, the plural of datum, is a single fact, number, letter, statistic, code, or item. Data can be collected and stored in a database. When data is processed into a group of like items, it becomes **information**. Information includes text documents, images, audio clips, software programs, and other types of data. In the healthcare environment, for information to be functional and of value, it must:

- be accurate and timely
- be specific and organized for a purpose
- be presented in a manner that is relevant and useful
- lead to an increased understanding of the subject matter

Table 6.2 illustrates the differences between data and information.

Table 6.2 Data versus Information

Data	Information
Raw facts	Data that is organized, summarized, or analyzed
No context	Processed data
Just numbers or text	Data in context of specific subject matter
	Used to make decisions

Without data, there is no information. In health care, many people at many different points collect data for many different purposes. Data is collected by physicians, nurses, pharmacies, healthcare organizations, and insurance companies for use in patient care, billing and reimbursement, and quality review.

A **data element** is a single fact with a single meaning, defined for the purpose of data processing. In the medical record, the patient name, birth date, and account number are all examples of data elements. A data element is defined by size (in characters) and type (alphanumeric, numeric only, true/false, date, etc.). A specific set of values or a range of values may also be a part of the definition. These data elements are stored in a **field**, the physical unit of storage in a computer record (see Figure 6.1).

Figure 6.1 Common Data Fields in an EHR Admissions Screen

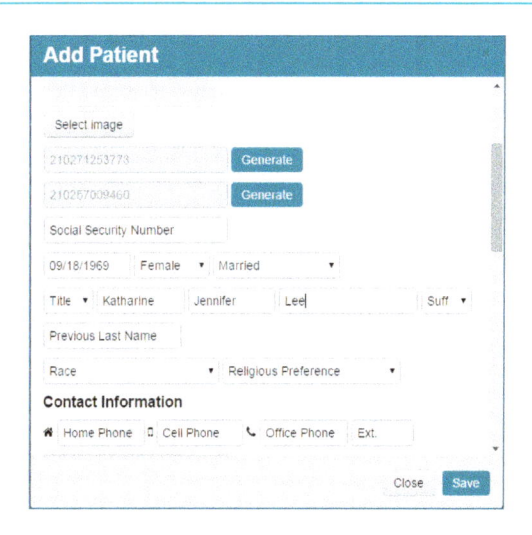

Data Standardization

In health care, there has been a historic lack of structured data or standardization of data elements. For example, one system may collect data elements on medications prescribed while others do not. However, with the implementation of electronic medical billing and the EHR, the need for data standardization is growing. In the 1990s, the Department of Health and Human Services commissioned the National Committee on Vital and Health Statistics (NCVHS) to develop a list of **core health data elements** and standard definitions to facilitate data sharing among providers and healthcare agencies. The committee recommended the 42 data elements (see Table 6.3). The data elements are divided into two groups: *personal/enrollment data* (such as date of birth, sex, and race) and *encounter data* (such as admission date, attending physician identification, and medications prescribed). Agreement has not been reached for all items on the list. List items identified with 1/ indicate that substantial agreement has been reached, but some amount of additional work is needed. Items identified with 2/ indicate that significant agreement has been reached, but considerable work is still needed. Items without a footnote indicate elements that are ready for implementation.

Table 6.3 Core Health Data Elements

Personal/Unique Identifier 2/	Operating Clinician Identification 1/
Date of Birth	Healthcare Practitioner Specialty 1/
Gender	Principal Diagnosis (inpatient)
Race and Ethnicity	Primary Diagnosis (inpatient)
Residence	Other Diagnoses (inpatient)
Marital Status	Qualifier for Other Diagnoses (inpatient)
Living/Residential Arrangement 1/	Patient's Stated Reason for Visit or Chief Complaint (outpatient) 2/
Self-Reported Health Status 2/	Diagnosis Chiefly Responsible for Services Provided (outpatient)
Functional Status 2/	Other Diagnoses (outpatient)
Years of Schooling	External Cause of Injury
Patient's Relationship to Subscriber/Person Eligible for Entitlement	Birth Weight of Newborn
Current or Most Recent Occupation and Industry 2/	Principal Procedure (inpatient)
Type of Encounter 2/	Other Procedures (inpatient)
Admission Date (inpatient)	Dates of Procedures (inpatient)
Discharge Date (inpatient)	Procedures and Services (outpatient)
Date of Encounter (outpatient and physician services)	Medications Prescribed
Facility Identification 1/	Disposition of Patient (inpatient) 1/
Type of Facility/Place of Encounter 1/	Disposition (outpatient)
Healthcare Practitioner Identification (outpatient) 1/	Patient's Expected Sources of Payment 1/
Provider Location or Address of Encounter (outpatient)	Injury Related to Employment
Attending Physician Identification (inpatient) 1/	Total Billed Charges 1/

When data elements with uniform definitions are grouped together for a particular use, it is called a **dataset**. In health care, datasets identify those data elements that must be collected for each patient and that provide uniform data definitions for each element. The Healthcare Effectiveness Data and Information Set (HEDIS) is one example of a dataset widely used in health care to measure performance. HEDIS consists of 81 measures across five domains of care and addresses a broad range of important health issues, including:

- asthma medication use
- persistence of beta-blocker treatment after a heart attack
- controlling high blood pressure
- comprehensive diabetes care
- breast cancer screening
- antidepressant medication management
- childhood and adolescent immunization status
- childhood and adult weight/body mass index (BMI) assessment

HEDIS measures are well defined, making it possible to compare health plan performance on an "apples-to-apples" basis. Many health plans report HEDIS data to employers and use the results to improve the quality of care and service. Employers, consultants, and consumers use HEDIS data, along with accreditation information, to help them select the best health plan for their needs. To ensure the validity of HEDIS results, certified auditors rigorously audit the data by using a process designed by the National Committee for Quality Assurance (NCQA).

Databases

A **database** is a collection of related data that is organized so that its contents can easily be accessed, managed, updated, and extracted. In a physician office, for example, individual data elements—such as patient birth date, insurance carrier, or the numeric value of a white blood cell (WBC) count—are collected in designated fields and stored in a medical database.

A **database management system (DBMS)** is a group of programs that manages the access and the retrieval of information from a database. The process of extracting specific data elements from individual patient files and combining those elements together is known as compiling **aggregate data**. Aggregate data is used for many purposes, including medical research, public health reporting, and trend analysis. For example, if a researcher wants to know the number of men between the ages of 40 and 62 who live in a specific geographical area, have a BMI over 35, and were admitted to a hospital during 2016 and 2017 with a diagnosis of myocardial infarction, the researcher might structure a query that includes these data elements:

1. myocardial infarction
2. male
3. age 40 to 62

4. BMI > 35
5. zip code = 65421
6. Admit dates between 1/1/16 and 12/31/17

Continuing the example above, by breaking down certain components of aggregated data, the researcher could gather additional information. For example, the researcher could structure a query to gather data for each year separately. Searching and analyzing large amounts of data in a database is called **data mining**. Data mining aids in the discovery of patterns, relationships, and trends.

Consumer Informatics

Digital tools and resources have become part of everyday life, allowing healthcare professionals and healthcare consumers greater access to patient data as well as to research and information on health issues and trends and opening the lines of communication between patients and providers. Eric Dishman of Intel Corporation calls the trend "the medicalization of consumer devices." Patients can research health conditions online and use smartphone and tablet applications (apps) to track personal health trends (e.g., weight, calories, exercise) and transmit health data (e.g., heart rhythms) back to their physicians.

> **BE AWARE**
>
> Not all health information available online is factual or from a reliable source, and some information can even be harmful. Patients should not try to self-diagnose or treat an illness from online information.

IT REALLY HAPPENS

Patient Sandra Adams could feel her heart racing, but when her physician ordered an electrocardiogram (EKG) to check her heart rhythm, the results were normal. Her cardiologist then suggested Sandra wear a cardiac event monitor, which continuously records the heart's rhythms, for three days. The monitor's sensors were attached to Sandra's chest with sticky patches. When she felt her heart race, she pushed a button on the event monitor. Once a day, Sandra transmitted data from the monitor to her physician via her cell phone. By the end of the three days, the monitor data showed an irregular heartbeat, which her physician diagnosed as atrial fibrillation, a dangerous condition that can cause blood clots or a stroke. The doctor then prescribed medication to normalize her heartbeat.

Data Security

The same technology that allows us to share data and information across the web and across the globe has also opened the door to a whole host of new cyber threats, including computer viruses, electronic theft, and accidental and unintentional security breaches.

It is important, therefore, to have safeguards in place to keep data secure. IT systems are subject to a number of threats, which can result in data theft or the unauthorized use, deletion, or destruction of data, software, and hardware systems. The Health

Insurance Portability and Accountability Act of 1996 (HIPAA) Security Rule (discussed in greater detail in Chapters 7 and 8) outlines requirements for maintaining the security of electronic health information. The HIM and IT departments work together to ensure that electronic health information is protected.

Data Threats

Malware and phishing are two of the most common types of data threats, but cookies can also be problematic to data security.

Malware is a malicious software program that is installed on a computer or a system without authorization. Malware is designed to gain access to the user's system in order to damage or disrupt data or programs or to steal sensitive information. This hostile and intrusive software comes in many forms: self-replicating **viruses** and **worms** that can damage data, destroy files, and infect entire networks and **Trojan horse** programs that masquerade as real programs but can damage or delete files and information when opened. A Trojan horse program can also be used to open a "backdoor" into a computer or a system, allowing hackers access to protected data.

Phishing involves sending fake emails designed to appear as if they are coming from a legitimate source, such as a bank, an employer, or an online shopping website. Phishing's purpose is to deceive users into surrendering private information (such as user names, passwords, and credit card information).

IT REALLY HAPPENS

In Tacoma, Washington, scammers used phishing to access the files of as many as 12,000 patients of the Tacoma Franciscan Health System. The scammers sent out an email that appeared to come from the health system's corporate office. In the email, employees were asked to click a link and then provide their computer login and password. About 20 of the company's employees did so, allowing scammers to access patient names, social security numbers, and some medical record information.

Read more about the Tacoma Franciscan Health System security breach at http://IntroHIM.ParadigmCollege.net/PhishingScam.

In the world of computer technology, just as in real life, cookies can be good or bad depending on the ingredients. A computer **cookie** is a small file that attaches to an individual's computer when the user visits certain websites. Cookies track users' information and activities, usually without their knowledge. Some cookies are helpful; they can be used to remember a user's identity and preferences on frequently visited websites. However, cookies can also be malicious, collecting user identities for the purpose of identity theft.

Prevention of Security Threats

There are a number of ways to defend against computer threats. One way is by utilizing **data loss prevention (DLP) software**: antivirus and anti-malware software and firewalls. Antivirus and anti-malware programs detect and remove computer viruses and malware. A **firewall** protects computer networks and individual computers from viruses and security threats by blocking or limiting outside users' access to data and systems.

Password security is another important element of data protection. A **password** is a secret code assigned to or chosen by an individual user. Organizations should require employees to use complex passwords, which are more difficult for computer hackers to break. For example, a password should not include the user's birth date or child's name. Employers should require users to change passwords frequently and on a regular basis, such as every 90 days, a procedure known as **password aging**.

To protect data from computer hackers, Microsoft offers a strategy for creating strong passwords that cannot be easily broken.

A **strong password** should:

- contain at least eight characters
- not contain the individual's user name, real name, or company name
- not contain a complete word
- be significantly different from previous passwords

A strong password should also contain characters from each of the four catagories in Table 6.4.

Table 6.4 Strong Password Elements

Category	Examples
Uppercase letters	A, B, C
Lowercase letters	a, b, c
Numbers	0, 1, 2, 3, 4, 5, 6, 7, 8, 9
Symbols found on the keyboard (all keyboard characters not defined as letters or numerals) and spaces	` ~ ! @ # $ % ^ & * ( ) _ - + = { } [ ] \ | : ; " ' < > , . ? /

Some companies and organizations use a **digital certificate** to protect data and computer systems. Also referred to as a *public key certificate*, a digital certificate is an attachment to an electronic message that provides identifying information about the sender. The digital certificate, also referred to as an *electronic passport*, allows a person, a computer, or an organization to exchange information securely over the Internet. A digital certificate issued by an official, trusted agency, contains identifying information and is forgery resistant.

To ensure that patient privacy is protected and patient health information remains secure, it is important for HIM professionals to stay informed about cyber security and new security threats and to work collaboratively with the IT department to prevent unauthorized access to computer systems and health data.

The Information Technology Department

The **American Recovery and Reinvestment Act (ARRA)**, signed into law in 2009, provided financial incentives to encourage healthcare organizations to adopt and use certified electronic health records to improve the quality of patient care and the exchange of health information. Since then, healthcare providers and organizations have made EHR implementation a priority, hiring additional IT staff and adding new positions to help develop, implement, and maintain these complex systems. Traditionally, the HIM department managed and maintained all patient health records in paper format, but with the transition to the EHR, the HIM and the HIT departments are moving into closer alignment and, in some cases, integrating staff and services. As an HIM professional, it is important to understand the IT department's organization, to know where HIM and HIT roles and responsibilities intersect, and to be aware of the career opportunities available in health information technology now and in the future.

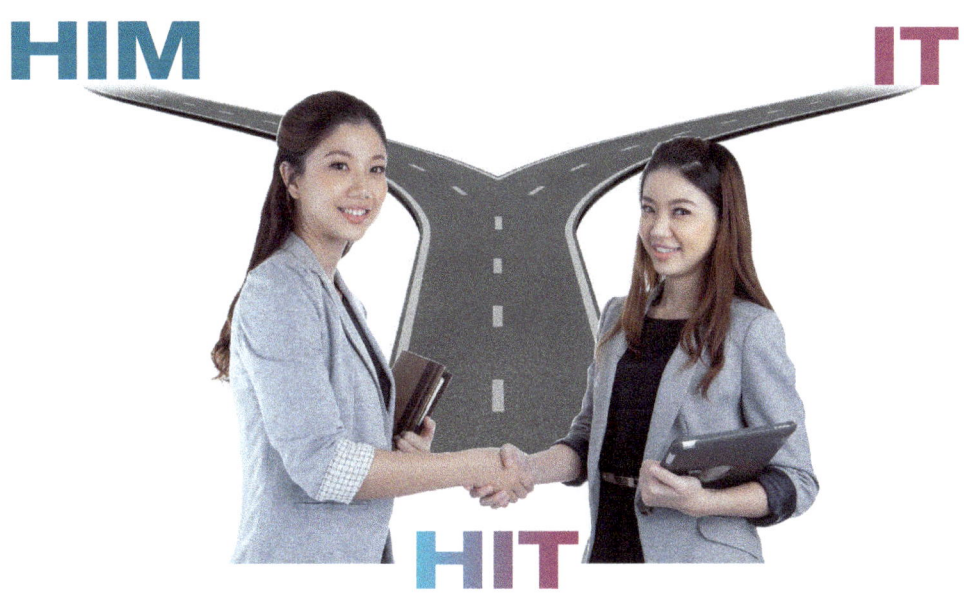

HIM and IT specialists join together to provide the HIT services needed to improve patient care.

The head of the IT department in most hospitals is a director-level position. The **IT director** oversees all hospital computer systems and **infrastructure** (hardware used to connect computers). The IT director is responsible for developing the facility's **strategic plan**, which documents the organization's IT goals, identifies the resources needed, and recommends the steps to take to achieve those goals.

Most IT departments are structured by function. Table 6.5 lists the areas of expertise and job descriptions for the positions commonly found in a hospital IT department. Hospitals may have more or fewer positions, depending on the size of the hospital.

With the adoption of electronic health records, the IT department has created several new positions, including those listed in Table 6.6.

Chapter 6 Information Technology in Health Care

Table 6.5 IT Positions and Functions

Area of Expertise	Job Description
infrastructure	installs and supports networks and servers as well as communication equipment including email, telephone systems, and remote access software (which allows users to access the computer system securely from outside of the facility); also responsible for IT security (the information security officer works here) and disaster recovery planning
user support	operates the help desk and assists users with software and hardware concerns, questions, and problems while also providing workstation support and repair and basic training for applications such as email and Microsoft products
systems and data architecture	writes and edits software programs, creates and maintains the data dictionary and databases, prepares reports, and provides data analysis
applications	participates in the selection of vendor-supplied software systems; provides system support, maintenance, and installation; installs upgrades and replacement software; and defines interface fields to integrate programs and systems
electronic health record	participates in the selection and the implementation of the EHR system; provides training and oversees the integration of other systems with the EHR; and maintains EHR and telemedicine technology

Table 6.6 New IT Positions

Job Title	Job Description
project manager	assists in determining the project's scope of work, objectives, budget, and schedule as well as the individual/team responsibility for each project component
clinical analyst	studies EHR workflow to improve efficiency and ease of use, designs and builds EHR forms, and screens order sets and other clinical content
clinical application coordinator	coordinates the integration of different applications in hospital systems that use software products by multiple/different vendors, and coordinates implementation and user training for new software
information security officer	works with the facility's privacy officer to ensure data security

EXPAND YOUR KNOWLEDGE

The American Health Information Management Association (AHIMA) publishes information regarding career opportunities that combine HIM and IT roles. To learn more, go to the AHIMA Career Map at http://IntroHIM.ParadigmCollege.net/CareerMap.

Career Opportunities in HIT

A number of HIT career opportunities are available for someone with a registered health information technician (RHIT) certification and an interest in healthcare technology. Table 6.7 lists a number of existing and emerging HIT career paths.

Table 6.7 HIT Career Opportunities

Current	Emerging
implementation support specialist	practice workflow and implementation specialist
data, application, or systems analyst	EHR implementation specialist
data architect	HIM and technology trainer
	HIT subspecialist

Students interested in healthcare IT can earn AHIMA certification as a healthcare technology specialist (CHTS). AHIMA offers six types of CHTS certificates (shown in Table 6.8) that demonstrate competency in the implementation and the management of electronic health information in these areas:

- assessing workflows
- selecting hardware and software
- working with vendors
- installing and testing systems
- diagnosing IT problems
- training practice staff on systems

Table 6.8 CHTS Certifications Offered by AHIMA

Certification Title	Responsibilities and Experience
Clinician/Practitioner Consultant (CHTS-CP)	This individual works in public health and clinical settings to address implementation problems, assists in vendor selection, and addresses workflow and data collection issues from a clinical perspective. Experience as a clinical or public health professional is recommended.
Implementation Manager (CHTS-IM)	This position involves the on-site management of mobile adoption support teams and the health IT system implementation process. It requires prior experience in health care, IT environments, and administrative or managerial positions.
Implementation Support Specialist (CHTS-IS)	This individual provides on-site user support during the health IT system implementation process. Previous background in information technology or information management is expected.
Practice Workflow and Information Management Redesign Specialist (CHTS-PW)	This individual uses health IT to help providers improve healthcare delivery. Those in this role may have a background in health care (for example, as a practice administrator) or in information technology, but they are not licensed clinical professionals.
Technical/Software Support Staff (CHTS-TS)	Staff in this role maintain systems in clinical and public health settings; this maintenance may include patching and upgrading software. Candidate backgrounds include information technology or information management.
Trainer Examination (CHTS-TR)	Those in this role design and deliver employee-training programs in clinical and public health settings. Experience as a trainer is desired along with experience as a health professional or a health information management specialist.

Source: AHIMA.org

Chapter Summary

As the HIM and IT departments continue to collaborate to meet the needs of the healthcare staff, physicians, and patients, it is important for the HIM professional to be familiar with the basic terms and digital technologies used in healthcare environments. Hardware is the term used to describe the physical equipment, such as computers, keyboards, and monitors. Software is the term used to describe the programs that run the hardware and process data. Computers can be networked to each other and to other devices by hardwire (Ethernet cables) or on wireless networks. When calculating organizational needs for digital storage, it is important to consider both access and processing speeds by looking at the megabytes of storage as well as the gigahertz speed rate available.

Digital technologies are making it easier for patients to become more involved and engaged in their health care, but the increasing reliance on web-based communications, smartphones, and other technologies raises security and privacy concerns. HIM professionals must stay up-to-date on information about electronic security threats, such as malware, Trojan horses, and phishing scams, and they must ensure that proper security measures, such as password aging and firewalls, are in place to reduce those threats.

Being familiar with the IT department and its roles and responsibilities will improve collaboration between the HIM and IT departments. HIM graduates who are interested in healthcare IT and electronic health records management have the opportunity to earn certification as a certified healthcare technology specialist.

HIM Review

Check Your Understanding

Test your understanding of the material covered in this chapter by completing the following multiple-choice questions. For each question, select the best answer from the choices provided.

1. ARRA was signed into law in _____
    a. 2005.
    b. 2006.
    c. 2008.
    d. 2009.

2. The _____ system tracks departmental inventory and supplies, provides ordering service for supplies, and tracks supply expenditures.
    a. MIS
    b. materiel management
    c. human resources
    d. scheduling

3. A _____ is smaller than a gigabyte.
    a. terabyte
    b. kilobyte
    c. megabyte
    d. b & c

4. A strong password _____
    a. is at least eight characters long.
    b. contains whole words.
    c. is easy to remember.
    d. is similar to previous passwords.

5. A data element is *not* defined by _____
    a. size.
    b. type.
    c. unit of storage.
    d. a specific set of values or a range of values.

Chapter 6   Information Technology in Health Care

6. _____ is malicious software that masquerades as a useful program.

   a. Spyware

   b. A Trojan horse

   c. A virus

   d. A worm

7. A _____ connects computers located in a geographically close area.

   a. LAN

   b. WAN

   c. WAP

   d. VPN

8. Microsoft Windows, DOS, and Mac OS X are examples of _____

   a. application software.

   b. operating systems.

   c. spreadsheets.

   d. database software.

9. Storing and accessing data and programs over the Internet is known as _____

   a. phishing.

   b. digital certificates.

   c. cloud computing.

   d. infrastructure.

10. The CHTS certification exams do not measure an individual's competency with regard to _____

    a. installing and testing systems.

    b. diagnosing IT problems.

    c. selecting hardware and software.

    d. programming software.

Think Critically

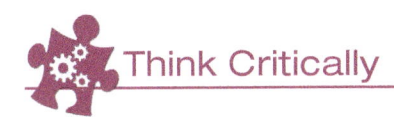

Consider the following real-world scenario and draft a response.

As the director of HIM for a new 200-bed hospital, you must prepare a hospital-wide policy for password selection and use. Your policy should explain the purpose and importance of passwords, identify the parameters for password-selection criteria and password aging, and detail the penalties for password sharing or misuse.

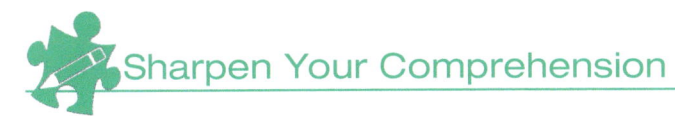

Sharpen Your Comprehension

Complete the following matching exercise by selecting, from the list provided, the answer that best matches each of the numbered statements. For each statement, only one answer is correct.

a. aggregate data
b. HL7
c. server
d. CPU
e. gigahertz
f. browser
g. HTML
h. DPL
i. data
j. data mining

1. _____ The brain of the computer
2. _____ When processed by a computer, becomes information
3. _____ Searching through and analyzing large amounts of data
4. _____ Application used to locate, retrieve, and display content on the World Wide Web (WWW)
5. _____ The programming language most commonly used for the Internet
6. _____ Extracting individual patient data from a medical database and combining it together
7. _____ Access speed of at least one billion cycles per second
8. _____ The exchange protocol used by most software programs in US health care
9. _____ Many computers connected together
10. _____ Software used to defend against computer threats

Chapter 6   Information Technology in Health Care

Connect Theory to Practice

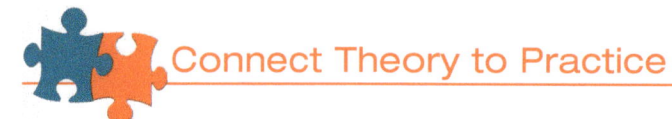

To help translate the concepts presented in this chapter to the workplace, complete the following exercise.

Watch this short video "Effective Healthcare IT Leaders" at http://IntroHIM.Paradigm College.net/LeadershipVideo.

After viewing the video, write a two- to three-page paper (not including cover or reference page) describing the traits of an effective IT leader, and identify which trait is the most important. In your paper, rate your skills as an effective healthcare IT leader based on the traits described in the video. Please be specific. Suggest three steps you could take to improve your IT leadership skills.

Student eResources

*To enhance your comprehension of the chapter material, go to **Navigator+** and complete the additional practice items as advised by your instructor.*

Chapter Terms

- access speed
- aggregate data
- American Recovery and Reinvestment Act (ARRA)
- application software
- bit
- central processing unit (CPU)
- cloud computing
- computer port
- cookie
- core health data elements
- data
- data element
- data loss prevention (DLP) software
- data mining
- dataset
- database
- database management system (DBMS)

- digital certificate
- domain name
- Ethernet
- external hard drive
- field
- firewall
- flash drive
- gigahertz (GHz)
- hard drive
- hardware
- health information technology (HIT)
- information
- information technology (IT)
- infrastructure
- interface
- Internet
- interoperable

intranet
IT director
local area network (LAN)
malware
megahertz (MHz)
memory chip
microcomputer
microprocessor
motherboard
networking
password
password aging
phishing
random access memory (RAM)
server

software
strategic plan
strong password
system software
Trojan horse
uniform resource locator (URL)
virtual private network (VPN)
virus
web browser
website
wide area network (WAN)
Wi-Fi
wireless access point (WAP)
wireless local area network (WLAN)
worm

" The HIM professional is best suited to assume critical roles in the management, use, privacy, security, and integrity of the EHR (electronic health record). "

—Health information technology (HIT) consultant James H. Braden

Career Tip

EHR Job Opportunities Are HOT

The federal Bureau of Labor Statistics estimates there will be a need for 272,000 medical record technicians in the United States by 2022, 85,000 more than a decade earlier.

Seventy-three percent of healthcare providers surveyed in 2013 by the global professional services company Towers Watson reported difficulty hiring individuals with specialized skills needed to meet new electronic medical record requirements.

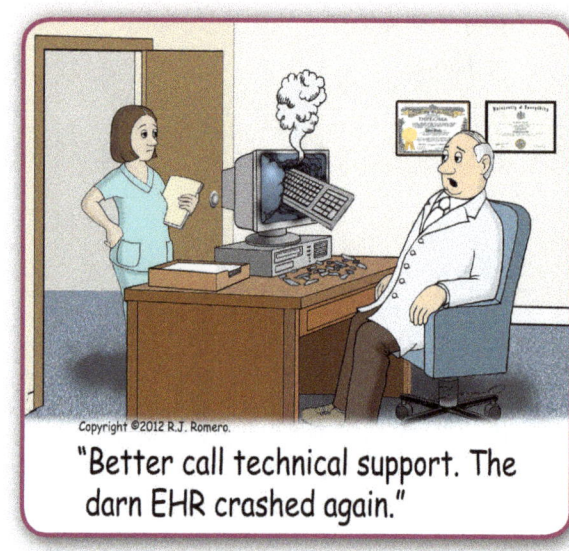

"Better call technical support. The darn EHR crashed again."

© R.J. Romero/hippacartoons.com

Fast Facts

In the past, health information management focused on manually assembling, analyzing, counting, and moving paper medical records. With the evolution of the electronic health record, it has become "a body of knowledge and practice that ensures the availability of health information to facilitate real-time healthcare delivery and critical health-related decision making for multiple purposes across diverse organizations, settings, and disciplines."

—American Health Information Management Association (AHIMA)

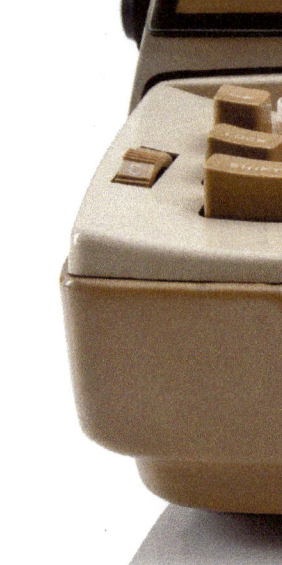

Chapter 7

Electronic Health Records

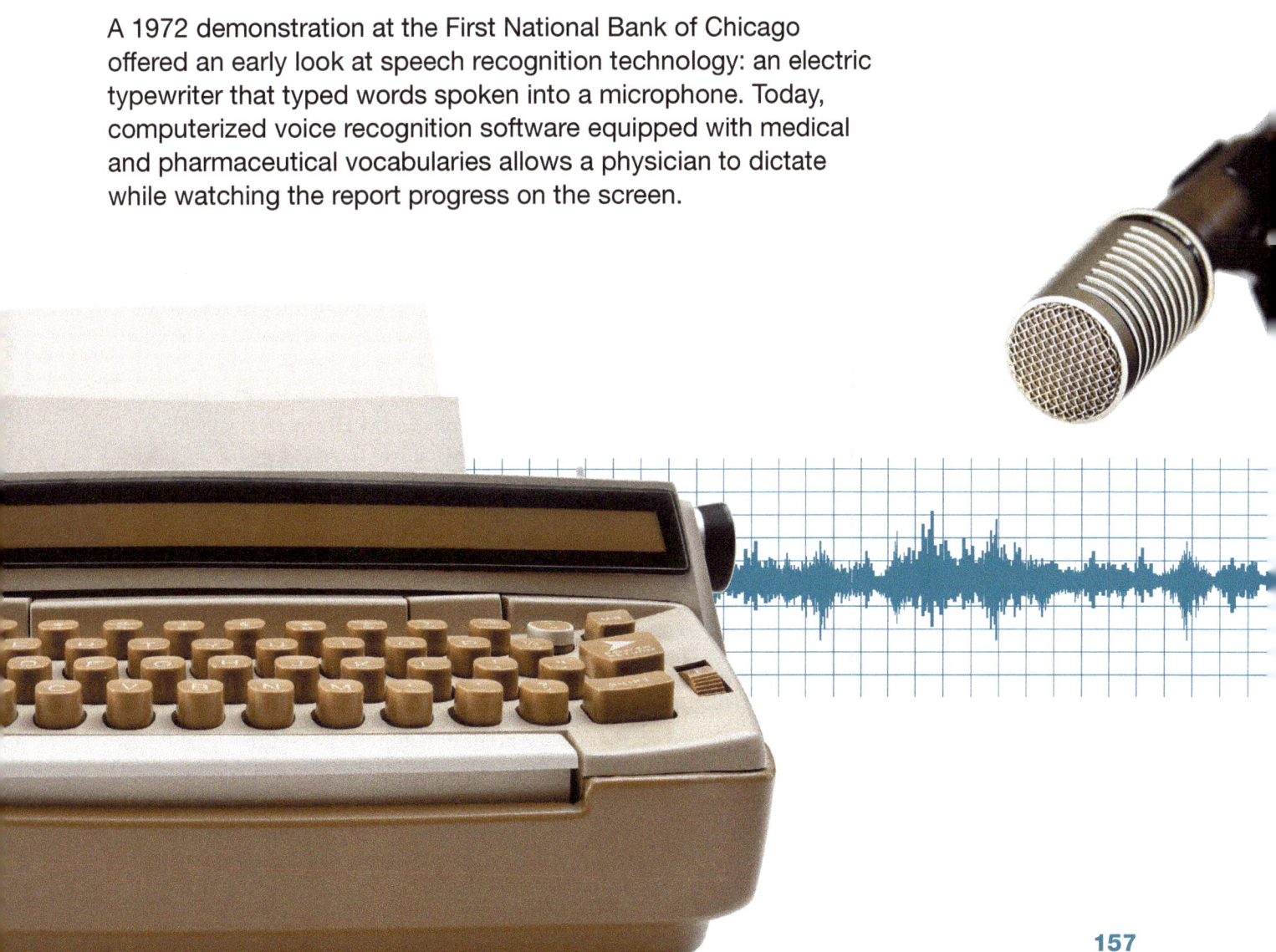

A 1972 demonstration at the First National Bank of Chicago offered an early look at speech recognition technology: an electric typewriter that typed words spoken into a microphone. Today, computerized voice recognition software equipped with medical and pharmaceutical vocabularies allows a physician to dictate while watching the report progress on the screen.

Learning Objectives

- Explain the functions and the organization of electronic health records (EHRs).
- Describe the advantages and the disadvantages of the EHR.
- Discuss the importance of EHR security.
- Distinguish between administrative, physical, and technical safeguards used to secure electronic personal health information.
- Describe the master patient index; admission, discharge, and transfer; practice management; and scheduling systems.
- Demonstrate disaster-preparedness and downtime procedures for the EHR.
- Understand the different systems used in a health information management (HIM) department.
- Examine how the EHR is changing HIM staff roles.
- Describe the benefits of the personal health record.

At a basic level, the **electronic health record (EHR)** is a record of all of a patient's health information for different episodes of care across time and healthcare organizations. The EHR is referred to as a **longitudinal record** because it incorporates all of the information from multiple sources gathered over a period of time.

An EHR is much more than the duplication of a paper record or a chart stored on a computer, however. The EHR also includes a number of computer-based functions that can improve patient care. **Decision support** software embedded within the EHR provides physicians with the most current information about diseases and treatment; **alerts** warn providers about potential medication interactions. The EHR enables providers to access a patient's **protected health information (PHI)**, individually identifiable health information that is protected by federal law, such as diagnostic results across time and between healthcare facilities. The EHR allows a physician to track a patient's progress over time; for example, the physician can review graphs that chart a patient's weight, blood pressure, cholesterol level, and glucose readings over several visits or even several years.

EHR Functions

No two electronic health record systems are created the same. An individual provider's EHR will be based on the specific needs of that provider and the capabilities of the vendor's software program. For example, a facility that operates an intensive care unit (ICU) would require an EHR system that can support complex flow sheets for patient monitoring. A small community clinic would not need such a complex EHR. Therefore, the EHR systems used by these providers would likely have different capabilities and features.

Regardless of the differences, however, most EHRs are designed to meet specific meaningful use objectives that will improve healthcare outcomes and efficiency. The Office of the National Coordinator for Health Information Technology (ONC) has grouped these objectives into five patient-driven domains, each connected to specific healthcare outcomes and policy priorities.

Improve quality, safety, and efficiency Some examples of patient care quality and safety improvements include the use of drug interaction checks, medication lists, and medication allergy lists. Efficiencies can be achieved by using automated patient reminders for tests and appointments, freeing staff to do other things.

Engage patients and families Patients will be able to access health information, including a clinical summary of the visit and educational materials, via a patient portal allowing them to be actively engaged in their care.

Improve care coordination The electronic exchange of health information between physicians will improve the coordination of the patient's care, regardless of how many different physicians or organizations are involved.

Improve public and population health Information will flow electronically to designated registries, such as the state's immunization or cancer registries.

Ensure privacy and security of PHI Every EHR will have privacy and security features to ensure that all patient health information remains confidential.

A System of Systems

An EHR system is a collection of computer systems with integrated applications (specific computer programs) that share information. This information sharing is referred to as *interoperability*. The Healthcare Information and Management Systems Society (HIMSS) defines **interoperability** as the ability of different information technology systems and software applications to communicate and exchange data within and across organizations and use the information that has been exchanged. The data should be accessible to clinicians, labs, hospitals, pharmacies, and patients, regardless of the application or application vendor.

Just as the human body contains many independent systems (e.g., cardiac, urinary, musculoskeletal) that must work together, the EHR system is made up of several different independent systems (e.g., admissions, laboratory, pharmacy, and radiology) that work together. The systems of the body share critical information with each other via the nervous, lymphatic, and circulatory (blood) systems. (Touch something hot and the nervous system alerts your brain to move your hand!) The EHR system uses a similar two-way communication system to relay information between different parts. For example, patient information entered by a care provider is automatically cross-referenced with decision support software in the EHR. If the information is in conflict—the patient has been prescribed two drugs that cannot be safely taken together, for example—the system generates an automated alert. As shown in Figure 7.1, a typical EHR system communicates between numerous independent systems that can be clustered into four broad categories: administrative, clinical, core EHR, and document management.

EXPAND YOUR KNOWLEDGE

There are three levels of interoperability in health information technology: foundational, semantic, and structural. Read more about interoperability at http://IntroHIM.ParadigmCollege.net/Interoperability.

Figure 7.1 EHR Systems Interface

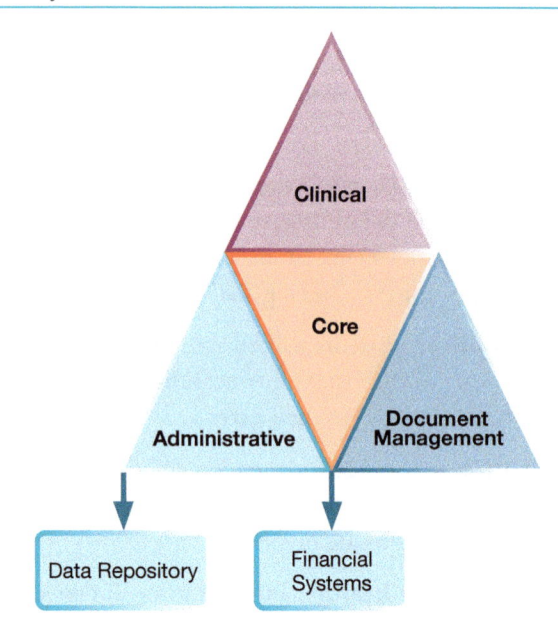

Core EHR

The **core EHR system**, also referred to as the **central system**, is most often purchased from a vendor, but in some cases, it may be developed independently by a hospital, a physician office, or another facility. The core EHR system performs several functions including medication ordering, referred to as **computerized provider order entry (CPOE)**, nursing documentation and flow sheets, and fill-in-the-blank forms or free-style writing notes for ancillary departments.

The core EHR system accepts data from patient monitoring devices (e.g., glucose monitors and telemetry monitors) and connects the information to flow sheets, eliminating the need for manual charting. This system accepts all information from the administrative and medical systems, including reference and alerts generated by each of these systems. Figure 7.2 shows an example of a reference and alert sent to the EHR about a patient allergy to penicillin-based antibiotics. Other alerts warn physicians about potentially hazardous drug interactions and include access to the *Physicians' Desk Reference* (*PDR*).

Figure 7.2 Medication Reference and Alert

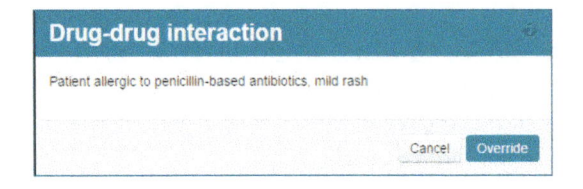

Administrative

In a hospital setting, the administrative systems that feed into the core EHR include the **admission, discharge, and transfer (ADT) system** and the **master patient index (MPI)**. The ADT system tracks patients from admission through departure, either by transfer, discharge, or death. The MPI is a component of the ADT system. It collects patient demographic information, including name, birth date, address, and phone number. A practice management system (PMS) is used to track patients in a physician practice. Other administrative systems receive data from the EHR that is used for billing or external reporting requirements, such as the Joint Commission indicators. These administrative systems also generate data on patient quality of care and patient outcomes for reporting to outside agencies.

Clinical

The **clinical system** receives and processes medical orders which, when completed, become the final results stored in the core of the EHR. Radiology, laboratory, pharmacy, cardiology, emergency department, and transcription are all examples of medical systems that work with the EHR through a two-way communication exchange called an **interface**. One example of an interface is an **electronic medication administration record (eMAR)**. The eMAR documents the time, dosage, and administration route for every medication administered to a patient in the hospital. The information is generated by a separate medical system (pharmacy) and electronically transferred to and stored in the EHR. The **picture archiving and communication system (PACS)** is another example of an interface. This system captures and stores radiology images and scans (such as computerized tomography [CT] scans), then interfaces with the core EHR to store the images and scans.

Document Management

In a true EHR environment, all information would be placed into the EHR electronically through an interface with another system or by someone typing directly into the patient record. Some information, however, cannot be added to the EHR in this fashion. For example, X-ray images or photographic images taken during a colonoscopy must be downloaded or scanned into the EHR using a document management system. A **document management system** manages pictures or images of scanned documents (see Figure 7.3). It can be a stand-alone system or a part of a package purchased with the core EHR product. Paper documents, such as records from another provider or a patient healthcare directive, can also be added to the EHR using a document scanner. Once scanned into the system, these documents are given a title, similar to the title of the paper form equivalent, and then stored in the designated location in the EHR.

Figure 7.3 Adding Documents to the EHR

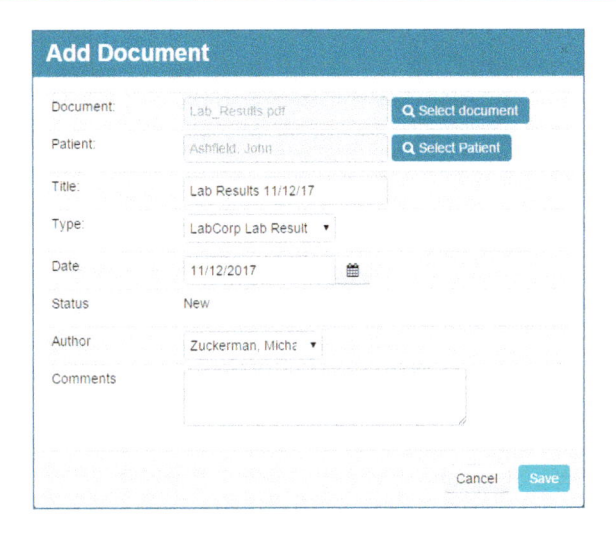

IT REALLY HAPPENS

Many patients who live in the northern part of the United States relocate during the winter to the milder climate of the southern states. These "snowbirds" arrive for medical appointments carrying handwritten treatment orders from their home physicians that need to be scanned into the document imaging system and stored in the EHR system under "orders."

Think Ethics!

Federal and state law prohibit healthcare organizations from basing medical decisions on a patient's ability to pay or medical coding on charges accumulated. This is one reason why it is important that patients' financial information not be stored with their clinical information.

Financial Systems

An EHR is a collection of all of an individual patient's clinical data. It is important to note that just like the paper medical record, the EHR should not contain *financial data* such as charges, bills, payments received, or debt due. In some settings, clinical and financial data may be forwarded to a data repository and integrated together for reporting to outside agencies, such as the Joint Commission, or for internal use by the healthcare leadership team. Integrated data may be used, for example, to analyze the cost of care by patient population.

EHR Advantages and Disadvantages

The move from paper to electronic health records offers healthcare providers and organizations both advantages and disadvantages. Electronic records bring efficiencies, improve patient care, help to reduce medical errors, and increase patient engagement. The most significant disadvantage of the electronic health record is cost, with regard to the initial investment and the ongoing expenses of maintenance and system upgrades. Nevertheless, as health care and technology continue to align, the EHR will become the standard across the industry. The following section discusses some of the EHR advantages and disadvantages in greater detail.

EHR Advantages

In healthcare organizations that rely on paper records, obtaining patient records can be a lengthy process. Consider the example of an emergency department (ED) physician who needs to see a patient's medical records before making a diagnosis or prescribing a drug. Without access to an EHR, the typical procedure would involve the physician asking the unit secretary to call or fax the request to the HIM department. HIM staff would then locate the record, sign it out to the ED, and either physically carry it to the ED or request a hospital runner to deliver it.

Of course, that is a best-case scenario. If the unit secretary has several STAT (immediate) orders—an electrocardiogram (ECG) for a chest pain patient, for example—the ED physician's records request may be delayed. If the HIM department is having difficulty finding the record or if the department is short staffed or closed, there will also be a delay in retrieving the record. In a busy hospital ED, fulfilling a physician's request for a paper record can take anywhere from 15 minutes to several hours. In an emergency situation, that is too long. The physician may end up treating the patient without seeing the record, resulting in extra expense if the physician duplicates a test that was performed days before, or injury to the patient if the physician orders a medication that is contraindicated by information in the patient record.

The EHR eliminates these types of delays. Physicians can access a patient's medical record immediately at the **point of care (POC)** by using a computer terminal at the patient's bedside.

Improved Patient Safety

To improve patient safety, point-of-care reminders and alerts embedded within the EHR display critical information to providers. The EHR may remind staff to elevate the head of a patient's bed or don gloves and a mask before entering a patient's room. Medication alerts can warn physicians about dangerous drug interactions. The EHR utilizes **clinical decision support (CDS)** software to analyze patient-specific information and generate reminders, alerts, clinical guidelines, diagnostic support, and relevant reference information. CDS tools may be purchased from the vendor or can be developed in-house to include facility- or practitioner-specific protocols.

Faster Diagnostic Results

The EHR also provides physicians with faster access to diagnostic test results and images. As discussed in the example above, paper records can lead to delays in patient care. Paper records can also be a source of confusion, especially if the record includes hard-to-read handwritten orders or information that requires clarification. For example, if a physician ordering a chest X-ray writes the word "chest" on a paper order, the radiology technician will need to clarify the type of chest X-ray requested before proceeding. If the physician is unavailable, this can result in a lengthy delay.

If the physician inputs the same order into the patient's EHR, a list of options stored under the default profile tab on the EHR will drop down automatically with details about the medical parameters necessary for each type of order (see Figure 7.4), prompting the physician to add additional required information. For example, X-ray—two views, Chest PA and Lateral. Once the chest X-ray is completed, the physician can get immediate access to the results via the EHR; in some systems, the results may be emailed directly to the physician's smartphone.

Figure 7.4 EHR Drop-Down Menus

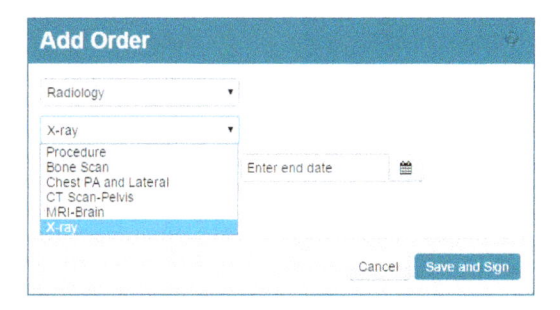

Fewer Duplicate Tests

When a physician cannot review the results of a diagnostic test (either because the results cannot be found or were not received when requested), he or she will order the test again. Performing duplicate tests causes patients stress, delays treatment, and increases costs. The EHR allows physicians to order tests electronically and receive results as soon as they are available. Some departments, such as radiology and cardiology, post draft diagnostic results in the EHR and then add the final results once they have been reviewed and electronically signed (e-signed) by the physician who interpreted the test. An **electronic signature (e-signature)** is a digital rather than handwritten signature, and it allows providers to approve and sign a document securely in an online system.

Simultaneous Access

Most people imagine that after a patient is discharged from the hospital, there is little need to access the patient's medical record. The opposite is true. Physicians, coders, auditors, and other hospital staff need access to the medical record to complete a number of important tasks under tight deadlines. With paper records, documentation is handed from one person to the next, and the record is in constant motion throughout the day. Unlike paper records, electronic records can be accessed by many individuals at the same time. Staff members can access the record by logging into the EHR system and providing an individual password. However, for security purposes, once a patient is discharged, care providers (except for the physicians on the case) should no longer have access to the patient's EHR. If additional review or study of the patient record is required, the HIM department retrieval clerk can provide staff with temporary access based on the organization's privacy protocols. However, anytime a patient returns to the facility for any reason, the previous record is automatically reactivated so that everyone involved in treating the patient can review the patient's medical history. Table 7.1 shows which staff members

Table 7.1 Access to Patient Information Following Discharge

EHR Users	Purpose	Timeframe for Use
All physicians and residents on record (1–20 individuals)	Complete required dictation and signatures	24 hours to 30 days after discharge, depending on the report type and state regulations
HIM personnel (1–5 individuals)	Assemble, analyze, and file transcribed reports, loose miscellaneous reports, and final diagnostic reports	24 hours
Medical coder	Codes and abstracts the final diagnosis and surgical procedures to send to the billing system	24–48 hours
Billing auditor	Review record documentation to support billing accuracy; this may be a routine process, performed per patient request, or performed in preparation for an insurance audit	As a routine process, two to three days before the bill is dropped. Per request or external audit, the time varies
Care coordinator (utilization review department)	Contact insurance company for approval of final day of hospital stay by providing justification from the medical record	Day after discharge before 5 p.m.
Follow-up call nurse	Call patients the day after discharge to see how they are doing; documents calls in the record	Day after discharge
Special review by infection control nurse, pharmacist, nurse manager, administrator, and others who may need to review the record (0-20 individuals)	May review the record for issues such as infection, medication error, or patient complaint	Immediately to 24 hours after discharge
Data collector—various departments (0-5 individuals)	Collect data to comply with mandatory requirements for reporting to the Joint Commission, cancer registry, trauma registry, cardiac registry, diabetes registry, and others	Varies for each reporting entity
Performance improvement coordinator	Review records for clinical indicators; selects records to review at medical staff meetings or by physician peer review	30 days
Release of information coordinator (HIM department)	Provide copies of record to requestors	Immediately for patient care; timeframe for other requests is based on the request type and on state and federal laws

need to access the patient record after discharge, for what purpose they need to access the record, and the approximate timelines for completing the work.

Legible Documentation

Most people have heard horror stories about physicians with terrible handwriting, but doctors are not the only providers with bad handwriting. As shown in Figure 7.5, notes in the record made by nurses, dieticians, case managers, and just about anyone else can be difficult to read or incomplete, which can cause delay and frustration. Both the Joint Commission and the Centers for Medicare & Medicaid Services (CMS) require all medical documentation to be legible, timed, dated, and authenticated to reduce medical errors and delays in care. In a fully functioning EHR system, all notes are typed into the record, and decision support functions prompt providers to produce more complete and accurate documentation.

Figure 7.5 Illegible Documentation in the Patient Record

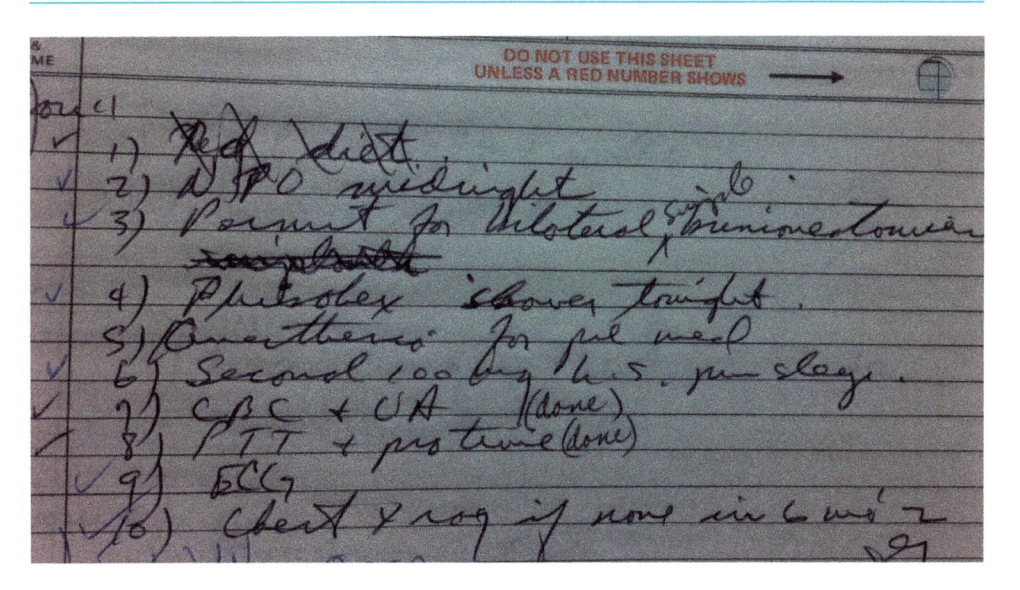

IT REALLY HAPPENS

Dr. Montoya received a call to perform a consultation on a patient in the hospital. The physician reviewed the consultation order and the progress notes but was unable to decipher the attending physician's poor handwriting. He asked several other healthcare workers, but none of them could interpret what the attending physician had written in the record.

When the consulting doctor contacted the attending physician's office for clarification, he was told the attending physician was in surgery all day. The consulting physician could not see the patient until the attending doctor was available. Thus, patient care was delayed due to illegible documentation.

Elimination of Lost or Misplaced Records

Important items get lost all the time—keys, wallets, and cell phones, to name just a few. Paper health records can also be lost or misplaced. Because electronic health records are stored on a computer server, it is impossible for an EHR to be misplaced, misfiled, or lost. Furthermore, EHRs are backed up on a secondary server that is usually located in another state to ensure that records are protected in the event of a natural disaster. Some EHR systems have real-time or redundant backup systems that allow the user to access information created only minutes before. This type of backup system is quite expensive, however, and is used more often by hospitals than clinics or physician offices.

Enhanced Privacy and Security

Protecting patient privacy is required under the federal Health Insurance Portability and Accountability Act of 1996 (HIPAA) and is an ethical obligation for all healthcare employees. An EHR offers greater privacy protection and better security than a paper record. Access to an electronic record is password protected, and every person who has access to it can be identified in an audit trail. An **audit trail** is a computer-generated report that identifies every person who accessed a computer system or an individual record and what action he or she took.

Paperless Referrals and Prescriptions

The EHR allows physicians to generate electronic prescriptions (a practice referred to as **e-prescribing** or **eRx**) and physician referrals, decreasing wait times, and eliminating lost documents (see Figure 7.6). Prescriptions can also be printed if a patient needs a hard copy for travel or for another reason.

Figure 7.6 Electronic Prescribing

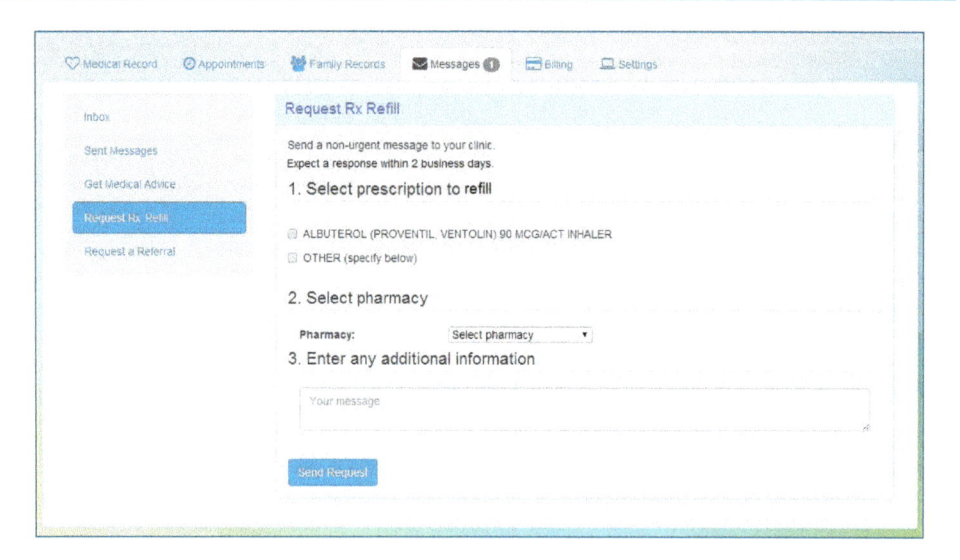

Improved Patient Engagement

Electronic health records offer patients access to their health information through a **patient portal**, a secure website that provides patients with convenient, 24-hour access to physician notes, diagnostic results, physical examination results, medications, and other information. Patient portals can improve communication between patient and provider, encourage better and more timely patient self-care, and improve patient satisfaction.

Reduced Record Storage

As discussed in Chapter 5, electronic health records require much less physical storage space than paper health records. As electronic health records replace paper records, healthcare facilities will require less space for paper record storage, freeing up space for other revenue-generating opportunities, such as additional patient rooms or new diagnostic equipment.

Data Sharing

A **clinical data repository (CDR)** stores individual data elements from all of the separate systems that comprise the EHR and, in many cases, combines clinical data from the EHR with the billing data related to a specific episode of care. These data elements can be shared with external reporting systems such as the Minimum Data Set (MDS) for long-term care and the National Cancer Data Base (NCDB) for acute care hospitals. The interface reduces staff time spent manually abstracting data and reduces the error rate as there is less need to input data manually. The reporting requirements are time sensitive; using an automated process for transferring data also accelerates processing time. Additionally, the EHR facilitates the sharing of patient health information electronically between physicians, pharmacists, patients, and other providers and healthcare organizations. This is known as **health information exchange (HIE)**, which is the standardized process of data exchange. HIEs allow patient information to be shared electronically in a secure format that improves the speed, quality, and safety of patient care while reducing costs.

> **EXPAND YOUR KNOWLEDGE**
>
> To learn more about the future of health information exchange, read the *Journal of AHIMA* article "ONC Issues Plans to Accelerate HIE Expansion" at http://IntroHIM.ParadigmCollege.net/HIE.

EHR Disadvantages

Disadvantages of the electronic health record can be classified into two categories: unavoidable and manageable. Some disadvantages, such as the high cost of implementing an EHR system, are unavoidable. Although there are some opportunities to negotiate costs when an institution is purchasing hardware and software, start-up will still be expensive.

Manageable disadvantages include such things as workflow changes for both administrative and clinical staff, staff resistance to change, poor planning that leads to improper installation, and inadequate training. The more these disadvantages are kept in mind during the planning process and properly managed during implementation, the more successfully the EHR will perform.

Implementation Costs

Investing in new technology or equipment is expensive, and healthcare providers want to see a return on that investment. **Return on investment** is the ability of an investment to pay for itself over time and generate a profit. If a hospital purchases a new MRI machine for the radiology department at a cost of $5 million, for example, it expects to see a return on that investment within a reasonable timeframe. In this example, the hospital calculates the new machine will perform 100 patient MRI scans per month, and the hospital will charge $3,000 per scan. Based on that estimate, the new MRI will generate $300,000 per month in additional revenue, or $3.6 million per year. Therefore, the return on investment for the new MRI machine would be achieved in 1.4 years.

The purchase of an MRI machine is one example of an investment that returns **hard dollars** (actual cash payments or savings). In a hospital setting, hard dollars can be generated in a number of ways: by increasing services (serving more patients), for example, or through cost savings, such as a reduction of staff or supplies. Implementing an EHR system, however, rarely provides a return on investment in hard dollars. Instead, an EHR generates a soft dollar return on investment. **Soft dollars** are non-monetary benefits and cost savings. The EHR reduces medical errors and can potentially reduce the number of malpractice suits. This is an example of soft dollar savings. Soft dollar savings are usually substantial and considered a desirable outcome in every healthcare setting. Table 7.2 shows the approximate costs associated with the implementation and maintenance of an EHR system for a hospital and physician group.

Table 7.2 EHR Implementation and Maintenance Costs

Hospital	Physician Group
$14,500 per bed	$25,000–$45,000 per physician
Annual operating/maintenance costs amount to $2,700 per bed per year.	Annual operating, licensing, and maintenance costs are $3,000–$9,000 per physician.

Source: Congressional Budget Office

To calculate the average cost of EHR implementation for a 250-bed hospital using the data in Table 7.2, you would first multiply the number of beds by the average cost per bed (250 beds × $14,500 = $3,625,000). Next, calculate the annual cost of operations, licensing, and maintenance (250 beds × $2,700 = $675,000). Adding the two together will provide a rough estimate of the EHR implementation cost.

The actual cost of implementing and maintaining an EHR system will vary, of course, depending on the size of the facility or the practice and the complexity of the EHR system.

Extensive Training

More than 75 percent of the employees in a healthcare facility will need initial training when an EHR system is implemented and ongoing training when the system is upgraded or changed. Physicians need training as well, even those physicians who have used another EHR system, because each system is unique. Training must accommodate learners at all levels of experience, from entry-level clerks to physicians. Training is also costly and time-consuming. Hospitals and large practices may even need to establish a department specifically for EHR training. Poor or ineffective training has and will continue to derail EHR success.

Documentation Quality

Ensuring **documentation integrity**—documentation that is complete and accurate with no mistakes, errors, or inconsistencies—has become a major concern with the adoption of the EHR, specifically because of the overuse of documentation shortcuts, such as cloning, templates, and macros added to EHR software to improve physician efficiency. When used inappropriately, the features described in this section can produce inaccurate documentation, medical errors, and fraudulent claims.

Cloning involves copying and pasting information from the documentation of one episode of care into the documentation of another episode of care or from one note to another. Cloning produces poor documentation because important updates or changes in a patient's condition are not recorded. Physicians sometimes clone information because it is faster and easier, but cloning negatively affects patient care, medical coding accuracy, and insurance/Medicare reimbursement.

Templates are fill-in-the-blank features built into an EHR. These pretyped reports require physicians to enter a few simple fill-in-the-blank answers from a drop-down screen. Although this can improve efficiency, it can also introduce errors and inaccuracies. Consider the case of a patient who visited an ophthalmologist with a complaint of blurred vision. The physician determined the patient had dry eyes and sought to document her findings in the patient's EHR by clicking on an arrow and then choosing from one of several programmed answer choices on a template. The form, however, did not have a diagnosis for blurred vision or dry eyes. Because the physician was required to select something in order for the patient to get his prescription and leave, she chose blindness. Such a diagnosis could cause problems for the patient in the future if he was trying to obtain a driver's license or employment, for example.

> **BE AWARE**
>
> According to the Centers for Medicare & Medicaid Services, "Medical decision making is a cognitive process that's hard to document with templates and macros."

Templates are quick and easy, requiring few keystrokes, but as this example shows, they can also lead to incomplete or inaccurate documentation. Most diagnoses require a more thorough description of the patient's condition. CMS cautions that templates are meant to prompt documentation, not to replace it.

IT REALLY HAPPENS

Patricia, a 42-year-old female was admitted to the hospital. The progress note on her first day read, "Patient is admitted with cough, fever, and shortness of breath. She has a temperature of 102 and rales in both lower lobes of her lungs."

The progress note on the second day stated the exact same thing. In fact, all of the progress notes in the patient's record read the same way until the day she was discharged from the hospital, and yet she was sent home without any medication or follow-up treatment plan.

Based on the EHR documentation, it did not appear that the patient was improving although her condition *had* improved (she was sent home). Rather than update the record, the physician had cloned the progress note entries.

The EHR also allows the use of **macros**, shortcuts that can produce words, sentences, paragraphs, or entire reports with a few keystrokes. Examples 7.1–7.4 illustrate the different types of macros used.

Example 7.1   Abbreviation Macro

Macros can be used to eliminate keystrokes for long medical terms. In this example, the typed abbreviation will be spelled out.

Key In	Result
F1 + EGD (Abbreviations will be spelled out.)	Esophagogastroduodenoscopy

Example 7.2   Standard Documentation Macro

Physicians can build their own specific macros that will insert standardized documentation that does not change, as in this example of patient discharge instructions.

Key In	Result
F5 + ins (Specific macro built for this physician's patients)	**Patient discharge instructions:** No lifting over 10 pounds. Diet as tolerated. Take Tylenol with codeine every 4 hours as needed. Make appointment to see physician in 3 days. Contact physician if fever more than 100 degrees or excessive bleeding from surgical site.

Example 7.3   Order Protocols Macro

Macros can be used when a group or department of physicians elects to follow the same order protocols, as in this example of admission orders for myocardial infarction (MI) patients.

Key In	Result
F5 + CCU2 (The Department of Cardiology for General Hospital has determined that this hospital will follow the following protocols for all new MI patients.)	**General Hospital admit orders for MI patients** Admit patient to CCU as observation ECG Stat Chest X-ray upon admission Cardiac Monitor/oximeter Oxygen @ 2L/min via nc Start IV with saline lock Bed rest NPO Vitals q4h for 24h then q8h Aspirin 4–81 mg PO Stat–patient to chew Then Aspirin 325 mg PO daily Sublingual Nitroglycerin 0.4 mg Heparin 60 U/kg bolus for 48 h Labs: CBC, PT, PTT, CKMB, and total CK, Troponin-T and Troponin-1

Example 7.4 Report Macro

Macros can be used for an entire report that has a regular or expected path of completion by allowing the physician to dictate the few miscellaneous components, as in this example of an operative report.

Key In	Result
jF5 + Richard Car Tun (Dr. Richard can dictate an entire operative report with a few fill in the blanks. In this case, the physician would dictate the word "left" for the blanks.) Although this macro may look like a template due to the fill in the blanks, it is not. A template provides the users choices of words or phrases from a drop-down menu.	**Operative Report** **Surgical Date:** 01/06/2016 **Patient:** Shauntel Dubois **Surgeon:** Harry Richard, M.D. **Anesthesia:** Regional Block **Complications:** None **Blood loss:** Minimal **Pre-operative diagnosis:** _____ carpal tunnel syndrome **Post-operative diagnosis:** Status post _____ carpal tunnel syndrome **Operative procedures:** _____ carpal tunnel release **History:** This is a 32-year-old black female diagnosed with carpal tunnel syndrome; treated with medication and physical therapy for the last year. Her condition has become progressively worse, with muscle wasting and continual numbness. **Operative note:** The patient was brought to the operating room and placed in the supine position. The _____ arm was prepped and draped in the usual fashion.

Because CMS audits have uncovered problems with the use of shortcuts in EHR documentation, the Office of the Inspector General (OIG) has developed a work plan to review:

- concerns about *upcoding* (insertion of a code for a procedure or a diagnosis that is more complex than the actual procedure or diagnosis, resulting in higher reimbursement)
- cloning patient data on subsequent visits
- auto population or "auto fill" features
- data cloned (pulled forward) without updates by the physician
- patient histories that are auto populated without evidence that the work was actually performed
- charts EHR systems have upcoded based on history and exam elements without the proper medical necessity

> **EXPAND YOUR KNOWLEDGE**
> To learn more about the problems related to cloning, templates, and macros, read "The Perils of Copy-Paste" in *For the Record* at http://IntroHIM.ParadigmCollege.net/CopyPaste.

Concerns about the accuracy and the validity of EHR documentation can result in reduced or denied payments to providers who may also be subject to false-claims investigations. These documentation concerns should be addressed as part of initial and follow-up training.

> **EXPAND YOUR KNOWLEDGE**
>
> For more information on the use of electronic health records in courts of law, read "EHRs Prove a Difficult Witness in Court" in the *Journal of AHIMA* at http://IntroHIM.ParadigmCollege.net/EHRCourt.

System Output Usability

A great deal of the development of electronic health records has focused on building the appropriate screens for data input. Far less consideration has been given to how that information is formatted for output. When an electronic record is printed, the print version usually does not match what is shown on the screen; for example, some elements may be missing, or there may be no organization or flow. Print versions of electronic records are also very difficult to read. The poor quality of the EHR printout can cause problems if those records are required as evidence in a lawsuit, for example, or need to be produced in response to a subpoena.

In legal proceedings, there is a saying: "If it isn't documented, it wasn't done." That holds true for documents that are unreadable, too. The paper output from an EHR is not only difficult to read but also cumbersome. A printed EHR document produces 10 times more paper than a regular paper record.

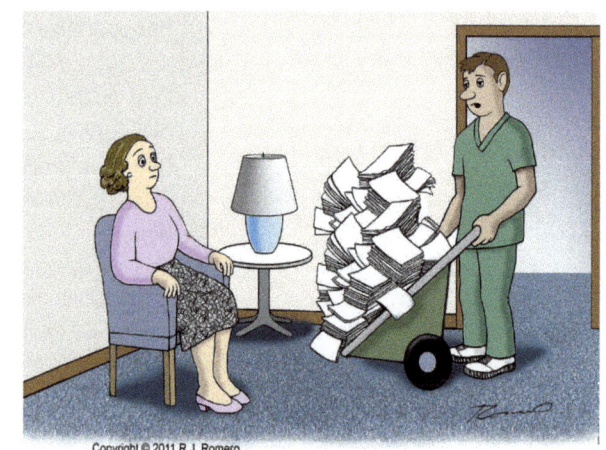

"Are you the lady that ordered a print out of her electronic medical record?"

© R.J. Romero/hippacartoons.com

An HIM professional can help to ensure the data is presented accurately when producing or printing the medical record.

Unintended Consequences

In addition to the disadvantages discussed previously, the success of the EHR can be hampered by unintended consequences, particularly in the implementation phase. The following are examples of unintended consequences.

During the transition from paper to electronic records, healthcare facilities can often end up with **hybrid records,** records that are part paper/manual record and part computerized/electronic records (see Chapter 5). A facility may choose to use a hybrid record for a variety of reasons: to reduce expenses (the facility can only afford one or two components of the EHR); to handle concerns about staffing and training (the facility can only support a limited number of installations at a time, which spreads out the implementation over years); or to accommodate physicians and staff members who are reluctant to give up paper documents. Hybrid record systems are quite cumbersome to use; these systems require two separate procedures for each record component. Hybrid systems also require greater diligence to maintain accuracy and proper management, and often require additional HIM staff.

Staff may resist or refuse to use the EHR. This lack of buy-in can be the unintended result of a lack of support at the top of the organization or of staff members feeling they have not had input into the design or development of the EHR system. There is always resistance to change, but when users do not buy in to a new EHR system, they tend to use the system inefficiently and even incorrectly.

A system that fails to meet the needs of users can also result in unintended consequences. For example, a system that does not allow users to type in *free text* (in the user's own words) may make fully describing a patient problem difficult and may result in incomplete or inaccurate documentation. A system that limits the amount and type of data that can be entered may leave healthcare providers open to possible malpractice lawsuits.

Poor system performance will also reduce user buy-in. No one wants to work on a computer system that is slow or experiences frequent periods of downtime, has poor vendor support, or creates inefficient workflow. One of the top reasons cited for discontinuing the use of an EHR system is the time required to input data, the result of a slow system-response time and/or a system that requires users to click through an excessive number of screens to input data.

IT REALLY HAPPENS

> While having occupational therapy on her hand at a rehabilitation hospital, a patient noticed that the staff had spent more than an hour documenting her medical history on paper forms. When she asked the staff if they were planning to switch to an EHR, the director of the department stated, "We've already tried, but it was too slow and had too many screens. We could not get the documentation we needed into the system, so we went back to paper, which is much faster."

Evolution of the EHR

Dr. Lawrence L. Weed first introduced the concept of an electronic medical record in the 1960s at the University of Vermont. Weed's work included the development of the **problem-oriented medical information system (PROMIS)** and the **problem-oriented medical record (POMR)**, which established standardized documentation formats (as discussed in Chapter 4). In 1970, the Medical Center of Vermont started using the POMR process to input data electronically. Over the next two decades, several electronic medical record systems were developed and refined to better meet the needs of healthcare providers and improve patient care.

Government Influence

In 2004, President George W. Bush called for the widespread use of electronic health information technology within the decade, outlining a plan to ensure that most healthcare facilities would adopt EHRs by 2014. That year he also established the **Office of the National Coordinator for Health Information Technology (ONC)**.

Five years later, in 2009, Congress approved and President Barack Obama signed into law the **American Recovery and Reinvestment Act (ARRA)**, an economic stimulus package intended to jumpstart the US economy. The ARRA included significant investments to improve health care and healthcare technology. The **Health Information Technology for Economic and Clinical Health (HITECH) Act,** a provision of the ARRA, promoted the adoption of meaningful use health information technology and strengthened the civil and criminal penalties for violations of the HIPAA security provision regarding the electronic transmission of health information. Figure 7.7 shows the evolution of documentation standards.

Figure 7.7 EHR Timeline

- **1919** The American College of Surgeons (ACS) develops standards for medical documentation.
- **1960s** Dr. Lawrence L. Weed develops the PROMIS and POMR systems.
- **1970–1980** The electronic medical record (EMR) is developed and refined.
- **2004** President Bush establishes ONC.
- **2009** President Obama signs ARRA and HITECH into law.
- **2011** CMS institutes initial meaningful use incentives.
- **2011-2012** Meaningful use Stage I: data capture and sharing
- **2014** Meaningful use Stage II: advanced clinical processes
- **2015** Providers who have not achieved meaningful use now face financial penalties.
- **2016** Meaningful use: Stage III: improve health outcomes

Among its provisions, the HITECH Act authorized CMS to offer eligible hospitals, critical access hospitals (CAHs), and eligible professionals (EPs) financial incentives to promote the adoption and "meaningful use" of certified EHR technology to improve patient care and public health according to specific criteria.

Meaningful Use

CMS defines **meaningful use** as the use of certified EHR technology to meet identified goals for improving patient and public health. The ONC develops the standards, implementation specifications, and certification criteria for the EHR. Meaningful use requirements are phased in over three stages. At each stage, providers must meet specific core objectives for all patients. As providers progress through the stages, some objectives may be increased, combined, or eliminated, as illustrated by the comparison of Stage 1 and Stage 2 objectives in Table 7.3.

Table 7.3 Meaningful Use: A Comparison of Stage 1 and Stage 2 Objectives

Stage 1 Objective	Stage 1 Measure	Stage 2 Objective	Stage 2 Measure
Use computerized provider order entry for medication orders directly entered by any licensed healthcare professional who can enter orders into the medical record per state, local, and professional guidelines.	More than 30 percent of unique patients with at least one medication in their medication list seen by the EP have at least one medication order entered using CPOE.	Use computerized provider order entry for medication, laboratory, and radiology orders directly entered by any licensed healthcare professional who can enter orders into the medical record per state, local, and professional guidelines.	More than 60 percent of medication, 30 percent of laboratory, and 30 percent of radiology orders created by the EP during the EHR reporting period are recorded using CPOE.
Implement drug-drug and drug-allergy interaction checks.	The EP has enabled this functionality for the entire EHR reporting period.	There is no longer a separate objective for Stage 2.	This measure is incorporated into the Stage 2 Clinical Decision Support Rule measure.

Source: Centers for Medicare & Medicaid Services

TAKE THE CHALLENGE

Go to http://cms.gov and look up the latest meaningful use requirements in either the eligible professional or eligible hospital category. Record each core objective and each menu objective required in the last "final rule" published. Document how each core objective benefits the patient.

Meaningful Use Incentives

The federal government has employed a "carrot-and-stick" approach of financial rewards and penalties to encourage the adoption of the meaningful use of electronic health records. In 2011, it began providing incentive payments to providers who met meaningful use objectives. These financial incentives are available for providers who treat Medicaid or Medicare patients. Providers may only participate in one of the financial incentive programs (Medicare or Medicaid). Eligible providers who adopted meaningful use in 2012, at the beginning of the process, have been rewarded financially each year since adoption, although incentive payments have decreased over time. Eligible hospitals and providers who bill for Medicare or Medicaid patients and are not certified by the final deadline, approximately 2015, will be penalized 1 percent of Medicare revenue for each year, up to a maximum of 5 percent, for failing to meet the meaningful use target objectives. Table 7.4 illustrates how the incentive payment process works for Medicare billing.

EXPAND YOUR KNOWLEDGE

For more about the implementation of the Medicare and Medicaid EHR Incentive Program on HealthIT.gov at http://IntroHIM.ParadigmCollege.net/EHRIncentives.

Table 7.4 Medicare EHR Incentive Payment Schedule for Eligible Professionals

Payment Amounts	First Payment in 2011	First Payment in 2012	First Payment in 2013	First Payment in 2014	First Payment in 2015
2011	$18,000				
2012	$12,000	$18,000			
2013	$8,000	$12,000	$15,000		
2014	$4,000	$8,000	$12,000	$12,000	
2015	$2,000	$4,000	$8,000	$8,000	
2016		$2,000	$4,000	$4,000	
Total Payment	$44,000	$44,000	$39,000	$24,000	

Source: Centers for Medicare & Medicaid Services

EHR Security

At home, doors have locks to keep possessions and loved ones safe, and shades can be drawn to keep others from looking in. We have pass-code protected security systems to alert us if someone tries to break in. In a similar fashion, one of the key responsibilities of an HIM professional is to guard the privacy and the security of patient health information.

HIPAA established national standards for the protection, privacy, and security of health information. The **Privacy Rule** established standards for the protection of individually identifiable PHI. The **Security Rule** established standards for the protection of health information that is held or transmitted electronically (**electronic protected health information** or **ePHI**) in three broad areas: administrative safeguards, physical safeguards, and technical safeguards.

The Security Rule defines **administrative safeguards** as administrative actions undertaken to meet security standards, such as developing policies and procedures; assigning personnel—such as the security officer—to be responsible for security, disaster, or downtime contingency planning; and developing security training plans for every person who has access to ePHI. Risk and management analysis is one of the most important requirements of the administrative safeguards. Administrative safeguards should be an ongoing process as organizations and technologies change. Table 7.5 lists the administrative safeguard standards and examples of implementation specifications.

Physical safeguards are the mechanisms required to protect electronic systems and equipment and the data they hold from environmental and human threats and damage. Physical safeguards include restricting access to ePHI, monitoring and recording hardware and software movement, and retaining off-site computer backups.

Some examples of physical threats include:

- technological threats—malware or computer viruses
- environmental hazards—fire or water damage
- unauthorized intrusion—theft or tampering (hacking)

Table 7.5 Administrative Safeguards

Standards	Implementation Specifications
Security management process	Risk analysis
	Risk management
	Sanction policy
	Information system activity review
Assign security responsibility	No separate implementation specification
Workforce security	Authorization and/or supervision
	Workforce clearance procedure
	Termination procedures
Information access management	Isolating healthcare clearinghouse functions
	Access authorization
	Access establishment and modification
Security awareness and training	Security reminders
	Protection from malicious software
	Login monitoring
	Password management
Security incident procedures	Response and reporting
Contingency plan	Data backup plan
	Disaster recovery plan
	Emergency mode operation plan
	Testing and revision procedures
	Applications and data criticality analysis
Evaluation	No separate implementation specification
Business associate contracts and other arrangements	Written contract or other arrangement

Table 7.6 lists physical safeguard standards and examples of implementation specifications.

Table 7.6 Physical Safeguards

Standards	Implementation Specifications
Facility access controls	Contingency operations
	Facility security plan
	Access control and validation procedures
	Maintenance records
Workstation use	No separate implementation specification
Workstation security	No separate implementation specification
Device and media controls	Disposal
	Media reuse
	Accountability
	Data backup and storage

Chapter 7 Electronic Health Records

Technical safeguards are automated processes that utilize software to protect and control access to data. They include using authentication controls to verify that the person signing onto a computer is authorized to access ePHI, providing audit capabilities, and encrypting/decrypting data as it is being stored and/or transmitted. Table 7.7 shows the technical safeguard standards and examples of implementation specifications.

Table 7.7 Technical Safeguards

Standards	Specification Implementations
Access control	Unique user identification
	Emergency access procedure
	Automatic logoff
	Encryption and decryption
Audit controls	No separate implementation specification
Integrity	Mechanism to authenticate electronic protected health information
Person or entity authentication	No separate implementation specification
Transmission security	Integrity controls
	Encryption

> **BE AWARE**
>
> Failure to provide required security for ePHI can result in substantial fines. In 2012, the Alaska Department of Health and Social Services was fined $1.7 million for violating the Security Rule.

The HIM Department's Role in EHR Security

The HIM and information technology (IT) departments must work hand in hand to ensure that ePHI remains private and safe. In a hospital setting, a facility's privacy officer is commonly an HIM professional. The privacy officer oversees all ongoing activities related to the development, implementation, and maintenance of the organization's privacy policies in accordance with applicable federal and state laws. In a hospital setting, the security officer is commonly an IT professional. In a physician office, these two positions may be combined and are most often the responsibility of the office manager.

The HIM department can implement a variety of safeguards to protect the privacy and the security of health information, including:

- developing a written policy that specifies by job description what ePHI access employees need to perform their job duties (administrative safeguard)

- ensuring computer monitors face away from customers and other staff; if a monitor must be stationed in a public corridor, it should have a security screen that allows only the person sitting in front of the monitor to view the data (physical safeguard)

- setting an automatic computer logoff if the user has not touched the keyboard for a specified length of time, approximately three to six minutes (technical safeguard)

Access Control

Controlling access to electronic health information is the first step in protecting PHI. *Access control* is an important security process that includes four components: identification, authentication, authorization, and accounting.

Identification is a unique user ID created for each individual. The user ID includes a name, number, or some combination of the two. For example, an employee named Mary Johnson might be issued the user ID mjohnson824.

Authentication is simply a password. Passwords should be a minimum of eight characters and contain both alpha and numeric characters. They should be difficult for someone else to figure out and changed periodically.

Authorization limits individual user access to the minimum data necessary to do the job. It can be challenging, however, to determine how much access an individual needs. Job duties can overlap and change over time. Each job description should include a designated level of access based on the minimum data necessary to perform the job. Table 7.8 provides examples of levels of access by job title.

Accounting requires conducting audits to ensure that only authorized personnel have accessed patient records. Audits should include a random sample of patient records from all units and departments in the facility. Audits should be conducted monthly, whenever there is a patient complaint, or when a patient in the facility could pose a high security risk. Security risks can include celebrity patients or patients with unique diagnoses (e.g., conjoined twins, avian flu).

Table 7.8 Levels of Access

Job Title	Access Level	Permitted Access
HIM director	1	Administrative access and all clinical information access
HIM supervisor	3	All clinical information access
Billing clerk	10	Demographic information only
Respiratory therapist	5	Demographics, orders, medical history, respiratory therapy notes and flow sheets, and lab results for current (not discharged) patients

WHAT WOULD YOU DO?

In 2007, actor George Clooney was hospitalized in New Jersey after a motorcycle accident. When the hospital's privacy officer conducted a privacy audit of the EHR, something that is routinely performed on the records of celebrity patients, the audit revealed that at least 27 doctors and other hospital employees not involved in Clooney's care had accessed his EHR. Within hours of the actor's hospitalization, a pop culture magazine had published accurate information on Clooney's location and his medical condition.

The review and the unauthorized release of George Clooney's medical records are clear violations of HIPAA. As an HIM professional, what recommendations would you make to the hospital chief executive officer for discipline of:

- the employee(s) who accessed the record to satisfy personal curiosity
- the employee(s) who leaked information to the press

What steps might you take to ensure that a similar leak would not happen again?

EHR Selection and Maintenance

Some healthcare facilities and providers are just installing their first EHR systems while others are already replacing existing systems with newer technology. Regardless of whether it is a new or replacement system, any EHR system will require ongoing support and maintenance. The HIM professional can provide expertise by recommending that a new or upgraded EHR system meet these criteria:

- It is ONC certified and meets the standards and the certification criteria adopted by the US Department of Health and Human Services (HHS).
- It has proven interoperability with other systems.
- Long-term storage capabilities allow records to be retrieved with current or future software applications.
- The system prompts users for additional information to ensure that the highest level of specificity (detail) is listed and permits unlimited freestyle writing.
- It is user-friendly in both electronic and paper output formats.
- It is easy to navigate and does not require users to enter and exit multiple screens to complete an activity.

Ensuring High-Quality EHR Documentation

Ensuring end users' needs are met requires that all information in the EHR is organized in a logical way. The HIM professional is the expert on complete, concise, and accurate documentation and should provide guidance in selecting which data elements are required or necessary and in eliminating documentation redundancy. **Documentation redundancy** occurs when the same data elements are collected and saved more than once by the same or different healthcare providers during the same patient encounter.

IT REALLY HAPPENS

Elaina Lopez was experiencing chest pain and called 911. When the emergency medical technicians (EMTs) arrived at her home, they asked her, "Do you have any allergies?" She was then transported to the ED where the triage nurse also asked if she had any allergies. Then, the ED physician who examined her asked if she had allergies. Mrs. Lopez was next sent to the observation floor. There, the nurse completing her admission assessment asked about allergies as did the technician performing her cardiac catheterization procedure. And the story goes on… At least seven more healthcare professionals asked Mrs. Lopez if she had allergies, documenting her answer on their own department screen or form.

The above situation is an excellent example of documentation redundancy. The patient was frightened and in pain, yet everyone kept asking her the same question. Can you imagine what she was thinking? *Don't they communicate with each other? Didn't they read the previous note? Does the right hand know what the left hand is doing? Am I safe being treated here?*

Not only does documentation redundancy take away valuable staff time and frustrate the patient, it can also cause medical errors if the information documented by two different providers is in conflict.

In the example above, the patient told the ED personnel that she was allergic to quinidine but forgot to tell the cardiac catheterization technician about her allergy (the fourth time she was asked). Therefore, the patient experienced an arrhythmia during catheterization because the doctor ordered and she was given quinidine. The patient had a serious allergic episode and had to be intubated. Her chest pain and arrhythmias increased dramatically.

To reduce documentation redundancy, the EHR implementation and maintenance team should develop a data dictionary. A **data dictionary** identifies the individual **data elements** recorded by each professional in a health record. Data elements may be recorded in an independent system (such as a master patient index or radiology department system) and downloaded to the EHR or typed directly into the EHR. Some examples of data elements include birth date, sex, weight, and height. Each department may need the same data, but each system may record this information differently. For example, birth dates may be recorded as October 15, 1989, 10/15/89, or 15-10-1989. The information may also be created in three different medical systems or screens in the EHR. The team responsible for EHR implementation and maintenance should determine in which format the data will be captured and stored.

One option is to develop the data dictionary based on data element formats specified by **Health Level Seven International** (**HL7**), a committee of members from more than 55 countries that is the global authority on the standards and the interoperability of health information technology. The HL7 format for birth dates is year-month-day (CCYYMMDD), which is different from all of the formats previously mentioned. The new format for birth date would be 19891015. A data dictionary is also used to provide formatting guidelines so that data can be translated into the required format for each system. For example, if a state reporting system requires that birth dates be submitted as MM/DD/YYYY, the interface protocols would export the HL7 data in the EHR as 10/15/1989.

Once a data dictionary has been established, the EHR implementation and maintenance team should determine which department "owns" each data element and which providers may update or edit each data element. Information entered during the initial patient encounter should be carried forward to all departments that record that information. Then, instead of asking patients to repeat information, subsequent providers would confirm it with the patient by stating, "I see that you are allergic to aspirin and quinidine; is there anything else you can think of?" Asking for verification saves providers time and reduces patient anxiety while prompting the patient to recall additional information.

> **BE AWARE**
>
> All healthcare systems in the United States that utilize an EHR must be HL7 compliant so that information can be easily shared with other healthcare systems.

Chapter 7   Electronic Health Records

Other Healthcare Data Systems

Healthcare facilities use other data systems in their day-to-day operations. These systems are separate from the EHR although some provide information to the EHR.

In hospital settings, all health records begin in the admitting department. These departments use an ADT system, which tracks patients from the point of arrival to discharge.

Master Patient Index

The MPI is one component of an ADT system. The admitting department maintains the MPI, which generates and stores one record for every patient. As shown in Figure 7.8, patient demographic information flows from the MPI to the ADT database and then to the EHR. The purpose of the MPI is to ensure that each patient is represented only once across all of the software systems used within the organization. The MPI contains key demographic information, such as name, date of birth, gender, and social security number, and may include other demographic information as well (see Figure 7.9). Each patient's MPI record has a unique identifier called the hospital or **medical record number (MRN)**. There should be only one record in the MPI per patient; however, patient records may include more than one patient encounter or visit designated by a separate account number (billing number) for each encounter. The MPI must be retained permanently, and this should be reflected in a facility's retention policy.

Figure 7.8 Information Flow from MPI to EHR

Patient demographic information is shared among systems. After the information is entered into the master patient index, it flows into the admission, discharge, and transfer database and then into the electronic health record.

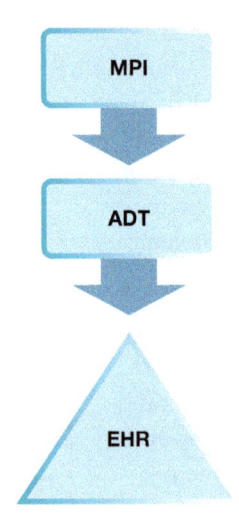

Figure 7.9 Master Patient Index

Duplicate Records

The MPI is used to determine if an individual has been a patient at the facility at any other time, and it is intended to eliminate the potential duplication of records. If a duplicate record is created, the HIM department must undertake a complex process to combine and eliminate the duplicate record. This process cannot be performed until the patient has been discharged from the hospital because current patient care will be connected to the wrong medical record number. Hospitals should seek to reduce or eliminate the problem of MPI duplicate records through training programs that emphasize the importance of specific procedures.

The following procedural steps can reduce the number of duplicate records created:

- Request patient identification.
- Always use the patient's social security number in searches.
- Ask a patient for *all* previous names used, including his or her name before marriage.
- Use the system alias (aka) features to add the patient's new name(s) to the record.

The HIM department should audit the MPI for duplicate records at least once each month. The systems will generate a report identifying potential duplicate records. Duplicate records should be merged into a single record, usually the record with the earliest date. Duplicate records may be created for a number of reasons. Some of the most common reasons include:

- The patient goes by a nickname (Kathy instead of Kathleen).
- The patient uses his or her middle name rather than legal first name. (J. Paul Stephens vs. Paul Stephens. It is important to know what the "J" stands for and use it as the first name in the record.)
- The patient has a hyphenated name but a portion of the name is not recorded (Mary Todd-Lincoln vs. Mary Lincoln).
- A typographical error (DOB 11/20/1960 instead of 11/21/1960 or Dianna instead of Diana).
- Confusion over names that are not gender-specific, such as Pat, Chris, or Kelly (Chris Ehdlund, M, 2/25/1949 and Chris Ehdlund, F, 2/25/1949).
- Name changes stemming from marriage, divorce, or other reasons.

Before merging duplicate records, make sure the records are for the same patient by comparing information—such as aliases, middle names, social security numbers, next of kin, or patient signatures—in both records. Also compare demographic information, such as addresses and phone numbers, but keep in mind that demographic information can change frequently.

Admission, Discharge, and Transfer System

Data from the MPI is used to populate the ADT system, which maintains the patient's dates of service and classification (inpatient or outpatient). These items must be accurate to ensure that coding and billing are compiled accurately. In Table 7.9 below, the patient was admitted to the medical floor and then transferred to the cardiac care unit (CCU). Since the CCU provides a significantly higher level of care, the daily room charge will be higher, too. The change in the ADT system automatically updates the charges on the patient bill in the patient financial system (billing system).

Table 7.9 Admission, Discharge, and Transfer System Tracking

Name	MR #	ACCT #	ADM	Hr.	Unit/Rm.	Disch	Time	Status
Joseph Russo	4532729	14-12987	10/22	1500	Med/109			IP
Joseph Russo	4532729	14-12987	10/23	0120	CCU/bed 3			IP
Joseph Russo	4532729	14-12987	10/28	1029	Med/220			IP
Joseph Russo	4532729	14-12987				10/30	1347	Transferred to skilled nursing home

The ADT system is a system for tracking patient movement during a hospitalization. In this example, if the lab department received an order on 10/22 for a morning blood draw, the phlebotomist would use the ADT system to determine the patient's current location.

The ADT system also generates daily reports, including unit census reports and admission and discharge lists, which provide all hospital departments with the information necessary for planning and staffing. The system provides the data used to compile statistics on patient days, births, deaths, average length of stay, and other items.

Admissions are keyed in by the admissions department. Discharges and transfers can be keyed in by the nurse caring for the patient or by the admissions department, depending on the organization's policy.

The HIM department uses a special feature in the ADT system to monitor delinquent medical records and to designate which physicians have lost admitting privileges due to delinquent records. For example, an HIM staff member may type the screen query "Have the physician's privileges been suspended due to delinquent records?" The default answer is "no." This answer may be changed to "yes" by authorized personnel in the HIM department.

If a registrar tries to admit or schedule a patient for a physician who has a "yes" next to his or her name, the computer will issue an alert. The registrar should then advise the physician that he or she cannot admit or schedule the patient until the records have been completed. Each facility has protocol to follow for emergencies and exceptions. These protocols are outlined in the medical staff rules and regulations and medical staff policies. Only authorized HIM personnel may change the designation back to "no" once a physician has completed all delinquent records.

Scheduling Systems

When a patient makes an appointment, whether with a physician office, an outpatient radiology center for a follow-up X-ray, or a surgery center for an upcoming procedure, the appointment is keyed into a **scheduling system**. The scheduling system includes a calendar with dates and times allotted for each event, the name of the practitioner or physician the patient will see, and the anticipated duration of the appointment. Surgical schedules include additional information, such as the type of surgery, location, anesthesiologist, and type of anesthetic that will be used. Based on the physician name and the surgery type, a surgical kit may be ordered for the day of surgery. Scheduling systems may be stand-alone or part of a supplemental package purchased with the core EHR system. Scheduling data does not become part of the permanent EHR but is an important tool used to keep patient flow smooth and organized.

Practice Management System

A **practice management system (PMS)**, sometimes referred to as a *medical practice management system*, is used in the outpatient setting, most often in physician offices. The practice management system traditionally includes programs for an MPI, scheduling, medical billing, insurance verification, and revenue cycle management. The programs included with the system vary by vendor. Many vendors now provide both practice management and EHR functionality in the same system.

Bed Control System

A *bed control system* is used as a patient flow system to monitor bed turnover in a hospital. A patient is likely to move many times during a hospital stay. The same patient may go from the emergency room to a standard patient care unit to the operating room to the critical care unit and then back to the standard patient care unit. The bed control system is used by the continuity of care department to ensure that patients move to the appropriate level of care on a timely basis and open beds are allocated to other patients who need them. The bed control system interfaces with the ADT and EHR systems to ensure that patient location is always up-to-date.

Disaster-Preparedness and Downtime Procedures

The Joint Commission and HIPAA require that all medical records be kept safe from fire, water damage, and theft. Although data stored in the EHR system is backed up, data cannot be accessed without hardware such as computers, monitors, and printers. The HIM professional must have procedures in place to protect the EHR hardware.

Natural disasters can occur at any time and with little or no warning and cause power outages, flooding, and other damage. Natural disasters are not the only threat to computer systems, however. Water pipes can suddenly burst, and power and equipment can fail. The HIM department must prepare in advance for all of these potential emergency situations.

If water threatens to damage computers containing patient information, HIM staff should shut down and unplug all equipment and then move it to a safe location. If equipment cannot be moved, it should be covered with heavy-duty plastic sheets or the plastic covers used for outdoor patio furniture. Equipment should not be uncovered or plugged back in until the biomedical engineering department has checked it for damage.

Since power outages are normally unscheduled, the HIM staff should identify in advance which systems need backup generator support during a power outage. Backup generators have limited capacity, however, and patient care applications are always the first priority. Most HIM applications, including MPIs and EHRs, will not remain accessible for long during a power outage. Therefore, backup batteries may be suggested for systems that are sensitive to power outages so that the systems can be shut down slowly.

When the EHR system is down, staff members use paper forms that emulate the EHR output for that section of documentation. Downtime procedures should clearly define what forms should be used, where the forms are located, and how these manual forms will be integrated into the electronic record after the event.

Downtime procedures should be reviewed with staff periodically so that they are prepared if and when the unexpected occurs. Table 7.10 is a timetable for implementing manual processes during EHR downtime.

Table 7.10 Schedule for Downtime Integration of Manual Forms

Estimated Downtime	Reason for Downtime	Manual Form Data Integration into the EHR
Less than 3 hours	Software upgrades and maintenance or short-term power outage	Staff use manual forms for record-keeping notes and enter the data into the system when it becomes available
3–24 hours	System or power outage	Staff use manual forms for record-keeping; manual forms are scanned into the EHR using the document management system when it becomes available
More than 24 hours to days or weeks	System or power outage	Staff use manual forms for record-keeping notes; temporary patient binders should be retrieved from storage to contain these manual forms Downtime scanning team (to be established as needed) should scan manual forms into the EHR using the document management system when it becomes available

WHAT WOULD YOU DO?

Good Samaritan Hospital is threatened by an approaching Category 5 hurricane. At a minimum, the hospital can expect flooding and water damage. Preparations are underway to transfer patients who can travel. As an HIM professional, what steps would you take in advance of the storm to protect patient information and computer equipment? Explain how would you ensure that the staff has continued access to patient records for those patients who will remain in the hospital during the storm?

Systems Used in HIM Departments

The HIM department is responsible for many processes. HIM staff members use a number of independent computer systems to maximize efficiency and ensure the accuracy of these processes. Each system is responsible for a specific function or a set of functions.

Release of Information

The **release of information (ROI)** system is a database that collects and stores information on all health records that have been requested, copied, and released. When a patient record is requested or subpoenaed, the HIM department releases a copy of the record in accordance with state and federal laws (discussed further in Chapter 8). The release of information must be recorded so that the privacy officer may refer to it at a later date should a patient ask for an **accounting of disclosures (AODs)**, a detailed list of the information released and to whom it was released. An ROI database collects the patient's name, medical record number, and billing or encounter number along with the name and the address of the person the information was released to, the date released, the specific documents released, and any charges levied for document reproduction.

The ROI system also generates standardized letters—for example, a letter explaining a delay in completing the release request or a letter requesting additional patient information, such as a birth date, to ensure that the correct record is released. The ROI system also produces invoices for document copying fees. In addition, the ROI system can generate reports to track the status of incomplete requests and provide statistical data on the number and the types of requests received.

Record Analysis

The **record analysis system** is an independent system that flags deficiencies in physician documentation in the health record. As discussed in Chapter 4, certain documents, such as history and physical examinations (H&Ps) or discharge summaries, must be dictated and signed before the record is considered complete. If a document has not been dictated, an HIM analysis technician can request the document be completed by inserting a "dictation needed" flag for that record. In a similar fashion, the HIM analysis technician can also flag verbal and telephone orders that need a manual or an electronic signature. The physician may electronically sign incomplete records via the analysis system and, in some cases, directly on the document in the EHR system. The analysis system notifies physicians of records due, tracks physician suspensions due to delinquent records, and maintains statistics by physician, medical department, and deficiency type for Joint Commission and medical staff credentialing.

Transcription and Speech Recognition

The **transcription system** is an enhanced word processing system similar to Microsoft Word that has special capabilities such as an ADT interface, an EHR interface, medical spell-check, template design, and statistical tracking for staff production and physician document volume.

The transcriptionist listens to a submission dictated by the physician into a **dictation system**, a digital or other recording device, and types the information into the appropriate report template. The transcriptionist then selects the patient from the ADT system and sends the report to the patient's EHR. Occasionally, if the patient has not yet been entered into the ADT system, as may be the case for a patient scheduled for a future surgery, an HIM technician will match the dictation to the ADT information at a later date. The technician will also ensure that all ADT information is accurately assigned to each report and correct blanks in the report before sending it to the EHR—at which point the physician will review the information and verify its accuracy. The physician then authenticates the report with an electronic signature.

Today's speech recognition systems, equipped with medical and pharmaceutical dictionaries that include commonly used medical phrases and abbreviations, are reducing the need for transcription. Speech recognition systems allow physicians to dictate directly into the medical record form, view the result in real time, and make any necessary corrections. These systems "learn" the user's pronunciation and vocabulary and increase in accuracy over time. Some medical specialty systems (e.g., gastroenterology, emergency department, and cardiac catheterization) are designed to produce forms and test values specific to each specialty. These specialty systems have received positive user feedback compared to generic medical speech-recognition systems that have yet to reach their full potential. These generic systems tend to be slow, and the learning curve for physicians can be high. Physicians can also dictate reports and choose to send the file to a **medical language editor** (previously called a *medical transcriptionist*) for editing.

Coding

Medical coding is the process of assigning alphanumeric codes to medical diagnoses and procedures to facilitate billing and reimbursement, research, and quality review. Coding is one of the functions of the HIM department. Coding can be done manually, using coding manuals to research and locate the appropriate codes, or using **encoder software**, a program that helps the coder to identify the correct diagnostic and procedural codes.

When using an encoder, the coder may type a key word or an abbreviation—PNA (pneumonia), for example—into the encoder program. The program will generate a series of queries, such as "Is the patient on a ventilator?" or "Due to bacterial infection?", prompting the coder to review the record for specific documentation in order to identify the code with the highest level of specificity. As the coder answers the questions or in some cases selects from a choice of options from the encoder menu, the final code is obtained. Once all diagnosis and procedure codes are entered, the encoder system calculates the diagnosis-related group (DRG) for inpatients or the ambulatory payment classification (APC) for outpatients.

Coders also use **computer-assisted coding (CAC)** software that analyzes typed physician documentation and diagnostic test results to identify specific data elements and recommend codes that may be applicable. Although CAC software can improve coder productivity and accuracy, it does not eliminate or reduce the need for trained medical coders. A **medical coding editor** (formerly called a *coder*) reviews the CAC's recommendations for accuracy and makes changes as necessary.

EXPAND YOUR KNOWLEDGE

Computer-assisted coding is intended to improve the efficiency and accuracy of medical coding, however, the results of a national pilot program using CAC with ICD-10 suggest the CACs programs are only as good as the humans collecting the data. To find out more about the benefits and challenges of CAC, read the article "Why CAC Can't Solve All Your ICD-10 Problems," at http://IntroHIM.ParadigmCollege.net/CAC.

Once selected, the medical codes and DRG/APC are moved from the encoding or CAC system to another system, usually a clinical data repository, that maintains the codes and allows for the addition of noncoded information. The data repository system also permits the coder to abstract optional data that may be required by insurers or governmental agencies and needed for statistical reporting purposes. For example, an obstetrics department may want to track APGAR scores (a test given to newborns to assess their *appearance, pulse, grimace, activity, and respiration*) by physician. This data can be captured in an **optional field**, a field in a database designed by the user for collection of specific data, and the HIM staff can run reports to retrieve the optional field information.

Cancer Registry (Tumor Registry)

The *cancer registry* collects and stores required data on every patient diagnosed or treated for cancer. The facility's cancer registrar(s) types the data into the system, assisted by computer prompts that ensure the data is as complete and detailed as possible. The registry may be a large independent system purchased from a vendor, often found in facilities accredited by the American College of Surgeons, for example, or it may be a small system supplied by the state to collect the minimum requirements of that state. (Every state requires reporting on cancer patients.) The larger cancer-registry systems have an integrated encoder to assist the cancer registrar in selecting International Classification of Diseases for Oncology (ICD-O) morphology and topography pathology codes. The larger systems are also capable of collecting more-detailed data elements, maintaining follow-up data on patients, collecting additional data for special studies, and preparing graphic information for cancer committees and annual reports. Cancer registries are discussed in greater detail in Chapter 11.

Changing Roles of HIM Staff

As the implementation of the EHR advances, HIM staff roles will continue to evolve. Entry-level positions such as file clerks, chart assemblers, and the clerks who pull records for requestors will no longer be needed. Instead, the HIM field will require higher-skilled professionals who have computer experience, customer service experience, and knowledge of medical terminology. These employees will be able to transition to new positions, such as data management scanners and EHR retrieval clerks. The HIM department will become smaller and more decentralized as positions such as record analyzer, coder, auditor, and transcriptionist are outsourced or become home-based. As the use of CAC and speech recognition grows, coder and transcriptionist jobs are evolving into coding editor and medical language editor positions, respectively. Some HIM professionals will transition to EHR **data integrity analyst** positions. These new professionals provide oversight and supervision for all of the electronic processes related to the EHR system (including HIM systems), record processing functions, and electronic master patient index processes related to ePHI. The demand for trained professionals to fill these positions will continue to grow, and HIM professionals will be well suited to filling these needs.

The Personal Health Record (PHR)

A **personal health record (PHR)** is a record created and maintained by the patient. It is used to organize and store information about medications, treatments, and other health-related information. It is up to the individual to decide what information to keep in the PHR and whether to store the information as a paper or computer-based record.

IT REALLY HAPPENS

Tom, a 75-year-old man, had been very healthy all of his life. He had no chronic diseases and was not taking any medications. Suddenly, he became very ill, suffering with unexplained, excruciating pain throughout his body. Tom saw many different physicians and underwent numerous lab and X-ray tests, but doctors were unable to diagnose the cause of his pain. He was prescribed a variety of pain medications. After a while, Tom's condition and the medications he was taking began to affect his memory. Overwhelmed by the amount of medical information he needed to track, he created a PHR. He gathered all of his diagnostic results, physician names and phone numbers, and medications and patient instructions and organized them in a three-ring binder. His wife, Abby, kept a spiral notebook to document all the discussions, questions, and answers from each appointment. As Tom continued to seek treatment, the PHR he'd created made it much easier to make sure that his physicians had all the information they needed to make sound medical decisions.

In this example, the patient chose to use the storage medium he was comfortable with—paper. Increasingly, however, patients are using computer technology to organize and track their personal health information. An electronic PHR may be stored on a home computer, a flash drive, a CD, or on a secure Internet-based or cloud-based site maintained by a third party. A **cloud-based application** can be accessed from a web browser or mobile app. The software and the patient's healthcare information are stored in a remote location in the cloud. The advantage of this type of storage is that the information is available to the individual from any Internet-access point.

Benefits of the PHR

The biggest benefit of the PHR is that patients feel more empowered to manage and organize their own health care. Patients can track test results, manage appointments, and make notes about issues they want to discuss with a physician. In an emergency, when memory can fail, the PHR can serve as a helpful reference for medication and health history.

The PHR provides immediate access to a patient's health information, reducing wait time for vital information and reducing the risk of adverse drug or treatment reactions. It is up to the patient to decide whether to share information contained in the PHR with an individual healthcare provider. By maintaining an up-to-date PHR, the patient can ensure that each physician, regardless of specialty, has a big-picture view of his or her conditions and treatments.

A PHR versus a Provider Record

The PHR is different than a record created by a hospital or a physician. The PHR belongs to the patient. He or she chooses what information it contains. The biggest difference between a PHR and a hospital or physician record is that the PHR is not considered PHI (protected health information) under HIPAA. Information contained in the PHR is not protected by law if, for example, the patient's personal computer is hacked. If PHR information is accessed and released without the patient's authorization, the patient has no legal recourse with the provider.

Electronic PHR Applications

Several PHR applications are available on the Internet. Some PHRs, such as Microsoft HealthVault, are free to users. Because HIPAA does not protect the privacy of PHRs, any PHR application should include industry-standard security and a strong password requirement, also known as an **authentication scheme**.

Any PHR application should also include a confidentiality clause as well as a consumer terms and conditions of use statement. The patient should control access and audit the record to see who has accessed information. The PHR should be easy to navigate and have the capacity to store provider reports and even X-ray images. Many national pharmacies and laboratories can send information directly to a patient's PHR.

Chapter Summary

The electronic health record is an integral part of modern healthcare delivery. EHRs benefit both patients and providers by improving efficiencies, reducing medical errors, and allowing patients to become more engaged in their care. Many patients now maintain their own personal health records and share information stored on the PHR with providers. As with any computerized system, the EHR has disadvantages, too. Most of those disadvantages can be overcome through adequate planning and training. A key requirement of the EHR is that it is interoperable and can maintain clinical data from a variety of healthcare providers. The HIM professional is the expert in quality documentation and should be actively involved in the selection and implementation of the EHR system and in training staff on the effective use of the EHR. The HIM professional also has expertise in the use of a number of department-specific systems, including transcription, coding, release of information, and cancer registry. As EHR technology advances, HIM professionals' skill, knowledge, and proficiency with data management will open the door to many new and exciting career opportunities.

HIM Review

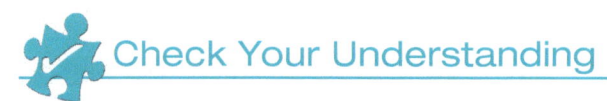

Check Your Understanding

Test your understanding of the material covered in this chapter by completing the following multiple-choice questions. For each question, select the best answer from the choices provided.

1. Which system is *not* included as part of the EHR?

    a. administrative

    b. accounting

    c. medical

    d. document management

2. The _____ is a component of an ADT system.

    a. management of technology

    b. major diagnostic category

    c. master information systems

    d. master patient index

3. A _____ is a central database that consolidates all of a patient's clinical information from separate sources into one location.

    a. clinical data repository

    b. central data repository

    c. clinical data dictionary

    d. central data dictionary

4. Which of the following statements does not apply to meaningful use requirements?

    a. All core objectives must be met.

    b. All menu objectives must be met.

    c. Each core objective has a predetermined percentage that must be met.

    d. Meaningful use requirements are established by the ONC.

5. Documentation redundancy is _____

    a. when different data elements are collected and saved.

    b. a problem encountered with the use of a data dictionary.

    c. one cause of medical errors.

    d. All of the choices are correct.

6. Which answer choice is not a disadvantage of the EHR?

    a. point-of-care reminders and alerts

    b. implementation costs

    c. quality of template documentation

    d. system output usability

7. _____ is the process of documenting physician orders electronically instead of on paper.

    a. eMAR

    b. PACS

    c. CPOE

    d. CDR

8. Sharing health information electronically across state, regional, and local areas is referred to as _____

    a. EDI.

    b. REC.

    c. HL7.

    d. HIE.

9. What law assesses monetary penalties for failure to use an EHR that meets meaningful use criteria?

    a. ARRA

    b. ONC

    c. HITECH

    d. None of the choices are correct.

10. A system that collects and stores information about health records that have been requested and released is called _____

    a. record analysis.

    b. release of information.

    c. a cancer registry.

    d. transcription.

Think Critically

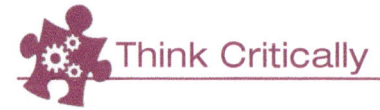

Consider the following real-world scenario and draft a response.

The healthcare facility at which you work is installing a new EHR system. The team members installing the system want to make sure there is physician buy-in, so they are recommending that physicians be able to cut and paste (clone) and fill in the blanks in the EHR as often as possible. Would you support the team's recommendation? Why or why not?

Sharpen Your Comprehension

Complete the following matching exercise by selecting, from the list provided, the answer that best matches each of the numbered statements. For each statement, only one answer is correct.

- a. interoperable
- b. audit trail
- c. longitudinal
- d. ADT
- e. alerts
- f. clinical
- g. simultaneous access
- h. records analysis
- i. practice management
- j. MRN

1. _____ This system receives and processes medical orders which, when completed, become the final documentation in the patient record
2. _____ Warns provider about potential medication interactions
3. _____ A record that incorporates all of the information from multiple sources gathered over a period of time
4. _____ The term for a system that has the ability to communicate, exchange data, and use the information that has been exchanged
5. _____ A computer-generated report that identifies who accessed a computer system or an individual record and the action taken
6. _____ The system that flags deficiencies in physician documentation in the health record
7. _____ Includes programs for an MPI, scheduling, medical billing, insurance verification, and revenue cycle management
8. _____ The unique identifier for each patient MPI record
9. _____ Allows electronic records to be accessed by many individuals at the same time
10. _____ Generates daily reports, including unit census reports and admission and discharge lists

Connect Theory to Practice

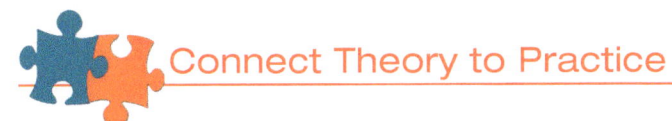

To help translate the concepts presented in this chapter to the workplace, complete the following exercise.

You are the privacy officer for a 250-bed hospital. It is your job to write a policy that specifies, by job title, the level of access to ePHI necessary to perform that job function. As part of that policy, you must create a spreadsheet listing the appropriate access level for each position.

Access levels
1. no access to ePHI
2. access to demographics, advance directives, consents, and physician orders
3. access to items listed in level two plus, H&P, operative report, and physician progress notes
4. access to items listed in levels two and three plus, MAR, vital signs, nurses notes, therapy notes and discharge planning notes
5. access to all record entries

For this assignment, create a two-column spreadsheet in Excel or as a Word table. In the first column of your spreadsheet, enter the job titles listed below. In the second column, enter the number (1-5) that best reflects, for each job title, level of access to ePHI required for that position. Submit the completed spreadsheet to your instructor.

Job title

admitting clerk
lab tech
dietician
nurse
treating physician
non-treating physician
maintenance worker
radiology tech
HIM coder
volunteer

patient representative
marketing director
physician assistant
member of the board of directors
physical therapy tech
anesthesia tech
CEO
nursing assistant
clergy
accounts payable clerk

Student eResources

*To enhance your comprehension of the chapter material, go to **Navigator+** and complete the additional practice items as advised by your instructor.*

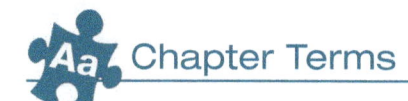

Chapter Terms

accounting of disclosures (AODs)
administrative safeguards
admission, discharge, and transfer (ADT) system
alert
American Recovery and Reinvestment Act (ARRA)
audit trail
authentication scheme
clinical data repository (CDR)
clinical decision support (CDS)
clinical system
cloning
cloud-based application
computer-assisted coding (CAC)
computerized provider order entry (CPOE)
core EHR system/central system
data dictionary
data elements
data integrity analyst
decision support
dictation system
document management system
documentation integrity
documentation redundancy
encoder software
electronic health record (EHR)
electronic medication administration record (eMAR)
electronic protected health information (ePHI)
electronic signature (e-signature)
e-prescribing (eRx)
hard dollars
health information exchange (HIE)
Health Information Technology for Economic and Clinical Health (HITECH) Act
Health Level Seven International (HL7)
hybrid record
interface
interoperability
longitudinal record
macros
master patient index (MPI)
meaningful use
medical coding editor
medical language editor
medical record number (MRN)
Office of the National Coordinator for Health Information Technology (ONC)
optional field

- patient portal
- personal health record (PHR)
- physical safeguards
- picture archiving and communication system (PACS)
- point of care (POC)
- practice management system (PMS)
- Privacy Rule
- problem-oriented medical information system (PROMIS)
- problem-oriented medical record (POMR)
- protected health information (PHI)
- record analysis system
- release of information (ROI)
- return on investment
- scheduling system
- Security Rule
- soft dollars
- technical safeguards
- templates
- transcription system

> "A personal choice to rise above one's circumstances and demonstrate the ownership necessary for achieving desired results—to See It, Own It, Solve It, and Do It."
>
> —Roger Connors and Tom Smith, cofounders of Partners in Leadership, from the article, "How to Create a 'Culture of Accountability'"

Professionalism Tip

Accountability

All Health Information Management (HIM) professionals are accountable for:
- ensuring that the patient health record is a sound legal document that is created, maintained, and used appropriately
- ensuring that the record is complete and accurate and supports continued patient care
- protecting the confidentiality, the security, and the privacy of patient health information

Fast Facts

Ninety-four percent of US hospitals reportedly experienced at least one security breach in the past two years; 45 percent reported more than five breaches, according to a 2012 study by the Ponemon Institute. The average economic impact of data breaches over the past two years for the 81 healthcare organizations participating in the study was $2.4 million.

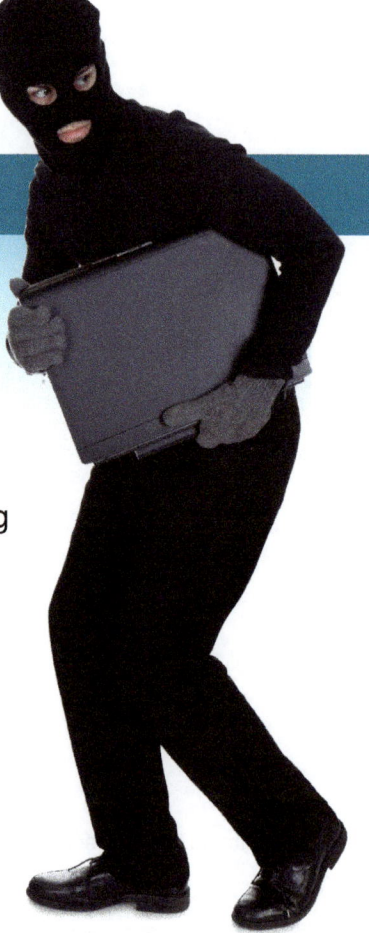

Chapter 8

Legal Aspects of Health Information Management

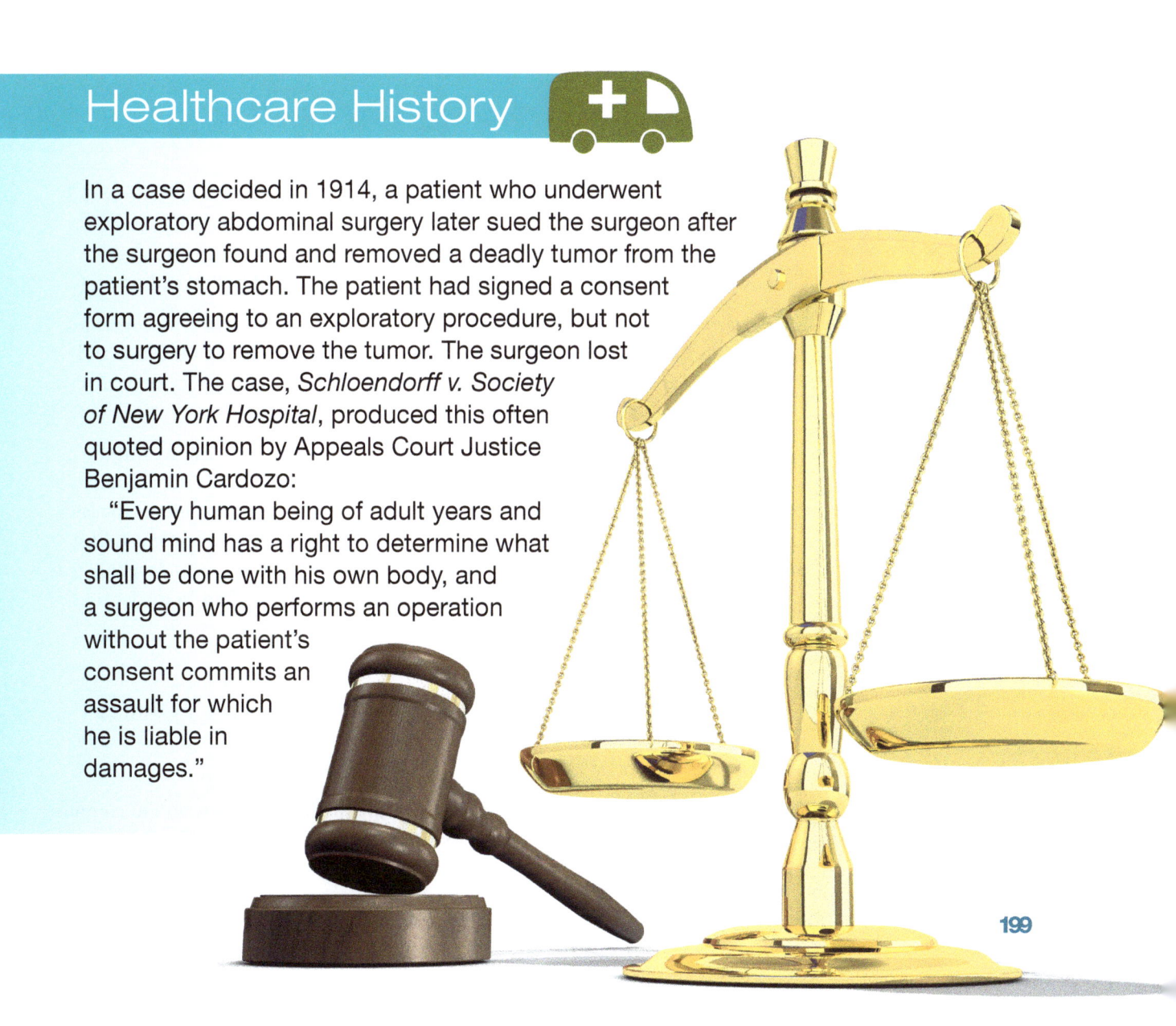

Healthcare History

In a case decided in 1914, a patient who underwent exploratory abdominal surgery later sued the surgeon after the surgeon found and removed a deadly tumor from the patient's stomach. The patient had signed a consent form agreeing to an exploratory procedure, but not to surgery to remove the tumor. The surgeon lost in court. The case, *Schloendorff v. Society of New York Hospital*, produced this often quoted opinion by Appeals Court Justice Benjamin Cardozo:

"Every human being of adult years and sound mind has a right to determine what shall be done with his own body, and a surgeon who performs an operation without the patient's consent commits an assault for which he is liable in damages."

Learning Objectives

- Understand the structure and function of the US legal system.
- Describe the components of the legal health record.
- Explain the different types of consent forms.
- Be familiar with other legal documents that may be included in a patient health record.
- Describe the major provisions of the Health Insurance Portability and Accountability Act of 1996 (HIPAA).
- Apply the HIPAA Privacy Rule and the HIPAA Security Rule to health information management (HIM).
- Explain the impact of identity theft on HIM.
- Demonstrate the steps in the release of information function.
- Differentiate among a subpoena, a deposition, a court order, and a warrant.
- Understand and be able to apply principles of ethical decision making.

Health care is a highly regulated field, and its practice is subject to myriad federal and state laws as well as to oversight by several governmental agencies, including the US Food and Drug Administration, US Department of Health and Human Services, Centers for Medicare & Medicaid Services, state departments of health, and others.

It is important for everyone involved in patient care and for everyone who comes in contact with patient information in a healthcare facility to understand the laws and regulations governing the documentation, use of, security of, and privacy of health information.

The **custodian** of the health record is responsible for the care, the custody, and the control of the patient record during the normal course of business. As the custodian of the record, it is the HIM professional's responsibility to know and to enforce the laws and regulations that govern the collection, storage, use, and release of patient health information. The health information management professional may also develop organizational policies and procedures and train care providers and others in the legal uses of the health record while also monitoring compliance.

More specifically, the HIM professional:

- conducts the release of protected health information in compliance with the Health Insurance Portability and Accountability Act of 1996 (HIPAA) and institutional policy
- monitors healthcare documentation to ensure that it is complete and in compliance with the institution's bylaws, policies, and procedures

- protects the privacy and the security of patient health information
- educates providers and other healthcare employees on the appropriate documentation, use, and maintenance requirements of the health record
- provides input into the design of electronic and paper record systems to create, use, store, and protect health information from unauthorized access or loss of information
- ensures that records are maintained according to legal standards, including the statute of limitations and the healthcare facility's records retention. (The **statute of limitations** is established by federal or state law and sets a time limit within which legal proceedings may be brought forward.)

The Legal System

The legal system in the United States is a complex organization of interconnected systems that includes the federal, state, and local governments and numerous state and federal regulatory agencies. The US Constitution is recognized as the supreme law of the land. Federal law is derived from constitutional law and includes the legal rights granted by the US Constitution. Statutory law is based on legislation passed by Congress or state legislatures. Case law is based on judicial decisions at the state or federal level. Each state has its own constitution that outlines the structure and the powers of the state government.

Sources of Law

In the United States, laws are derived from a variety of sources:

- *Constitutional law* is based on the US Constitution.
- *Statutory law* refers to law created by legislative statute (Congress or state legislatures).
- *Treaties* are formal agreements between two or more countries, as in reference to peace and trade.
- *Administrative regulations* are rules created by governmental agencies, such as the US Department of Health and Human Services, that carry the force of law. Regulations can be created at the federal, state, and local levels.
- *Common law* (which includes case law) is derived from *legal precedent* when no statute relating to the issue exists (i.e., law established from rulings in previous court cases).

Just as laws are created and enforced at all levels of government, Congress, state legislatures, and local governments all have the authority to regulate certain aspects of health care. Figure 8.1 shows how a bill becomes a law at the federal level. State laws follow a similar process.

Figure 8.1 How a Bill Becomes a Law

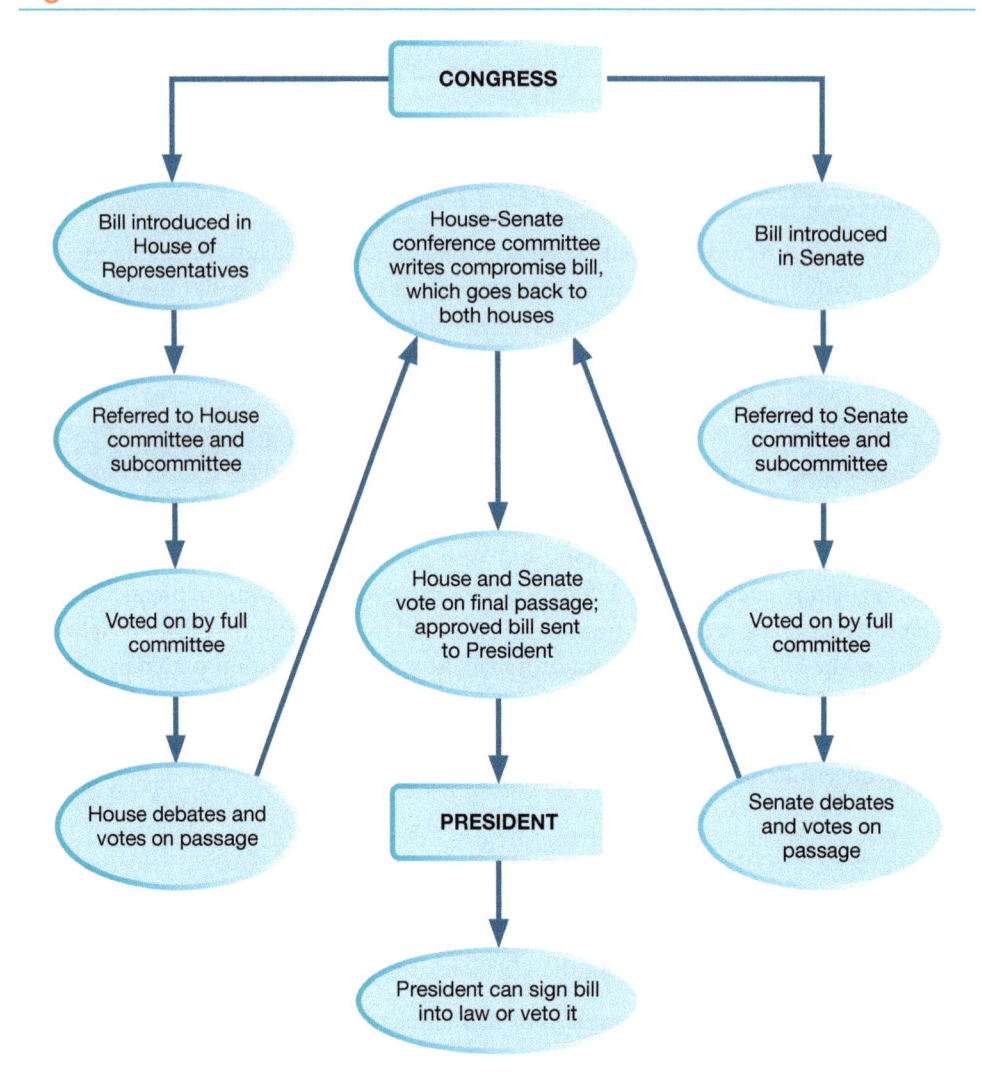

```
                          CONGRESS
          ┌──────────────────┼──────────────────┐
          ▼                  ▼                  ▼
   Bill introduced     House-Senate         Bill introduced
     in House of    conference committee      in Senate
   Representatives  writes compromise bill,
                    which goes back to
                       both houses
          │                                     │
          ▼                                     ▼
   Referred to House                     Referred to Senate
    committee and                         committee and
    subcommittee                          subcommittee
          │                                     │
          ▼                                     ▼
    Voted on by full                      Voted on by full
       committee                             committee
          │                                     │
          │         House and Senate            │
          │       vote on final passage;        │
          │        approved bill sent           │
          │           to President              │
          ▼                                     ▼
    House debates and      PRESIDENT      Senate debates
    votes on passage                      and votes on
                                            passage
                              │
                              ▼
                      President can sign bill
                       into law or veto it
```

Federal, State, and Local Law

The federal courts have jurisdiction over cases involving federal laws and regulations. **Jurisdiction** is the authority, the power, or the right to govern or legislate. **Regulations** are rules created by a governmental agency to explain how the agency intends to carry out a law. For example, Congress approved Public Law 104-191, HIPAA, but the US Department of Health and Human Services is responsible for drafting regulations and enforcing the law. A number of federal agencies have the authority to regulate some aspect of health care, including the manufacture and the sale of prescription drugs, the protection of public health, and the security and the protection of patient health information.

The federal court system hears cases involving the US Constitution, federal statues or regulations, federal land or facilities, and disputes between parties from different states. Cases may be related to:

- immigration
- bankruptcy

- Social Security and Supplemental Security Income (SSI) laws
- violations of federal antidiscrimination and civil rights laws (laws prohibiting discrimination based on race, age, gender, or disability)
- patent and copyright violations
- federal crimes, such as Medicare and insurance fraud

State courts have jurisdiction over state laws that are derived from the state's constitution, the state legislature, and from regulations established by state agencies. State laws must be consistent with, and in most cases cannot supersede, federal laws and regulations. When federal and state laws or regulations are in conflict, federal law takes precedence in most cases. One notable exception is the HIPAA Privacy Rule, which stipulates that if state laws protecting **individually identifiable health information** (information that can be used to identify the patient and/or treatment, such as address or date of birth) are more stringent than HIPAA, the more stringent state law should be followed.

State courts handle cases related to:

- criminal matters, except for federal crimes
- divorce and family issues
- real estate and other property matters
- business contracts
- welfare, public assistance, or Medicaid fraud
- wills, inheritances, and estates
- personal injury and most medical malpractice lawsuits
- workers' compensation claims

At the local level, states delegate some lawmaking on local issues (e.g., public safety and traffic enforcement, zoning, and permitting) to local agencies, townships, counties, cities, and special districts. These local rules are commonly called *ordinances*.

Laws governing patient health information include federal laws such as the Health Information Technology for Economic and Clinical Health (HITECH) Act, Meaningful Use criteria, the HIPAA Privacy and Security Rules, and regulations for reimbursement for federal programs such as Medicare. State laws include healthcare facility and provider licensing laws, confidentiality, privacy, and security regulations, and guidelines for the retention of health records. For example, federal guidelines for critical access hospitals require that patient records be retained for six years from the date of the last entry, or for a longer period if required by state statute, or if the record may be needed in any pending proceeding.

Numerous other healthcare regulations directly impact the use, storage, and release of patient information. The US Department of Health and Human Services (HHS) is responsible for healthcare insurance programs (Medicare and Medicaid), public health programs, social service programs, and research for the advancement of health care to support the HHS's mission "to help provide the building blocks that Americans need to live healthy, successful lives."

> **EXPAND YOUR KNOWLEDGE**
>
> For more information on regulations in your state, visit your state's department of health website or its equivalent, and look up the regulations for the use, retention, storage, and release of patient information.

Ownership of the Health Record

Who owns the patient health record?

The patient "owns" the information contained in the record. The patient has the right to review the record and verify the accuracy of the information in the record. The patient also has the right to request changes to the record, receive a copy of the record, and know who has viewed the record.

The healthcare facility or provider owns the physical record and the medium on which the information is stored, whether that medium is paper, microfilm, or an electronic record stored in a computer system.

Consistent with provisions of the HIPAA Privacy Rule, all healthcare facilities must have procedures in place for allowing patients to access their health information, regardless of the medium on which the record is maintained. A patient can make a request to the department or the office where the records are permanently stored to review the record, to request that documentation errors be corrected, and to request a copy of the record. In a hospital or other inpatient care facility, the health information or medical record department would handle these requests. In a physician office or other outpatient setting, such requests may be handled by the medical record department, an office manager, or front office personnel.

To obtain a copy of his or her medical record, a patient may be asked to complete an authorization for release of information form indicating the information requested, the purpose, and the dates of service. The patient is also required to provide identification. Most requests require several days to process, and most facilities charge fees for copying records. Many states, however, have established maximum allowable charges for copying medical records. Fees must be reasonable and consistent with the actual cost of providing the records. Some facilities allow patients to review the original records. A staff member, preferably a healthcare provider, should be present during the review to answer questions and explain the clinical information contained in the record. Although HIM professionals have knowledge of disease processes and diagnostic and treatment means, the HIM professional *should not* answer patient questions about the content of the health record. Only a direct care provider should answer these questions. HIM professionals can answer general questions. The HIM professional should ensure the record is not altered during the review.

Patients can access some of their medical information through patient portals. A **patient portal** is a password-protected online site where patients can obtain summary reports of information contained in the health record. The features and the information available in the patient portal vary considerably from one provider to another, but there are some common elements. These include:

- dates of recent doctor or hospital visits
- current medications and dosages
- immunization records
- known allergies

- test results
- discharge summary information from hospital stays (e.g., reason for admission, diagnostics, treatment, medical condition throughout stay and on discharge, and discharge instructions and follow-up care)

Some patient portals also allow patients to:

- email the provider
- request prescription refills
- schedule routine appointments
- update personal contact information
- submit payments
- download forms to schedule visits, to request copies of records, or for other purposes

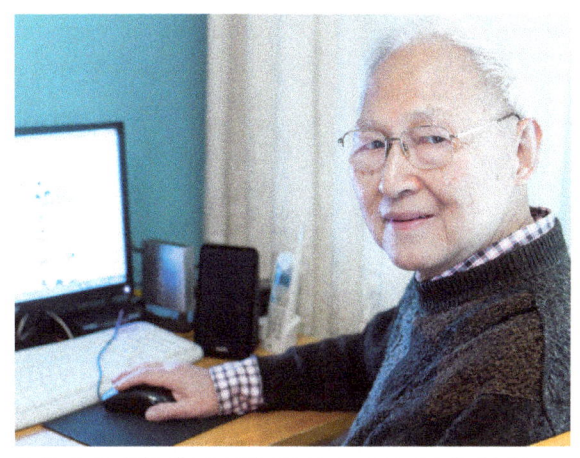

Patient portals allow patients to access medical information and prescription records anytime and from any Internet connection. The use of patient portals has the potential to improve patient engagement with providers and improve patient health.

The Legal Health Record

The **legal health record** is the official business record of a healthcare organization. It is a record of medical care provided to the patient, and it is used to substantiate the care provided for legal purposes, most notably as evidence in court proceedings.

HIPAA introduced another term, **designated record set**, for defining the patient record. The designated record set includes all protected health information, as well as all information contained in the legal health record, in billing records, and the information used to support care decisions, such as provider notes, resources, and established protocols. Table 8.1 illustrates the differences between the legal health record and the designated record set.

Table 8.1 The Legal Health Record and the Designated Record Set

Documentation	Official Business Record	Record of Medical Care Provided	Legal Evidence Subject to Subpoena	Billing Records	Documents to Support Decision for Care
Legal Health Record	X	X	X		
Designated Record Set	X	X	X	X	X

A **protocol**, or clinical-care guideline, is a preestablished plan for a course of medical treatment that is grounded in **evidence-based medicine**. Evidence-based medicine integrates the provider's expertise with external evidence, such as medical research or clinical trials, to support clinical decision making. A plan is established by studying patients with the same condition from a number of different facilities to determine the most effective treatments. For example, the treatment protocol for a patient with diabetic foot ulcers might include testing the patient for other symptoms of diabetes, measuring the wound on a weekly basis, evaluating blood flow to the legs, cleaning the wound, administering antibiotics, and instructing the patient not to put weight on the affected area.

This external evidence, found in literature and study reports, can become a part of the designated record set if the information is used in determining patient treatment and if there is no patient identifying information attached to it. The protocol itself would not be a part of the legal health record, however, because it does not document actual care provided. Each healthcare facility must determine what information constitutes the designated record set as well as the subset of information that makes up the legal health record.

The American Health Information Management Association's e-HIM task force on the legal health record has identified several purposes for the legal health record:

- to support the decisions made in patient care
- to support the reimbursement from third-party payers
- to document the services provided as legal testimony regarding the patient's illness or injury, response to treatment, and caregiver decisions
- to serve as the organization's business and legal record

As custodians of the legal record, HIM professionals should work in collaboration with the information technology department, hospital administration, and direct patient-care providers to determine the contents of the legal health record. Various licensing, accreditation, and certification standards must also be considered when determining the content and the scope of the legal health record.

Depending on the implementation status of the electronic health record (EHR), the legal health record may be a paper record, an electronic record, or a **hybrid record** that combines electronic and paper records or records from two or more electronic systems.

The process of defining the legal health record for an individual facility requires multiple steps. First, it is important to identify the applicable laws, regulations, policies, and standards that dictate what must be maintained in the legal record. This first stage includes identifying licensing and HIPAA requirements, HHS and other agency regulations, facility bylaws, and accreditation standards, such as this Joint Commission requirement: "H&P (history and physical) must be completed and documented within 24 hrs. following admission of the patient, but prior to surgery or a procedure requiring anesthesia services (including moderate sedation)."

Next, consider whether the information is a part of the **business record**. If the information is standard documentation and its inclusion in the patient record is required by the facility's policies and procedures, then it is a part of the business record, and therefore a part of the legal record. Some documentation, such as nurse notes that communicate the status of patients from one nursing shift to the next, are not a part of the official documentation required for treatment. Therefore, these notes are not a part of the business record. It is a good idea to mark documentation that is not part of the legal record as such, especially in paper records.

Finally, identify each form or type of information in the record and determine whether it is subject to release if requested or subpoenaed by a court. Table 8.2 is an example

Table 8.2 Decision Matrix Used to Identify Forms in the Legal Health Record

Form/Information Included in the Patient Health Record	Required in All Records?	Subject to Release per Request or Subpoena?	Part of the Legal Health Record?
Physical exam form (completed on admission)	Yes	Yes	Yes
Copy of physical exam (completed at another facility; copy sent for review)	No	No	No
Consent forms	Yes	Yes	Yes
Nurse notes of care (provided during shift)	Yes	Yes	Yes
Nursing worksheets (information gathered while treating the patient)	Yes (during hospitalization until the formal notes of care are completed; not part of the permanent record)	No	No

of a decision matrix that can be used both to identify the forms and information that may be included in a patient's health record and to determine which items are subject to release. Only those items that are subject to release if requested or subpoenaed constitute the legal health record. If the form is not subject to release, it is not a part of the legal record. A matrix, or decision matrix, is a helpful tool for comparing and assessing documents and information contained in the patient record and presenting that information in a useful format.

In the past, it was fairly simple to determine what comprised the legal health record. It was the paper chart or the medical record of treatment provided to a patient during his or her visit or inpatient stay. Defining the legal health record is now complicated by a number of factors:

- the increased use of electronic health records to maintain health information over time and from multiple visits
- patients and providers using the Internet to acquire and transmit health information
- the incorporation of patient-provided personal health information into the health record

All of these changes have resulted in additional, new information being included in the record of care. An electronic health record is no longer simply an individual record of an episode of care. Once the information is recorded in digital format in an electronic health record system, it can be compiled in a variety of formats—for example, a report showing a patient's medication history across several visits, a graph illustrating a trend line of the patient's blood pressure readings over time, or evidence-based medicine clinical support documentation used in treating the patient.

EHRs raise questions about what should be included in the legal health record. For example: Should information acquired from the Internet by either the patient or the provider be included in the legal record if it was used as the basis for a treatment decision? Should instructions from the provider or an updated medical history sent by the patient to the provider be part of the record?

Patients are being encouraged by many physicians, patient advocacy groups, and insurance companies to maintain a personal health record. A **personal health record (PHR)** is a health record generated and maintained by the patient. The patient chooses the record's format, contents, and means of storage. The PHR could be a simple list of current medications or past surgeries, or it could include lab test results, pathology reports, health information from multiple providers, or anything else that the patient chooses to retain.

Should a physician accept this information generated and compiled by the patient as part of the legal or permanent health record? Is the information compiled in the PHR correct, current, and complete, or did the patient exclude some information that he or she did not want to share? Unlike a record generated and maintained by a provider, a PHR does not fall under HIPAA guidelines and is not considered protected health information. However, if information in the patient's PHR is incorporated into the patient record maintained by a physician office or a hospital, then it could become a part of the legal health record and would then be subject to subpoena and covered under HIPAA. Healthcare organizations should establish policies and procedures regarding incorporation of PHR information into the legal health record.

Confidentiality

Confidentiality is the obligation to keep information known by two or more people secret or private. Maintaining the confidentiality of patient health information is critical to the patient-provider relationship. Providers need patients to be open about their health concerns and supply complete and accurate information. Patients need to trust that the information shared with care providers will be kept confidential. Federal laws and regulations have been enacted over a number of years to protect the confidentiality of patient health information.

Since HIPAA became law in 1996, much attention has been given to protecting patient confidentiality. As discussed in Chapter 7, the HIPAA Privacy Rule stipulates what is protected health information, how that information can be used, and how it can be disclosed. **Protected health information (PHI)** is individually identifiable information about the health status, the provision of care, or the payment for health care that can be linked to or used to identify a specific patient. The HIPAA Security Rule governs the use and the protection of protected health information in electronic form—**electronic protected health information (ePHI)**. Healthcare organizations must ensure the confidentiality of all PHI, whether or not that information is a part of the legal health record.

Other information collected from the health record, such as datasets or reports compiled from **aggregate data**—data compiled from multiple patients in which no individual patient can be identified—is not protected health information. Data in which all identifying information has been removed is referred to as **de-identified information**. De-identified data cannot contain any patient names, dates of birth, Social Security numbers, addresses, hospital numbers, names of next of kin or responsible parties, or any other identifying information.

Figure 8.2 shows a copy of a pulmonary function test in which all identifying information has been obscured from view. *Redact* is another term for removing all identifying information. To redact something is to edit or censor it.

Figure 8.2 De-identified Information

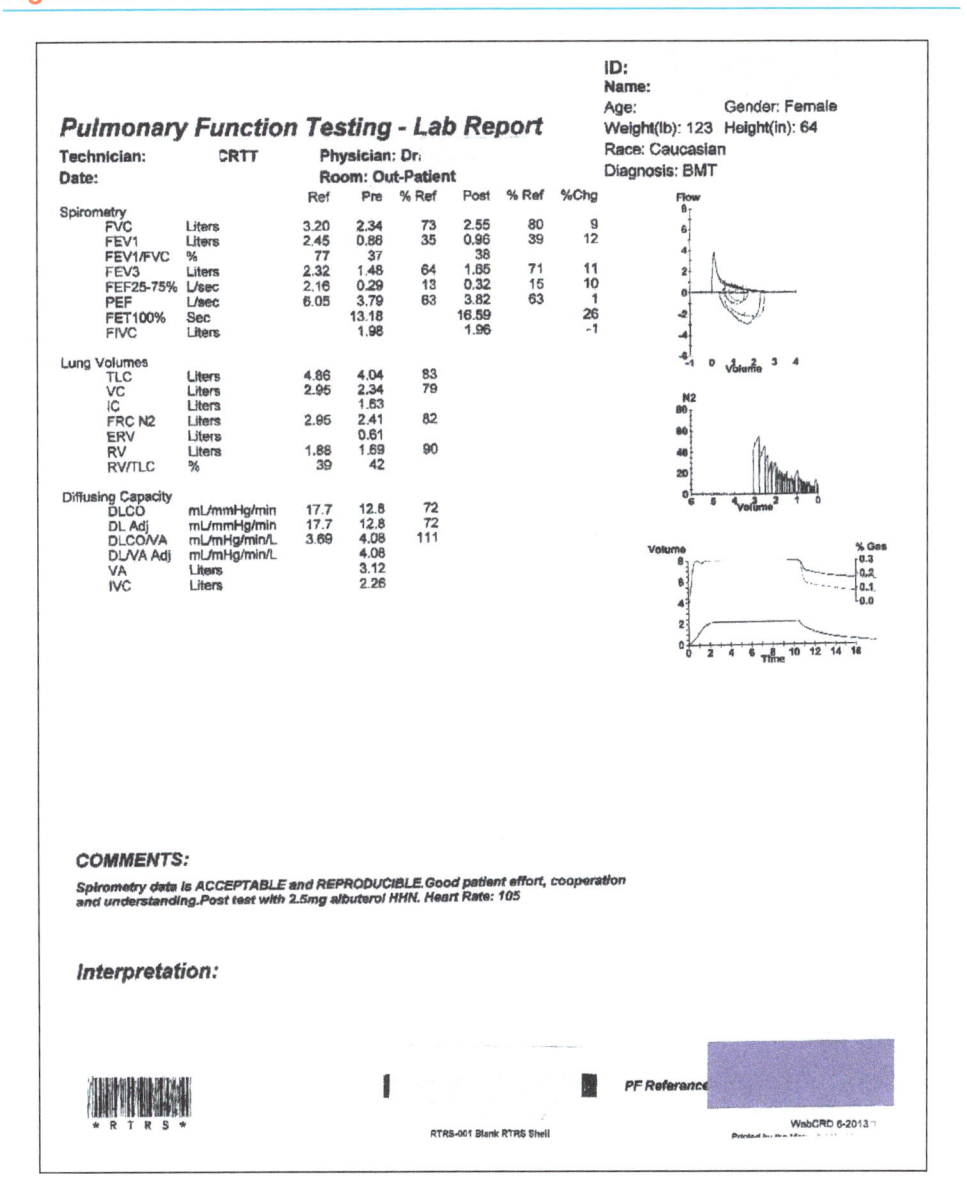

[Pulmonary Function Testing - Lab Report with de-identified ID, Name, Age fields blank; Gender: Female, Weight(lb): 123, Height(in): 64, Race: Caucasian, Diagnosis: BMT]

To further illustrate these two types of data, de-identified and aggregate data, consider the health information maintained for patients with AIDS. The information in each individual patient chart must be kept confidential. If all identifying information and anything in the chart that could lead to patient identification have been removed from the record, the medical information can be shared. De-identified patient information is often shared for educational purposes—for example, supplied to medical students so they may examine the record of care. If data is gathered from the medical records of a group of AIDS patients and compiled into a facility's statistical report, it is considered aggregate data. Aggregate data might include statistical information such as the following: the average length of stay for the AIDS patients is 18 days, the average age of the AIDS patients is 35, 12 percent of the AIDS patients have comorbid medical conditions, and 56 percent of the patients with AIDS are male. Because no patient can be identified from this type of statistical data, it is not protected health information.

Chapter 8 Legal Aspects of Health Information Management

Other examples of health information that is not protected under HIPAA include statistical reports, committee minutes, quality improvement data, and research study documentation. **Quality improvement** is the continuous process of monitoring and analyzing healthcare delivery to improve the timeliness, the efficacy, and the efficiency of patient care. The use of de-identified health information is vital to healthcare organizations in that such use supports the delivery of quality care and administrative functions.

Protected Health Information Documentation

The types of documents that are typically considered protected health information are numerous and vary from facility to facility depending on the nature of the facility and the care or the services provided. The majority of the documents are directly related to the provision of care, including:

- patient history and physical examination records
- allergy records
- care plans
- diagnostic reports (lab, X-ray, etc.)
- assessment reports (physical therapy, nursing, etc.)
- monitoring reports (vital signs, fluid intake/output, etc.)
- reports related to surgical intervention (anesthesia, operation and pathology, etc.)
- progress notes by the physician and other providers
- therapy reports (physical therapy, respiratory therapy, speech therapy, etc.)
- physician orders
- discharge reports (discharge summary and discharge orders)

Two factors must be considered when determining whether a document is protected health information under HIPAA. First, is the information related to the direct care of the patient during an encounter? An **encounter** is a specific interaction with a healthcare provider and can be either an outpatient visit or an inpatient stay. A single visit to a physician office could include several encounters. The interaction with the nurse taking the vital signs (temperature, pulse, blood pressure) and performing the initial assessment is one encounter. A lab technician drawing blood for a test is another. The physician exam and consultation and a nurse administering a flu shot would each constitute additional encounters. An inpatient stay includes numerous encounters throughout the patient's time in the facility. Encounter data is used internally to assess and improve the delivery of care.

The second factor to consider in determining whether a document is protected health information is whether it would be released in response to a request for the legal health record. If the document is related to the direct care of a patient, and if it would be released in response to a request for the legal health record, the information is protected health information under HIPAA.

Remember that other healthcare documents containing patient information, such as copies of health records from other providers, must also be kept confidential. A physician, for example, may always request a copy of the hospital discharge summary for his office records when one of his patients has been in the hospital, whether under his care or the care of another physician. The copy of the discharge summary is then filed along with the records of care provided at the physician office to ensure that all patient information is available when providing office care. Since the discharge summary does not document an encounter with the physician or his staff at the medical office, it is not a part of the legal health record for the physician office. It is PHI, however, because it contains patient identifiable information.

Documents Not Considered Part of the Legal Health Record

A number of administrative documents are not a part of the legal health record. These include:

- patient authorizations for the release of information
- copies of birth and death certificates
- financial or insurance-related forms
- databases supporting physician credentialing, statistical reporting, admission and discharge logs and other administrative functions
- logs commonly maintained for specific acts of care, such as a surgery log or a blood transfusion log (*Logs* include basic information such as name, date, time, and physician. Logs are becoming less common, however, with the increased use of electronic health records since this information can be queried from the patient record.)

Administrative records are confidential because they contain patient identifiable information. Administrative records are not released in response to a request or a subpoena except for patient authorizations, which may be subject to subpoena or discovery. Only the legal health record is subject to release.

Consents for Treatment

Consent for treatment involves the communication between the physician and the patient for the purpose of providing information about a proposed medical intervention. A **consent form** is used to document a patient's approval, assent, or permission to receive care. Providing medical treatment without the consent of the patient could be considered *battery*, a civil offense involving unlawful physical contact. Anyone who has been admitted to the hospital or an outpatient surgery center for a surgical procedure has been asked to sign a surgery consent form. Hospitals require signed patient consent forms for admission and treatment and for the release of a patient's record to an insurance company for billing purposes. During a hospital stay, a patient may need to sign additional informed consents for surgery, for example, or for a blood transfusion or participation in a clinical research study. The requirements for obtaining patient consent vary by state, but all states require that a consent form be completed in accordance with the organization's policy and signed by the patient and a witness. These consent forms become a part of the legal health record.

Types of Consents

Consents can be categorized in different ways. One of the most common is by the method used to obtain the consent. Methods used to obtain consent are implied consent, express consent, third-party/designee consent, individual consent, and informed consent. Table 8.3 provides definitions and examples of each type of consent.

Table 8.3 Type and Method of Obtaining Patient Consent

Type of Consent	Method of Obtaining Consent
Implied consent	Can be inferred either from the patient's actions (a patient goes to a clinic for a flu shot and does not object when the provider administers the shot) or from the situation (an unconscious patient admitted to the emergency department needs lifesaving intervention immediately and no family is present to give consent)
Express consent	An explanation given to the patient verbally, nonverbally, or in writing with understanding and agreement expressed by the patient (a physical therapist explains and demonstrates the use of equipment and then the patient uses the equipment)
Third-party/designee consent	When consent is provided by a patient's legal designee (a parent providing consent for a minor child or a legally designated representative providing consent for an incapacitated patient)
Individual consent	Specific to a certain treatment (to receive anesthesia, to decline use of blood products) or for granting permission for one to give consent for another (authorizing a relative or a friend to sign consents for a minor in the parents' absence or authorizing a camp counselor to sign consents when the minor is at camp)
Informed consent	Required for most surgeries, complex medical procedures, vaccinations, some blood tests, and for the protection of human subjects participating in research studies or clinical drug trials. **Informed consent** provides the patient with full disclosure and knowledge of the risks and the benefits of the intervention. Informed consent should include: • the specifics of what is to be done • an explanation of the procedure by the physician • potential consequences (risks and benefits) of the planned intervention • the possibility that observers (students) may be present • how the specimen (tissue removed as a part of a surgical procedure) will be disposed of • what steps will be taken if complications arise during the procedure • the patient's signature attesting that the patient received sufficient information about the procedure before signing the consent, understands the procedure to be performed, and consents to the physician performing the procedure

TAKE THE CHALLENGE

Go to http://IntroHIM.ParadigmCollege.net/ConsentForm and print out a copy of the surgical consent form. On the form, identify each of the elements of an informed consent as listed in Table 8.3.

Obtaining Consents

Before obtaining patient consent, the physician needs to explain the procedure in such a manner that the patient understands the reason for the procedure, the expected benefits, any potential **unintended consequences** (side effects or complications that could occur during or as a result of the procedure), and any alternative treatment options. In some circumstances, procedures will be performed when a patient is unable to consent—if emergency or lifesaving treatment is needed and no family member is present, for example.

Other Legal Documents in the Health Record

The patient record is a legal document, but the information contained in the record is primarily medical in nature. The record includes narrative reports that explain the onset of the patient's condition, the diagnostic means used, and all of the various aspects of treatment. For many years, the only types of legal information routinely contained in the record were the consent forms for admission and treatment.

Since the patient record is such a vital legal document, the record must demonstrate that the patient has agreed to be treated, that the patient has assigned any insurance benefits for payment to the facility, and that the patient received the facility's **notice of privacy practices**. Required by the HIPAA Privacy Rule, the notice of privacy practices explains how the patient's protected health information may be used or disclosed, and explains the patient's rights with regard to the use of protected health information. Advance directives and the Medicare beneficiary notice are examples of other forms that are just as important and may be included in the patient record if the patient supplies them.

In the paper record environment, many insurance-related forms and copies of records from previous visits or other healthcare facilities are also filed in the folder with the patient record. These items, however, are not a part of the legal health record.

These extraneous forms are either not medical related or not compiled as a part of a single episode of care. The nonmedical forms (e.g., insurance documents or correspondence regarding the patient) are not a part of the legal record. Medical-related forms may become a part of the legal record, however, if the forms provide documentation related to the episode of care—for example, a recent lab test that is sent from another facility, is specific to the condition the patient is being treated for, and reflects the onset of the illness. A different lab report, for example, a lab report from before admission for this episode of care, would not become a part of the legal record if it concerned an unrelated condition or was not considered a part of the diagnostic testing related to the current stay.

Increasingly, other types of legal documents are being added to the patient file. Medical science advancements, medicine's ability to prolong life, and concerns for the quality of life at the end of life are changing the way patients and physicians approach medical decision making. As medicine's ability to prolong life improves, family members have been taking on much of the burden of making difficult medical decisions. In turn, a number of legal instruments have been created to relieve families of the responsibility of making medical decisions for loved ones and to give patients greater control over the care they receive.

Advance Directives

An **advance directive** is a legal document with a set of written instructions that is prepared by a patient and that spells out the patient's wishes with regard to medical treatment in the event that he or she becomes unable to make such decisions. The most common types of advance directives are the living will, the durable power of attorney, and the do not resuscitate order. As long as the patient is of sound mind, he or she can change an advance directive. Laws regarding advance directives vary by state in terms of defining what constitutes a "terminal illness," the extent of instructions that can be outlined in the directive, and which forms will be accepted. These legal forms are intended to provide guidance for the healthcare team. Advance directives are kept with the health record and are similar to orders written by a physician. An advance directive is invoked in consultation with other healthcare providers and the patient's family. If a doctor refuses to follow a patient's advance directive, the physician may be obligated to transfer the patient to another physician or even to another hospital so that the patient's wishes can be carried out.

Living Will

A **living will** outlines a patient's wishes with regard to medical treatment if he or she is unable to make decisions. A living will generally includes the designation of a **healthcare proxy**, an individual legally entitled to make medical decisions for the patient when the patient is unable to do so. A living will is commonly used by terminally ill patients to instruct the medical team to withhold certain types of care at the end of life, such as tube feedings and use of ventilators. A living will takes effect once a physician has evaluated the patient and determined that an end-of-life situation exists, consistent with state law.

Durable Power of Attorney for Health Care

Durable power of attorney for health care gives an individual designated by the patient the legal power to make decisions about care and treatment if the patient is unconscious or incapacitated. In many states, a medical determination is required before the durable power of attorney can be invoked. A decision to invoke the power of attorney should be well documented in the patient record.

Do Not Resuscitate

A **do not resuscitate (DNR)** order is a legal document instructing all providers not to provide cardiopulmonary resuscitation (CPR) or any other heroic measure to prolong life when the heart or breathing stops. If a DNR has not been completed or is not included in a patient's chart, the healthcare team will attempt to revive the dying patient unless a physician determines such an attempt would be futile. DNR orders are accepted in all 50 states. The DNR order is the earliest form of advance directive.

Think Ethics!

All hospitals and care facilities have an **ethics committee** (or a committee that performs a similar function) that reviews cases and provides guidance on the implementation of advance directives. The ethics committee comprises representatives from different disciplines. Its purpose is to provide both guidance and support to providers and administrators with regard to ethical decisions and to assist in resolving conflicts.

The Health Insurance Portability and Accountability Act of 1996

As discussed in Chapter 7, the **Health Insurance Portability and Accountability Act of 1996 (HIPAA)** is a broad federal act that includes multiple provisions governing insurance coverage and provides federal protection for individually identifiable health information held by covered entities and their business associates (BAs).

The key provisions of HIPAA address:

- the transfer and the continuation of health insurance coverage when an individual changes or loses a job—the **portability** part of the act
- healthcare fraud and abuse
- standards for healthcare information with regard to electronic billing and other processes
- the protection and the confidential handling of protected health information

Two key components of HIPAA, known as the *Privacy Rule* and the *Security Rule*, address the protection and the confidential handling of PHI and directly impact the patient record and the functions of the HIM department.

One legal definition of **privacy** refers to the right to prevent the nonconsensual disclosure of sensitive, confidential, or discrediting information. Under HIPAA, the **Privacy Rule** specifically outlines the requirements for the protection of confidential patient information. The **Security Rule** specifically outlines protections for health information that is created, maintained, and received or transferred electronically, referred to as *ePHI*, or electronic protected health information.

The legal definition of information **security** is protecting information and information systems from unauthorized access, use, disclosure, disruption, modification, or destruction in order to provide integrity, confidentiality, and availability. As discussed in Chapter 7, the Security Rule addresses the administrative and physical safeguards that must be in place to protect PHI and ePHI.

Sections 261–264 of HIPAA mandate standards for the electronic exchange of and the privacy and the security of health information. In 2003, the US Department of Health and Human Services added provisions to the HIPAA Privacy Rule mandating that covered entities (health plans, healthcare clearinghouses, and healthcare providers who conduct standard healthcare transactions electronically) adopt federal protections for individually identifiable health information. The provisions address patients' rights to their health information, outline procedures for the exercise of those rights, and identify authorized and required uses and disclosures of patient information. The Privacy Rule requires healthcare providers to provide patient health information in a timely manner, and to develop a plan to ensure access to patient information during natural and human-made disasters.

> **EXPAND YOUR KNOWLEDGE**
> HIPAA established, for the first time at the federal level, national standards for the protection of patient privacy. Before 1996, states set standards for protecting the confidentiality of patient information, and standards varied greatly between the states.

> **BE AWARE**
>
> When federal law and state laws differ, in most cases, federal law preempts, or takes precedence over, state law. However, the HIPAA Privacy Rule specifically states that with regard to PHI, providers must follow the most stringent law. Each component of HIPAA must be compared with the state law, and the most stringent law must be followed.

The Office for Civil Rights (OCR) is responsible for the implementation and the enforcement of the Privacy Rule. The OCR investigates complaints and conducts compliance reviews. If a covered entity is found to be noncompliant, the OCR works with the covered entity to achieve voluntary compliance and may impose corrective action and/or a resolution agreement if necessary. Civil monetary penalties may be imposed if satisfactory action is not taken.

Since the implementation of HIPAA and the Privacy Rule, modifications to the rule continue to be made.

Privacy and Security of Health Information

One major focus of the Privacy Rule is the protection of PHI held or transmitted by a covered entity or its business associate, regardless of whether the information is transmitted electronically, on paper, or verbally. HIPAA defines a **covered entity (CE)** as any health plan, healthcare clearinghouse, or healthcare provider that electronically transmits any health information in connection with transactions for which HHS has adopted standards (usually for the billing and the payment of services). HHS further defines these CEs this way:

- *Health plans* are individual or group plans that provide for or pay the costs of medical care.

- *Healthcare clearinghouses* are entities that process information received from another entity (e.g., billing services, community health information systems).

- *Healthcare providers* are providers of medical or health services and any other person who furnishes, bills, or is paid for health care in the normal course of business.

The Security Rule sets national standards for the protection of electronic health information that is created, stored, or used by a covered entity (as defined by the Privacy Rule) and spells out technical and nontechnical safeguards that CEs must put in place to ensure the protection of ePHI. The Security Rule also allows the use of new technologies to improve care and control the cost of care.

Examples of Security Rule safeguards include written policies and procedures, employee awareness training, access and audit controls, and transmission security, such as those listed here:

- Written policies and procedures can include access management, device and media controls, security incident reporting, protection from malicious software, and sanctions for noncompliance with the policies. HIPAA defines a **security incident** as "the attempted or successful unauthorized access, use, disclosure, modification, or destruction of information or interference with system operations in an information system."

- CEs must provide initial awareness training as a part of an employee orientation program, and conduct general refresher training once a year. In addition,

- CEs should conduct periodic training whenever there are changes, such as new policies and procedures, new or updated software or hardware, or changes to the Security Rule.

- CEs must limit access to and the use of ePHI by implementing controls, such as requiring user names and passwords and restricting individual users' access to specific levels of information.

- CEs are required to put into place physical safeguards for all workstations that access ePHI. Safeguards can include measures such as locating workstations in a secure area and implementing policies governing the use of portable devices such as laptops, electronic tablets, and portable backup disks and drives.

- Audit controls can record and examine system activity and generate audit logs to track and identify security issues.

- Transmission security protects against unauthorized access to PHI that is transmitted electronically.

While similar in intent, the Privacy Rule specifies what information must be protected, and the Security Rule provides the means of protection—the administrative, physical, and technical safeguards.

Privacy Officer

Under HIPAA, covered entities are required to designate a **privacy officer**, an individual responsible for monitoring and enforcing HIPAA policies and procedures. In smaller facilities, the privacy officer responsibilities may be added to those of an existing employee, often a credentialed professional in the HIM department.

The privacy officer's responsibilities include:

- serving as the facility's public contact for privacy-related issues
- developing the CE's notice of privacy practices, an explanation of patient privacy rights and how patient health information is used within the facility, and ensuring the notice is distributed to patients
- providing information on policies and procedures to internal and external constituents
- providing orientation and continued training for all employees and volunteers
- monitoring activities for compliance and recommending changes in policies and procedures, training, etc., to improve compliance
- serving as the facility's contact when HIPAA violations occur
- investigating complaints/breaches, following up with appropriate reporting or other actions, and recommending any changes in policies, procedures, or training needed to address the issue(s)
- working with the Office for Civil Rights to review complaints and potential breaches

Business Associate Agreements

The Privacy Rule extends to **business associates (BAs),** defined by HIPAA as another person or organization that acts on behalf of a covered entity and requires access to protected health information. When a covered entity, such as a hospital or a physician office, uses a consultant, contractor, or vendor service company to perform activities that involve the use of or the disclosure of PHI, it executes a business associate agreement. The **business associate agreement** specifies in writing what safeguards need to be in place to ensure the proper handling and disclosing of PHI. Changes to HIPAA in 2013 increased business associates' liability in the event of an unauthorized disclosure of PHI. Examples of unauthorized disclosures by a business associate include allowing a nonauthorized individual access to patient information, faxing information to the wrong fax number, or losing a portable storage device containing protected health information—the same kinds of breaches that are common for a covered entity.

Business associates are directly liable for noncompliance and can be subject to corrective action plans or monetary penalties. Covered entities are required to conduct a HIPAA compliance assessment to determine potential risks and to develop monitoring plans both for their own facility and the BA. Both the covered entity and the BA are accountable for maintaining the privacy of the PHI made available to the BA.

Monitoring Disclosures

HIPAA prescribes specific guidelines for monitoring the disclosure of patient identifiable information. Requirements include the following:

- Covered entities must implement policies and procedures to limit the information disclosed to the **minimum necessary** to comply with the request. Reasonable steps must be taken to limit the use of, the disclosure of, and the requests for protected health information to the minimum necessary to accomplish the intended purpose. The request must specifically identify the information requested and the purpose of the request.

- Individuals have a right to an **accounting of disclosures** of their PHI. Covered entities must develop a process for recording all disclosures of patient identifiable information, including the person or entity to whom the information was disclosed and what information was provided. These disclosures are not related to information made available within the facility for **treatment, payment, or operations (TPO)** activities. TPO activities are those things that a facility must do to carry out its operations, such as providing patient care and treatment, billing and reimbursement, risk management, and quality improvement.

Security Processes and Monitoring

The Security Rule requires that CEs implement "reasonable and appropriate" administrative, technical, and physical safeguards for the protection of electronic protected health information. Specifically, covered entities must do the following:

- ensure the confidentiality, integrity, and availability of all ePHI that is created, received, maintained, or transmitted

- identify and protect against reasonably anticipated threats to the security or integrity of the information

- protect against reasonably anticipated, impermissible uses or disclosures

- ensure compliance by their workforce

Breach Notification

A **breach** occurs when a covered entity or a business associate commits an unauthorized or impermissible use or disclosure of health information protected under the Privacy Rule. When a breach occurs, it can compromise the privacy or the security of protected patient information. Some breaches are the result of employee actions while others result from system and policy failures. Here are some examples of breaches that have occurred over the past few years:

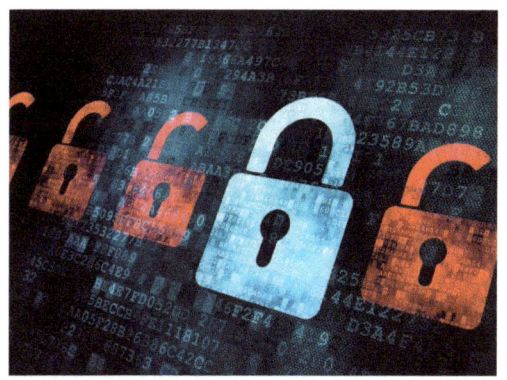

Covered entities are also responsible for the security of ePHI accessed remotely on a tablet or smartphone and ePHI stored on USB devices and other types of portable storage devices.

- A patient who had multiple births sued a hospital for disclosing the news to a reporter. The patient's file was also sent to all hospital employees in an attempt to make them aware of the situation. This case has not yet been resolved.

- A nurse was investigated for using patients' first names on Facebook during what she thought was a private chat. The chat was observed by others.

- Six records identifying patients' ages, dates of birth, and medical visit details were inadvertently faxed to an auto repair shop. The resolution is unknown.

- Five hospitals were fined after employees at those facilities accessed patient records without authorization. The largest fine, $250,000, was assessed after employees received unauthorized access to 204 patient records. It is not known what sanctions were placed on the employees. In most facilities, such actions by an employee would be grounds for suspension or dismissal.

- There have been numerous reports of hospital employees snooping in the records of celebrity patients, including Britney Spears, Farrah Fawcett, and Maria Shriver. One facility was fined $865,500 for selling information about a celebrity patient to a national publication.

- A $4.3 million civil penalty was assessed against a hospital that denied 41 patients access to their health records. While this is not a privacy breach, HIPAA requires that CEs provide patients with access to their health records.

Once a privacy breach has occurred, the covered entity is required to notify the affected individuals and the office of the Secretary of Health and Human Services. In some cases, the covered entity must also notify the media. If the breach affects 500 or more individuals, the CE must notify the affected individuals and the prominent media outlets. If the CE does not have sufficient contact information for 10 or more patients whose PHI has been breached, it must provide a substitute means of notification, such as posting the notice on the provider's website home page or in major print or broadcast media. If fewer than 10 patients are affected by the breach, notification can be made in writing, by telephone, or through some other means.

Notice made via print or broadcast media must include a toll-free contact number that individuals can call to determine if their PHI was involved in the breach.

In the event of a breach, the CE must be able to demonstrate that it has notification policies and procedures in place, to document employee training, and to document its policies outlining sanctions against employees who fail to comply with the Privacy Rule and notification guidelines.

In most cases, breaches of protected health information are not malicious. More often, the breach occurs inadvertently, such as when information is left in a public area where others can see it or take it, when an employee loses a laptop or a storage device that contains medical information, or when a fax with patient health information is received in an unstaffed, unsecured area.

IT REALLY HAPPENS

In August 2013, Affinity Health Plan, Inc. agreed to pay the US Department of Health and Human Services more than $1.2 million after a breach of protected health information. The OCR's investigation showed that "Affinity impermissibly disclosed the protected health information of some 344,579 individuals when it returned multiple photocopiers to a leasing agent without erasing the data contained on the copier hard drives."

The investigation also revealed that Affinity had failed to "incorporate the electronic protected health information stored in [the] copiers' hard drives in its analysis of risks and vulnerabilities as required by the Security Rule, and failed to implement policies and procedures when returning the hard drives to its leasing agents."

EXPAND YOUR KNOWLEDGE

Read more about the settlement agreement between Affinity and the US Department of Health and Human Services Office for Civil Rights at http://IntroHIM.ParadigmCollege.net/Breach.

All employees and volunteers are required to attend orientation to learn about patient confidentiality and privacy rules under HIPAA and to sign a confidentiality statement.

Under HIPAA, curious employees accessing information about a patient who is not in their care is considered a breach of the HIPAA Privacy Rule. There have been many instances of employee snooping, especially if the patient is a celebrity, well known, a relative, a friend, or a coworker. In many of these cases, employees have been fired for unauthorized access to patient information, consistent with the policies and the procedures of the facility. For example, several employees, including a contract worker (business associate), were terminated for accessing the records of former Congresswoman Gabrielle Giffords of Arizona after she was shot in 2011. Hospital employees not involved in her treatment did not have the right to access information about her condition, but several employees viewed her electronic medical record, a violation of the Privacy Rule. The employees were caught because the audit logs in the EHR system had recorded the login information of everyone who accessed patient information along with the date, the time, and the records accessed. The audit logs are monitored routinely and more frequently when a high-profile patient is in a facility.

Sometimes, an information breach is malicious. In 2008, an Arkansas nurse was sentenced to two years' probation and 100 hours of community service after accessing and disclosing a patient's health information for personal gain. The nurse copied private health information from a patient record and then gave the information to her husband, who was involved with the patient in a lawsuit related to an auto accident. The husband told the patient he intended to use the information against him in court. The patient immediately reported the husband's threat to the medical clinic where the nurse worked and to the local office of the US attorney. The nurse was fired the following day. She was later charged under federal law for violating HIPAA's privacy protections.

EXPAND YOUR KNOWLEDGE
Read more about the Arkansas nurse convicted of violating the HIPAA Privacy Rule at http://IntroHIM.ParadigmCollege.net/HIPAAViolator.

Identity Theft

Medical identity theft is a relatively new and rapidly growing issue in health care. **Medical identity theft** occurs when personal information (such as name, insurance number, or Social Security number) is stolen and used to secure medical care, buy drugs, or falsify medical claims for payment. Medical identity theft also includes the falsification of patient records for financial gain or to obtain medical care. In many cases, the patient is unaware of this theft, and it may be some time before the theft is discovered. The consequences for the victims of medical identity theft can be significant. Patients can be billed for false claims, and if incorrect medical information is comingled in the patient's chart, it can result in life-threatening treatment errors. The consequences of medical identity theft also extend to providers, insurance companies, and other third-party payers. Insurers may not pay any related medical claims if an identity theft has occurred.

Many more facilities are working to prevent medical identity theft by developing proactive programs to enhance identification processes, train staff to recognize and mitigate identity theft, increase reporting when identity theft occurs, and determine the role of each department in preventing theft.

According to a 2013 survey conducted by the Ponemon Institute, in 2012, medical identity theft affected an estimated 1.84 million Americans and cost victims $12.3 billion in out-of-pocket medical expenses.

HIM staff members play a vital role in preventing medical identity theft, preserving data integrity, and cleaning up documentation inaccuracies after a theft to ensure patient safety and quality of care. HHS defines **data integrity** as data or information that has not been altered or destroyed in an unauthorized manner. Data integrity is essential for the delivery of patient care and important for ensuring the accuracy of data for research, public health reporting, quality improvement, regulatory review, and auditing.

During an identity theft investigation, HIM staff may need to contact the patient and request a signature sample or a copy of a driver's license, a Social Security card, a passport, or another form of photo identification to keep on file for identification purposes. HIM staff will also be involved in clarifying the patient record, including creating separate new records for the patient and the individual who stole the patient's identity—even if that individual's identity is unknown.

Information that cannot be connected to either patient is kept for further review. Both the record belonging to the original patient and the record of the person who assumed the patient's identity are flagged to alert staff to monitor any future activity.

WHAT WOULD YOU DO?

As an HIM chart analyst, you are reviewing the hospital's electronic health records of discharged patients. At one point, you notice some discrepancies in a patient's EHR. In one area, the record states that the patient has "no known allergies." Another area of documentation indicates that the patient is "allergic to penicillin."

You check recorded names, dates of birth, and reasons for hospitalizations in all of the documentation, and all of the information seems to refer to the same patient. However, a few other areas show inconsistency or poor documentation, such as the difference in the patient's height during different hospitalizations, no mention of a preexisting chronic illness in the latest history report, and the conflicting documentation on the penicillin allergy—information that could be critical to future care.

What steps would you would take to follow up on these discrepancies? Explain how you would determine if all of the information in the record is from the same patient, and whether the discrepancies are the result of identity theft or improper documentation or if records for another patient have been comingled with the original patient.

Liability and Safety

The scenario above highlights a potential safety issue for the patient. An allergy to penicillin can cause a severe, sometimes life-threatening condition. That is why patients' drug allergies are prominently recorded in the record. Cleaning up a patient's medical record after medical identity theft has occurred can be quite difficult. Both the patient and the person who has assumed the patient's identity may have used the same name, date of birth, and insurance number along with other identifying information. Straightening this out can take quite some time. During this period, use of the record may be restricted, delaying patient care, release of information, and payment of claims. A patient's credit report may also be affected if claims for services provided at the time the identity was stolen go unpaid. Other departments in the facility, such as the patient accounting department and the risk management department, will be notified when the incident is reported. The goal of **risk management** is to proactively prevent errors and injury to patients, staff, and visitors and mitigate financial losses if a problem occurs.

Providers should encourage patients to take simple precautions to minimize the risk of medical identify theft:

- Review insurance documentation (Explanation of Benefit [EOB] statements) and credit card reports for charges for services that were not received.

- Never open email attachments from unknown individuals asking for personal identification information.

- Keep insurance cards and any other cards that display a Social Security number or other pertinent identifying information in a secure location.

- If concerned that medical identity theft has occurred, request a copy of medical records and review these records for inaccuracies.

Red Flags Rule

The federal **Red Flags Rule** is a part of the Federal Trade Commission's Fair and Accurate Credit Transactions Act (FACTA) of 2003. It is intended to prevent medical identify theft by requiring businesses and organizations, including physicians, hospitals, and other care providers, to develop theft detection and prevention programs.

Businesses and organizations covered by the law are required to conduct a risk analysis to identify potential vulnerabilities (i.e., red flags). A patient who presents an insurance card that appears to be altered is one example of a red flag. Every facility must have a security incident response team to investigate and mitigate instances of possible medical identity theft. Every facility must have an effective training program for employees in all departments identified in the risk assessment, including admissions, insurance, emergency, and health information, as well as a training program for the facility's privacy and security officers.

Red flags are potential patterns, practices, and specific activities that may indicate identity theft, such as a fraud alert on a credit card transaction or the use of a Social Security number that is listed on the Social Security Administration Death Master File.

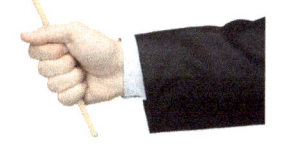

Release of Information

The HIM department is responsible for handling all **release of information (ROI)** requests. Requests for information from patient records may come from patients, other providers, insurance companies, or attorneys. The HIM department is required to comply with HIPAA guidelines when releasing patient information. The facility's ROI procedures should be outlined in a step-by-step format and in clear language that is easy to follow. The HIM department should respond to all requests in a timely manner.

It is also the responsibility of the HIM department to ensure that patient confidentiality is protected. HIPAA provides these general guidelines for releasing information about patients in a hospital:

- Unless a patient specifically requests that the information be withheld, or the patient is receiving drug- or alcohol-related treatment, the condition and the location of the patient in the facility can be released when the patient is identified by name. The patient's medical condition is maintained in a facility directory and generally reported in one-word, commonly accepted terms:
    - *Undetermined*   The patient is still awaiting assessment.
    - *Good*   The patient's vital signs are stable and within normal limits, and the patient is conscious and comfortable; indications are excellent.
    - *Fair*   Vital signs are stable and within normal limits; the patient is conscious and possibly uncomfortable, and indications are favorable.
    - *Serious*   The patient's vital signs are possibly unstable and not within normal limits; the patient has an acute condition with questionable indications.
    - *Critical/unstable*   Vital signs are not within normal limits, and the patient may be unconscious with unfavorable indication.

- The patient's location can be described as outpatient, inpatient, or emergency department.
    - Unless the patient requests otherwise, location information is available in the hospital directory and can be provided to friends and family and for deliveries.
    - Patient location information is not routinely given to the media. HIPAA does not prohibit the release of patient location information to the media but does recommend that facilities put in place a policy requiring patient authorization for release of information to the media. News media requests for such should be turned over to facility administration.
        — Any member(s) of the media visiting a patient should be accompanied by hospital personnel. Care must be taken to protect the privacy rights of other patients.
- Clergy may request a patient's name, location, general condition, and religious affiliation unless the patient has requested that information not be released to clergy.
- The death of a patient must be reported to law enforcement authorities when required by law. The patient's physician may release information about the cause of death if the family approves the release of that information.

Authorized Release of Information

Patient information may be released to others if the patient requests it and completes an **authorized release of information** form. Patients typically authorize this kind of release in order to have copies of medical records sent to another provider, an attorney, or an employer. Providing copies of records in response to legally required authorizations, such as a subpoena, is also considered an authorized release of information.

HIPAA has established federal regulations for the authorized release of information. Many states also have their own laws. As discussed earlier in this chapter, HIPAA requires that when federal and state regulations conflict, the most stringent requirements be followed. That means HIM professionals in some states will follow HIPAA regulations for certain aspects of ROI. In other states, state regulations may take precedence in some instances. Table 8.4 lists the federal requirements that must be included in a valid authorization for the disclosure of patient health information.

Additional state and federal requirements must be met when authorizing the disclosure of sensitive or restricted health information in specific categories:

- mental health or behavioral health
- alcohol or other drug abuse
- developmental disability
- HIV test results
- other: sexual abuse, child abuse, elder abuse, etc.

Table 8.4 HIPAA Requirements for Authorization to Disclose Patient Health Information

Authorization is written in plain language.
Authorization identifies the name of the patient whose PHI is being disclosed.
Authorization identifies the type of information to be disclosed.
Authorization identifies the names or the classes of persons or types of healthcare providers authorized to make the disclosure.
Authorization identifies the names or the classes of persons or types of healthcare providers to whom the organization is authorized to make the disclosure.
Authorization identifies the purpose of the disclosure.
Authorization contains the signature of the patient or the patient's authorized legal representative.
If signed by an authorized legal representative, the authorization identifies the relationship of that person to the patient.
Authorization includes the date on which the authorization is signed.
Authorization identifies the time period for which the authorization is effective and the expiration date or event.
Authorization contains a statement informing the individual regarding his or her right to revoke the authorization in writing and a description of how to do so.
Authorization contains a statement informing the individual about the organization's ability or inability to provide treatment, payment, enrollment, or eligibility for benefits.
Authorization contains a statement informing the individual about the potential for information to be redisclosed and no longer protected by the federal Privacy Rule.
Authorization contains a statement clarifying that if an organization is seeking the authorization, a copy must be provided to the individual signing the authorization.
Authorization contains a statement that the individual may inspect or copy the health information disclosed.
Authorization includes a statement regarding the assessment of reasonable fees for copy services.

Figure 8.3 is a copy of an authorized ROI form for the release of information related to alcohol/drug treatment, mental health, and confidential HIV/AIDS-related information. Note that the authorization does not permit redisclosure of the information released.

Figure 8.3 Authorized Release of Information

Authorization for Release of Health Information (Includes Alcohol/Drug Treatment and Mental Health Information) and Confidential HIV/AIDSrelated Information

STATE DEPARTMENT OF HEALTH

Name of Patient	Date of Birth	Patient Identification Number

Patient Address

I, or my authorized representative, request that health information regarding my care and treatment be released as set forth on this form. I understand that:

1. This authorization may include disclosure of information relating to ALCOHOL and DRUG TREATMENT, MENTAL HEALTH TREATMENT, and CONFIDENTIAL HIV/AIDS-RELATED INFORMATION only if I place my initials on the appropriate line in item 8. In the event the health information described below includes any of these types of information, and I initial the line on the box in Item 8, I specifically authorize release of such information to the person(s) indicated in Item 6.

2. With some exceptions, health information once disclosed may be redisclosed by the recipient. If I am authorizing the release of HIV/AIDSrelated, alcohol or drug treatment, or mental health treatment information, the recipient is prohibited from redisclosing such information or using the disclosed information for any other purpose without my authorization unless permitted to do so under federal or state law.

3. Unless withdrawn, this authorization will expire 180 days from the date of signature. A photocopy of this form will be considered as valid as the original.

4. Signing this authorization is voluntary. I understand that generally my treatment, payment, enrollment in a health plan, or eligibility for benefits will not be conditional upon my authorization of this disclosure. However, I do understand that I may be denied treatment in some circumstances if I do not sign this consent.

5. I can request a copy of this form after I sign it.

6. Name and Address of Provider or Entity to Release this Information:

7. Name and Address of Person(s) to Whom this Information Will Be Disclosed :

8. Purpose for Release of Information:

9. Unless previously revoked by me, the specific information below may be disclosed from: _____ until _____
   START DATE   EXPIRATION DATE OR EVENT

   ☐ All health information (written and oral), except:
   _____

For the following to be included, indicate the specific information to be disclosed and initial below.	Information to be Disclosed	Initials
☐ Records from alcohol/drug treatment programs		
☐ Clinical records from mental health programs*		
☐ HIV/AIDSrelated Information		

10. If not the patient, name of person signing form:	11. Authority to sign on behalf of patient:

All items on this form have been completed, my questions about this form have been answered and I have been provided a copy of the form.

_____   _____
SIGNATURE OF PATIENT OR REPRESENTATIVE AUTHORIZED BY LAW   DATE

Witness Statement/Signature: I have witnessed the execution of this authorization and state that a copy of the signed authorization was provided to the patient and/or the patient's authorized representative.

_____   _____   _____
STAFF PERSON'S NAME AND TITLE   SIGNATURE   DATE

Chapter 8 Legal Aspects of Health Information Management

Fees for Copying and Other Records Services

Healthcare facilities and providers may charge for copying patient medical records. Fees are established by hospital policy and must be reasonable while allowing the facility to recoup some of the expense of providing these services. Some facilities choose not to charge if the request requires copying just a few pages. In some states, maximum allowable fees are established by state regulation. In those states, fees cannot exceed the maximum amounts.

The ROI staff are often responsible for copying records for workers' compensation claims and Medicare audits. Fees for copying these records vary depending on the organization that requested the records and by state.

Special Circumstances

In special circumstances, patient authorization may not be required for the release of information. These circumstances vary by state. In general, information can be released without patient authorization:

- during a coroner's investigation
- when reporting to state driver and licensing agencies seeking to determine an individual's fitness to drive
- when it is in the public interest to protect the patient and others from harm, such as when controlling the spread of communicable diseases
- in the course of a criminal investigation (e.g., during an investigation into fraudulent medical billing, a physician's fitness to practice, or a coroner's inquest); in these cases, an attempt is made to get the patient's authorization, but disclosure may proceed without it

ROI Restrictions

Requests for patient information are commonly made by the patient, family members, medical providers involved in the patient's care, other healthcare facilities where the patient may be seeking treatment, insurers and other third-party payers, attorneys, and law enforcement officials. Some patient information may be subject to special restrictions, including records related to alcohol/drug abuse (Drug Abuse Office and Treatment Act of 1972), HIV/AIDS, adoption, involvement in a lawsuit, mental illness, and genetic testing. The Genetic Information Nondiscrimination Act of 2008 (GINA) prohibits discrimination on the basis of genetic information with respect to health insurance and employment.

ROI requests in these cases require the care provider to determine the applicable state and federal laws and procedures pertaining to the specific restriction. In some cases, such as those involving mental health care, the health care provider may need to be consulted. In unusual cases, hospital legal counsel may be consulted to determine what information is a part of the legal health record. Documents not considered a part of the legal health record are not released without a court order. The HIM credentialed employee performing the ROI function must be able to determine which cases should be referred for a legal opinion.

An ROI log can be used to track the filing and processing of information requests from the time of receipt of the request until the information is released. Typically, an ROI log records the number of requests made and processed, the status of unfilled requests (e.g., noting valid request needed, chart incomplete), the requests that are backlogged or in process, and the fees collected or due. Under HIPAA, care providers are required to account for disclosures of information, and the patient has the right to request this information.

Outsourcing ROI

Some HIM departments choose to outsource the processing of ROI requests to an outside vendor or to contract employees. Contract employees may work on-site or from a remote location. When fulfilling ROI requests by insurers, timeliness is an issue. The sooner the ROI request is filled, the sooner the care provider receives payments. A cost/benefit analysis should be done to determine whether to use in-house employees to fulfill the ROI function or contract the work to a vendor. Outsourcing has both advantages and disadvantages.

Outsourcing Advantages

- Improved efficiency: The process and the tracking of ROI requests are streamlined, ensuring that all steps in the process are completed without duplication of effort.

- Increased productivity in the HIM department: The ROI function includes a lot of busy work. By outsourcing the ROI function, HIM departmental staff can focus on more productive tasks (coding, data analysis, quality improvement, etc.).

- Increased morale: ROI involves a lot of repetitive work, which most employees do not enjoy.

- Increased security: Contract employees are trained extensively in ROI best practices to ensure compliance with HIPAA and state regulations.

- Reduced labor time and cost: Records are digitized for the release function, reducing both paper and copying costs.

Outsourcing Disadvantages

- The HIM department will experience adjustments as new procedures are implemented and contract staff begin working within the department.

- The department will need to complete a HIPAA-compliant contract between the vendor (business associate) and the facility.

- The HIM department should conduct a cost/benefit analysis that includes the cost of staffing, equipment, and supplies, and any monetary benefit that results from completing ROI requests in a timely manner.

Releases for Legal Purposes

In some situations, patient records must be released even if the patient has not authorized the release. These are referred to as **obligatory disclosures of information**, and often the request is part of a legal proceeding.

A **subpoena** is a legal document, most often issued by a judge, ordering that a person, document, or record be produced in court. It is not unusual for the HIM department to receive a **subpoena duces tecum**. This type of subpoena is used to compel an individual to produce documentary evidence in court—in this case, a patient record. Medical records are most often subpoenaed in civil disputes; in cases related to injuries resulting from a car accident, an altercation, or abuse; in divorce proceedings; and during custody disputes or family disputes over a will. Subpoenas related to malpractice suits against a healthcare facility or its personnel are less common; legal counsel should be advised if such a subpoena is received. The person receiving a *subpoena duces tecum* is legally referred to as the *custodian of the patient record* and will be required to swear to the authenticity of the record.

A **subpoena ad testificandum** is an order to appear in court and testify. This type of subpoena compels the custodian of the record, an HIM professional, to produce the record in court, testify that the record was kept "in the regular course of business," and answer any additional questions regarding the creation and maintenance of the record as per state regulations. Testimony is limited to matters within the custodian's knowledge, and the custodian is not required to testify as to the medical or financial information within the record. The HIM professional should bring a complete copy of the original record and request that the court accept the copy in lieu of the original record.

If the record is maintained in an EHR system, a copy of the record is printed out and taken to court. In some special circumstances, the record custodian will go to the courtroom in response to a subpoena and request that the judge review the record away from the courtroom in the judge's chambers. This is referred to as an **in camera review**. Such a request might be made in states where the law does not permit courts to subpoena mental health records. If necessary, the record custodian should be prepared to present a copy of the law pertaining to the release of mental health information to the judge for reference. Figure 8.4 shows the elements that are generally included on a subpoena.

A **deposition** is sworn oral testimony given before trial by a witness or a party in a criminal or civil proceeding. Depositions often take place in a law office and are part of the discovery process during which evidence is gathered for trial. An HIM employee asked to give a deposition would likely answer questions about the care provider's procedures for maintaining records. Just as in a court proceeding, an HIM employee would not answer questions about the medical information contained in the record or the medical treatment provided to a patient.

A **court order** is issued by a judge during a court proceeding. A court order may be used to define the relationships of parties in a civil court proceeding or to compel someone to do something or restrict him or her from doing something. Court orders can be issued for many reasons: to set a trial date, in response to an attorney's motion, to render an interim decision, to invoke a durable power of attorney, or to permit a noncustodial parent to have contact with his or her child. Court orders may be issued in oral or written form and are documented in the transcript of the court proceeding.

Figure 8.4 Sample Subpoena

1. The name and the jurisdiction of the court or administrative body that issued the subpoena
2. The title of the case and the case number
3. The names of the plaintiffs and defendants
4. The name of the person being ordered to appear
5. A list of the documents that must be presented if a subpoena compels the production of evidence
6. The time when and the place where the subpoenaed recipient must appear

230   Chapter 8   Legal Aspects of Health Information Management

A **warrant** is a written order directing law enforcement personnel to perform an act in support of the administration of justice. The most common warrants are arrest warrants and search warrants. A warrant can also be used to force a reluctant witness to appear in court. On rare occasions, a warrant may be issued to seize a patient record. In these cases, the provider's attorney should be notified. The original record(s) must be turned over to the warrant officer. The HIM personnel should request time to make a copy of the record to keep onsite.

> **BE AWARE**
>
> Incident reports and quality review/improvement documents should never be released. The facility's legal counsel should be notified if there is a request for this information.

Other types of disclosures that fall into the category of the obligatory releases of information were mentioned earlier, including records requested as a part of a coroner's investigation or used in determining an individual's medical fitness to drive, records required to protect the patient or others from harm, and records used for reporting on communicable diseases.

WHAT WOULD YOU DO?

As the custodian of patient health records at your facility, you have been served with a subpoena to appear in court with a copy of a patient's record from a previous hospital stay. The patient has not signed an ROI authorization form. The subpoena appears to be complete and to have the required signatures, but the patient's date of birth (DOB) and the dates of hospitalization are incorrect. All other patient identifiable information, such as name, address, Social Security number, and insurance number is consistent with that of the patient who stayed in the facility. The incorrect dates on the subpoena are similar to the documentation in the facility record and appear to be typos or transposed numbers.

1. Would you honor the subpoena and provide a copy of the record? Explain why.
2. If you decide not to honor the subpoena, what action would you take and why?

Remember, this is a subpoena for a record in a legal proceeding. Ignoring the subpoena is not an option.

Ethical Issues in HIM

Ethics is a set of principles of right conduct and a system of moral values. Ethical decisions often arise in the health information environment. HIM staff are responsible for protecting patient information and for doing the right thing for patients, coworkers, employers, the profession and its professional associations, the public, and themselves. Ethical decision making requires considering the values of all involved as well as any formal requirements (laws, professional standards, etc.).

> "Even the most rational approach to ethics is defenseless if there isn't the will to do what is right."
>
> —Aleksandr Solzhenitsyn, Nobel Prize winning author and historian

When considering the ethical implications of a situation, it is helpful to process the decision through a series of steps. These include defining the problem, gathering facts and information, investigating the values of those involved, discussing options, and evaluating all of the information in an attempt to find the best solution.

Some ethical issues are easier to resolve than others. Some of the more difficult cases occur when the ethical choice is in conflict with the law or a facility's rules or regulations. One example of such a conflict is the practice of upcoding. *Upcoding* is a fraudulent billing practice that is both illegal and unethical. It occurs when a diagnostic, procedural, or service code for a service or procedure is changed (upcoded) to a code that is similar but reimbursed at a higher rate in order to increase a facility's revenue.

Numerous ethical issues arise, however, when the action or the decision does not violate any law or regulation but does challenge individual or institutional principles and values.

Consider a situation in which an HIM employee is reviewing records and comes across the medical record of a relative. The employee knows that the patient omitted a history of drug abuse. This information may or may not affect the condition that the patient is being treated for at the time, but the patient record is incomplete.

Should the employee disclose that the information is incorrect, either to the HIM supervisor or the care provider who took the history report? Should the employee confront the relative and tell him or her to correct the information with the provider?

The first principle in the American Health Information Management Association (AHIMA) Code of Ethics states: "Advocate, uphold, and defend the individual's right to privacy and the doctrine of confidentiality in the use and disclosure of information." (See Appendix C for the AHIMA Code of Ethics.)

The guidelines supporting this principle state that the HIM professional has a responsibility to "safeguard" and "protect the confidentiality of all information obtained in the course of professional service."

The ethical dilemma here revolves around the patient's right to privacy and the confidentiality of the information provided by the patient. In these cases, there is not always a right or wrong way to respond. The course of action would be to carefully examine the situation, consider the values of all involved, consider the intent of the Code of Ethics, and from this choose the one best course of action.

The facility's ethics committee could provide support in working through this process of determining options and deciding what should be done.

WHAT WOULD YOU DO?

The healthcare facility where you work is preparing for a Joint Commission (JC) survey. The facility's administration and compliance committee has identified physicians' timely completion of incomplete health records as a priority area. The facility still uses paper records. Dr. Jones, in particular, is delinquent in completing documentation as well as in authenticating orders and reports. When notified that his delinquent records would be subject to review by the JC survey team, Dr. Jones requested that the HIM staff simply change the dates to indicate the reports were completed in a timely manner and before the delinquent date.

1. Is there an ethical issue here? If so, describe the issue.
2. What facts should the HIM supervisor consider before making a decision?
3. What are the values of all those involved (Dr. Jones, the HIM staff, the patient, the facility, etc.)?
4. Are there any extenuating circumstances or other information that should be considered in order to make a thorough and fair decision?
5. As one of the HIM staff members asked to make the changes requested by Dr. Jones, what would you do and why?
6. How might this situation be different if the facility were using electronic health records instead of paper health records?

Compliance

In the HIM environment, federal and state laws and regulations govern the handling of patient information as well as who has access to that information and for what purpose. There are many other laws, regulations, professional standards, and best practices that guide the provision of health care and the maintenance of patient information. Healthcare organizations and the HIM professionals who work for those organizations must comply with all laws and regulations, document their compliance, and have plans and procedures in place to ensure ongoing compliance. **Compliance** is to act in accordance with established guidelines or requirements.

Under HIPAA, healthcare organizations are required to protect the privacy and the security of patient health information and to have an established process for monitoring the organization's compliance with the law. A compliance officer or someone else may be charged with the responsibility of monitoring. Monitoring activities include:

- ensuring that the related policies and procedures are complete and up-to-date
- reviewing facility records to confirm that all new employees received the required orientation on security
- reviewing continuing education records to ensure that all employees, volunteers, and students attend a security training session annually
- reviewing reports documenting security issues to make sure that any issues have been evaluated appropriately, any required corrective action has been taken, and that all issues have been resolved
- conducting a facility "walkabout" to look for potential security breaches (e.g., making sure that computers displaying patient information cannot be read by unauthorized people passing by and privacy screens have been installed on computers in public areas)
- reviewing EHR audit logs to see what information has been accessed, by whom the information has been accessed, and if those individuals accessing the information had the required level of access
- listening to conversations in elevators, the dining room, and other public areas to determine if employees are discussing patient information in an environment where others can overhear them; remember, security covers verbal PHI as well as PHI in electronic and written form

The HIM professional privacy or security officer should evaluate information gathered through the monitoring process to determine if changes (in procedures, the location of equipment, or employee education, etc.) could improve compliance and enhance the quality of patient care. By conscientiously monitoring and making adjustments to ensure compliance, the facility is practicing **due diligence**—taking action to meet the intent of a law or guidelines. If a breach of information should occur, monitoring and compliance documentation would demonstrate the organization's good-faith efforts to comply with all aspects of the law.

Chapter Summary

It is necessary for an HIM professional to have a basic understanding of the legal system, to know how laws are created and enforced, and to be aware of the sources of legal information in order to keep up with changes in the law.

The health record, whether in paper or electronic form, is a legal document and is frequently used in court proceedings. Consent forms completed by the patient before the delivery of care become a part of the health record. While there have been laws protecting the confidentiality of patient information for a number of years, the adoption of HIPAA significantly changed the healthcare environment with regard to the privacy and the security of patient information. All healthcare employees, volunteers, and business associates must comply with privacy and security measures.

Medical identity theft is an emerging issue that has consequences for patients, providers, and insurers if patient financial or medical information becomes corrupted by theft.

Although much emphasis is placed on protecting the privacy and the security of patient information, in some circumstances, patient information must be released in compliance with the laws and the standards of patient care.

HIM Review

Check Your Understanding

Test your understanding of the material covered in this chapter by completing the following multiple-choice questions. For each question, select the best answer from the choices provided.

1. _____ is comprised of all protected health information, including the legal health record, billing records, the information used to support care decisions, and established protocols.

    a. The legal health record

    b. The designated record set

    c. The electronic health record

    d. None of the choices are correct.

2. The primary purpose(s) of the legal health record _____
   a. is to support the decisions made in a patient's case.
   b. is to support the revenue sought from third-party payers.
   c. is to document the services provided as legal testimony regarding the patient's illness or injury, response to treatment, and caregiver decisions.
   d. All of the choices are correct.

3. A record that combines electronic and paper records is _____
   a. an electronic health record.
   b. a designated record set.
   c. a hybrid record.
   d. a comprehensive patient record.

4. Which factor determines if a form is a part of the legal record?
   a. It is subject to release.
   b. It is subject to a subpoena.
   c. It is a part of the designated record set.
   d. It is generated during a patient's hospitalization.

5. _____ is any information about the health status, the provision of care, or the payment for health care that can be linked to or can identify a specific patient.
   a. The legal health record
   b. The designated record set
   c. The patient health record
   d. Protected health information

6. Which type of form is used to document a patient's approval, assent, or permission to receive care?
   a. authorization
   b. consent
   c. advance directive
   d. admission

7. Security safeguards include _____
   a. policies and procedures.
   b. employee awareness training.
   c. access and audit controls.
   d. All of the choices are correct.

8. A _____ is an unauthorized use or disclosure of information protected under the Privacy Rule.

   a. release of information
   b. lack of security
   c. disclosure
   d. breach

9. _____ is when personal information is stolen and used to secure medical care, buy drugs, or falsify medical claims for payment.

   a. Medical identity theft
   b. The Red Flags Rule
   c. A breach
   d. None of the choices are correct.

10. _____ reflects data or information that has not been altered or destroyed in an unauthorized manner.

    a. Data security
    b. Data integrity
    c. Protected health information
    d. The personal health record

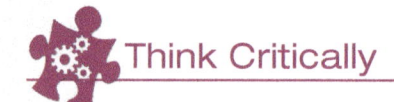

Think Critically

Consider the following real-world scenario and draft a response.

Compare and contrast the Privacy Rule with the Security Rule. Describe the focus of each rule and explain what it covers. For each rule, provide five examples of items that a healthcare facility would need to have in place in order to be in compliance.

Sharpen Your Comprehension

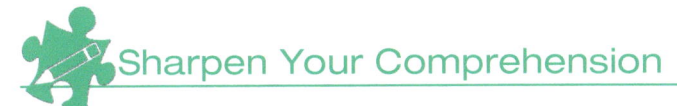

Complete the following matching exercise by selecting, from the list provided, the answer that best matches each of the numbered statements. For each statement, only one answer is correct.

a. advance directive
b. confidentiality
c. court order
d. deposition
e. durable power of attorney
f. judiciary
g. privacy
h. security
i. subpoena
j. warrant

1. _____ Right to prevent the nonconsensual disclosure of confidential information

2. _____ Decision or court order issued by a judge during a court procedure

3. _____ Legal document ordering that a person, a document, or a record be produced in court

4. _____ Keeping something secret or private

5. _____ Written order directing law enforcement personnel to perform an act to support the administration of justice

6. _____ Gives an individual designated by the patient the legal power to make decisions about care and treatment if the patient is unconscious or incapacitated

7. _____ Protecting information and information systems from unauthorized access

8. _____ A legal document prepared by the patient with instructions regarding medical care in the event that the patient is unable to make such decisions

9. _____ The court system and judges as considered collectively

10. _____ Sworn oral testimony given before a trial by a witness

Chapter 8 Legal Aspects of Health Information Management

Connect Theory to Practice

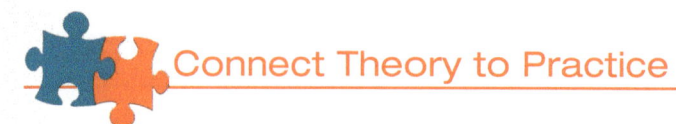

To help translate the concepts presented in this chapter to the workplace, complete the following exercise.

Test your knowledge of privacy and security regulations by playing the US Department of Health and Human Services, training game "CyberSecure: Your Medical Practice." Go to http://IntroHIM.ParadigmCollege.net/TrainingGame. Click the "continue" tab and select "new user." Create an identity. Once you have created an identity, you will be placed in a physician's office, where you will answer questions and respond to scenarios. Your job is to keep secure the protected health information collected by your office. Points are awarded based on your responses to the questions and the situations presented. Complete all three rounds of play and record your score for each round. Write down and present to your instructor any questions prompted by the scenarios and any concepts you do not understand.

Student eResources

*To enhance your comprehension of the chapter material, go to **Navigator+** and complete the additional practice items as advised by your instructor.*

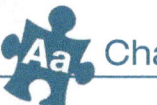

Chapter Terms

- accounting of disclosures
- advance directive
- aggregate data
- authorized release of information
- breach
- business associate (BA)
- business associate agreement
- business record
- compliance
- confidentiality
- consent
- consent form
- court order
- covered entity (CE)
- custodian
- data integrity
- de-identified information
- deposition
- designated record set
- do not resuscitate (DNR)
- due diligence
- durable power of attorney for health care
- electronic protected health information (ePHI)
- encounter
- ethics
- ethics committee
- evidence-based medicine
- Health Insurance Portability and Accountability Act of 1996 (HIPAA)
- healthcare proxy
- hybrid record

in camera review
individually identifiable health information
informed consent
jurisdiction
legal health record
living will
medical identity theft
minimum necessary
notice of privacy practices
obligatory disclosures of information
patient portal
personal health record (PHR)
portability
privacy
privacy officer
Privacy Rule

protected health information (PHI)
protocol
quality improvement
Red Flags Rule
regulation
release of information (ROI)
risk management
security
security incident
Security Rule
statute of limitations
subpoena
subpoena ad testificandum
subpoena duces tecum
treatment, payment, or operations (TPO)
unintended consequences
warrant

"Until recently, the biggest challenges in electronic health information management were first to be able to collect the data, then to sort through the high volume of data coming from a variety of systems.

Tomorrow's challenge will be to use that information—packaged and delivered to the right person at the right time—to drive decision making and improve the quality of care. Think of this as business intelligence for health care, or 'health intelligence.'"

—American Health Information Management Association (AHIMA) President Angela C. Kennedy, EdD, MBA, RHIA, "EHR in Place? Now the Real Work Begins," *Journal of AHIMA*, March 2014

Fast Facts

Healthcare Fraud
- Annual US healthcare expenditures: $3 trillion
- Estimated annual financial losses due to healthcare fraud: $90 billion–$210 billion
- Amount recovered for every $1 spent fighting civil healthcare fraud: $16
- Annual increase in federal prosecutions for healthcare fraud from 2003 to 2013: 9.9 percent
- Amount recovered through fraud enforcement efforts in 2013: $4.3 billion

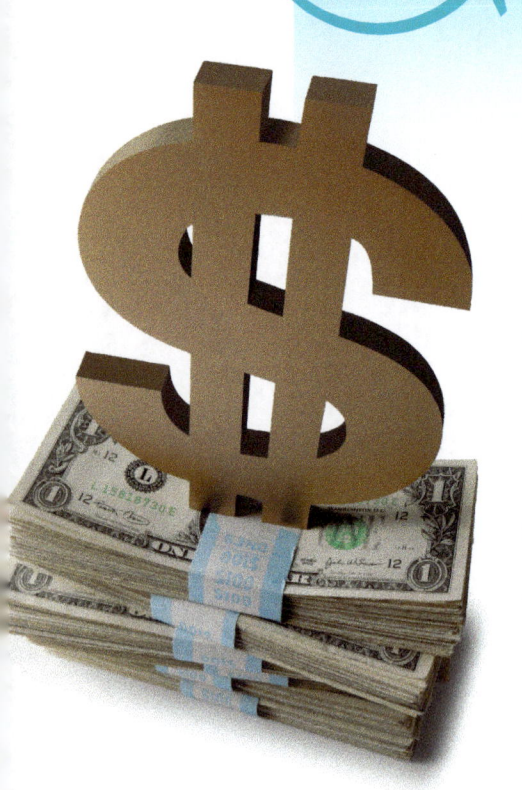

Think Ethics!

Health Information Management (HIM) professionals have an ethical responsibility to ensure that care providers have access to current, complete, and accurate patient information to support clinical decision making.

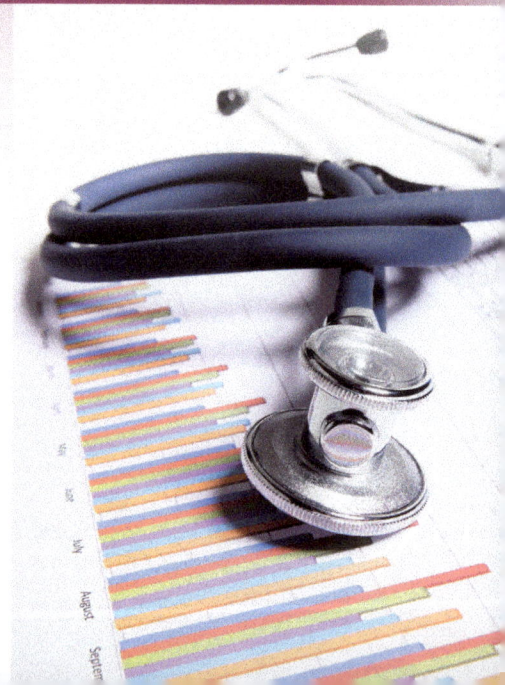

Chapter 9

Classification Systems and Reimbursement

The word *nomenclature* is commonly associated with the scientific classification of plants and animals. But nomenclature is the process of naming. For example, the nomenclature "tuxedo" derives from the fact that the jacket first became popular among the social elite who frequented the resort area of Tuxedo Park, New York.

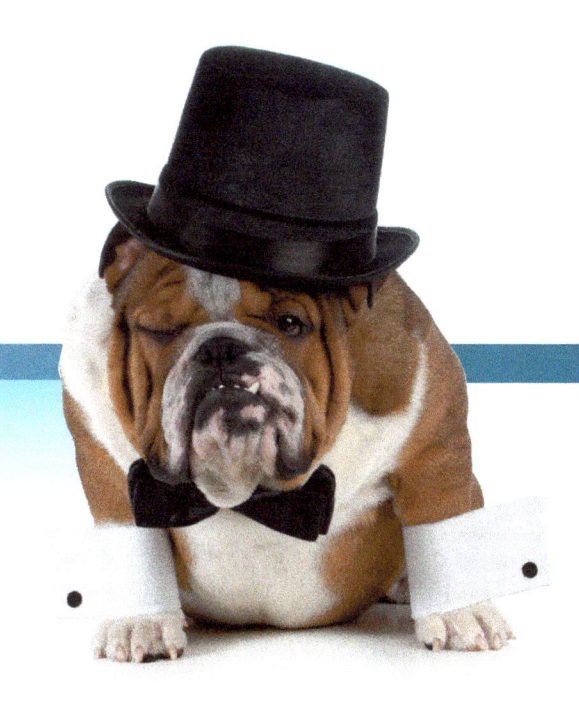

> " Fraud in any sector wastes scarce resources, but [with respect to] health care it has a direct negative impact on human life—with people waiting longer for treatment, people not being able to afford the treatment that they need, and some people never receiving the quality of patient care that is possible. "
>
> —Dr. David Evans, director of health systems financing,
> World Health Organization

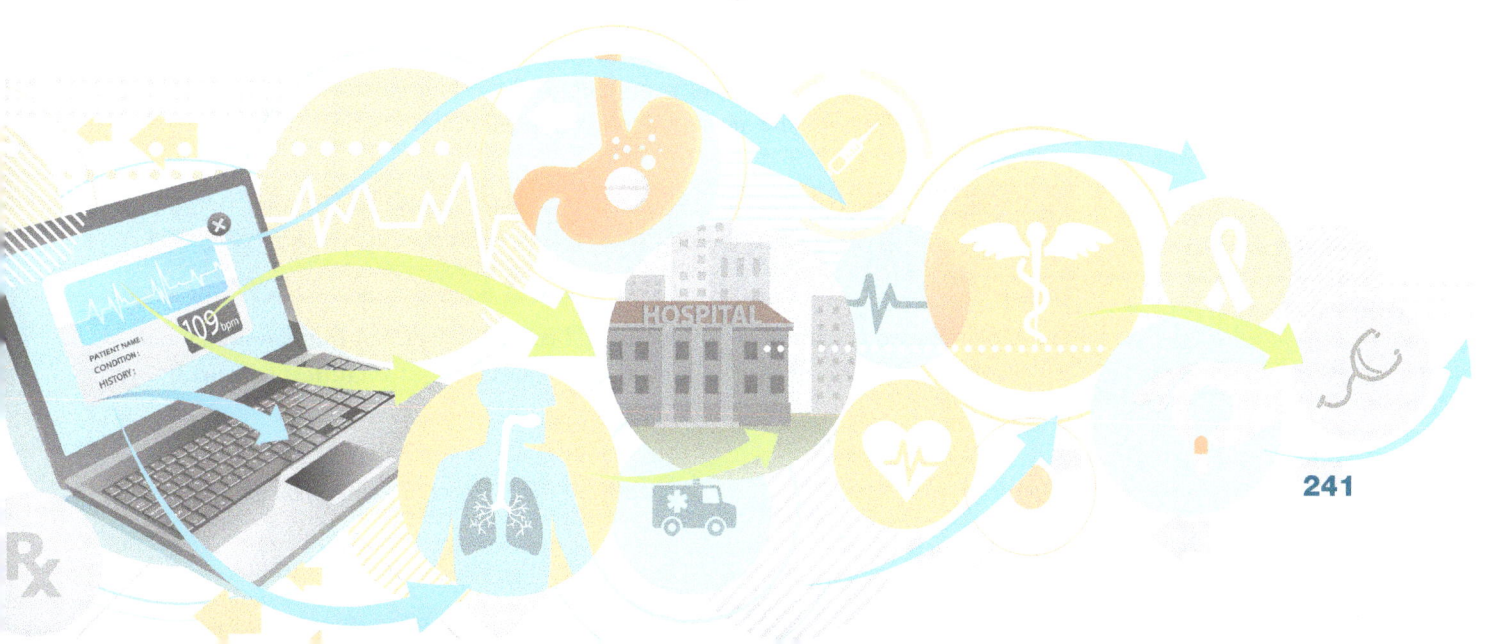

Learning Objectives

- Recognize clinical terminologies and nomenclatures.
- Explain the purpose of nomenclatures and classification systems commonly used in health care.
- Be familiar with the medical coding process.
- Compare and contrast ICD-9-CM and ICD-10-CM/PCS coding systems.
- Understand healthcare payment methodologies.
- Explain case mix index.
- Understand billing processes and procedures.
- Recognize the importance of revenue cycle monitoring.
- Be familiar with federal fraud laws and surveillance activities.

Ask for a soda in a restaurant in Georgia or Alabama, and the server will likely bring you a Coca-Cola. Ask for a soda in Minnesota, and you are liable to be served unsweetened, carbonated water. The term "soda" clearly means something different depending on where you are.

In medicine, often more than one term can be used to describe a specific disease or condition. But medical researchers, physicians, and other care providers need to be able to effectively communicate with each other across different medical settings, different medical specialties, and even across different languages. To avoid error and to ensure the continuity of patient care, providers have come to rely on a recognized standard medical language, also referred to as a *clinical vocabulary*.

The healthcare industry also relies on classification systems that group together similar diseases and conditions to make it easier to sort and organize healthcare data for the purposes of providing patient care, obtaining reimbursement, and conducting research.

Examples of the most commonly used classification systems include Current Procedural Terminology (CPT), used to identify medical, surgical, and diagnostic services; the Healthcare Common Procedure Coding System (HCPCS), used to identify medical services, supplies, and equipment; and the International Classification of Diseases (ICD), used internationally to classify mortality and morbidity data. These clinical classification systems provide the means for translating medical terms into medical codes.

Clinical Terminologies and Nomenclatures

The patient record contains a wealth of useful healthcare data, but translating that data into useful information requires a standard medical language, or **clinical (medical) terminology**.

Hospitals and physician offices use data from the patient record to support requests for reimbursement from third-party payers. Governments use healthcare data to track diseases and improve public health. In order for the data to have meaning, all parts of the healthcare system need to use the same terminology.

A **nomenclature** is a system of naming things within a particular group. In science and medicine, nomenclatures are used to categorize and classify plants, animals, biological organisms, diseases, and surgical procedures, among other things. The two primary medical nomenclatures currently in use are the Systematized Nomenclature of Medicine—Clinical Terms and the Logical Observation Identifiers, Names, and Codes.

Systematized Nomenclature of Medicine—Clinical Terms (SNOMED CT)

SNOMED was created in 1965 as the Systematized Nomenclature of Pathology as a way to organize information from pathology reports. Since then, it has undergone several revisions. The current version, the **Systematized Nomenclature of Medicine—Clinical Terms (SNOMED CT)**, was released in 2002. It is a nomenclature of clinical terms and multilingual health terminology that is considered the most comprehensive in the world. This system creates a standardized vocabulary to support communication between providers and facilitate the retrieval of data in an electronic health record. SNOMED CT data can be accessed electronically, implemented in a wide range of applications, and used for clinical decision support reporting (see Table 9.1).

Logical Observation Identifiers, Names, and Codes (LOINC)

Logical Observation Identifiers, Names, and Codes (LOINC) is a universal coding system used for tests, measurements, and observations that provides a common language to facilitate the exchange of clinical data between providers and between

Table 9.1 Nomenclatures

Nomenclature System	What It Does	How It Is Used
Systematized Nomenclature of Medicine—Clinical Terms	SNOMED CT is a recognized system of preferred terminology for naming disease processes. SNOMED CT contains more than 300,000 medical concepts, divided into hierarchies such as body structure, clinical findings, geographic location, and pharmaceutical/biological product. Each concept is represented by an individual number, and several concepts can be used simultaneously to describe a complex condition.	SNOMED CT is one of a suite of designated, standardized nomenclatures used by the US government and healthcare systems for the electronic exchange of clinical health information; it is also a required standard for interoperability certification.
Logical Observation Identifiers, Names, and Codes	LOINC was developed to provide a definitive standard for identifying clinical information in electronic health records. LOINC provides a set of universal names and identification codes for identifying laboratory and clinical test results and facilitates the exchange and the pooling of results for clinical care, outcomes management, and research.	LOINC is used in ordering or reporting laboratory tests and observations. Healthcare providers are required to use LOINC codes when reporting disease results to state and federal public health laboratories.

countries. It is designed for use with electronic health records systems at the **point of care** (the location where services are delivered, such as an exam room or a test site). LOINC provides a universal standard for identifying laboratory observations (see Table 9.1). There is currently no governmental mandate to use LOINC, but its use is slowly increasing.

Classification Systems

A **classification system** organizes groups or terms into categories. Medical coding classification systems group together diseases and procedures using corresponding numeric or alphanumeric codes to make it easier to organize and retrieve medical data. For example, one coding system identifies the diagnosis of diabetes mellitus without mention of complication by the number 250.00; the code for diabetes mellitus with ketoacidosis is 250.10. In the healthcare environment, classification systems have a variety of uses, including:

- as a standard system for the reimbursement of health care
- as an **index** (a list arranged alphabetically by author, subject, or keyword) of data on treatment outcomes; a disease index may be used to identify patients with a certain condition
- in determining, collecting, and reporting statistical data for internal facility use and to external agencies
- in developing databases for clinical, administrative, demographic, and statistical data
- in monitoring for fraud, abuse, and other compliance and regulatory issues
- to support quality and performance efforts

The translation of words into numerical codes can be difficult to understand. In coding systems, each number represents a term, an action, a concept, a timeframe, etc. Not all coding systems use the same translations. Several coding classification systems are currently in use in the United States. The most common are:

- International Classification of Diseases, Ninth Revision, Clinical Modification (ICD-9-CM)
- International Classification of Diseases, Tenth Revision, Clinical Modification (ICD-10-CM)
- International Classification of Diseases, Tenth Revision, Procedure Coding System (ICD-10-PCS)
- Current Procedural Terminology (CPT)
- Healthcare Common Procedure Coding System (HCPCS)

International Classification of Diseases

The International Classification of Diseases, designed and maintained by the World Health Organization (WHO), is the classification system used by many countries around the world to translate diagnoses, diseases, and other information into codes.

The system is used to record, analyze, interpret, and compare **morbidity** (disease state or symptom) and **mortality** (state of being mortal, subject to death) information.

ICD coding also captures **complications** and **comorbidities**. A complication is a disease or injury that arises during treatment for another condition (e.g., a patient in a hospital for a hip-fracture repair develops pneumonia). A comorbid condition is a coexisting medical condition or disease process that is present as an additional diagnosis (e.g., the patient with the hip fracture also has hypertension and diabetes).

ICD-9-CM

The **International Classification of Diseases, Ninth Revision, Clinical Modification**, widely referred to as **ICD-9-CM**, is used in the United States to code inpatient and outpatient diagnoses and inpatient procedures. These alphanumeric codes identify diagnoses, symptoms, procedures, and causes of death. There are approximately 13,000 codes available in the ICD-9 code set. Codes are three to five characters. For example, the ICD-9 code for the suture of an artery is 39.31.

ICD-9-CM is published in three volumes. Volume 1 is referred to as the *Tabular List of Diseases*, and it contains the numeric codes for diseases and injuries. Volume 2 is an alphabetic index of all of the codes listed in Volume 1. Volume 3 is an index of procedural codes.

ICD-10-CM

The **International Classification of Diseases, Tenth Revision, Clinical Modification**, or **ICD-10-CM**, is not just an update of the ICD-9 code set but represents a fundamental change in the structure and the theory of the ICD coding system. The tenth revision greatly expands the number of available codes from 13,000 in ICD-9-CM to more than 68,000 in ICD-10-CM and increases the number of digits in each code, allowing for greater specificity. Changes to the ICD-10-CM coding structure also allow for greater flexibility in adding codes for new diseases and diagnoses.

ICD-10-PCS

The **International Classification of Diseases, Tenth Revision, Procedure Coding System**, or **ICD-10-PCS**, is a new coding system that replaces ICD-9-CM, Volume 3, the index of procedural codes. The ICD-10-PCS is a list of codes for surgical procedures and is the companion to ICD-10-CM. Together, these two systems will replace ICD-9-CM. Table 9.2 shows some of the differences between ICD-9 and ICD-10 code sets.

Table 9.2 Comparison between ICD-9 and ICD-10 Diagnostic Codes

ICD-9	ICD-10
3–5 characters in length	3–7 characters in length
Approximately 13,000 available codes	Approximately 68,000 available codes
First digit may be alpha (E or V) or numeric; digits 2–5 are numeric	Digit 1 is alpha, digits 2 and 3 are numeric, and digits 4–7 are alpha or numeric
Limited space for adding new codes	Flexible for adding new codes
Lacks detail	Very specific
Lacks laterality	Has laterality (i.e., codes identifying the right and the left sides of the body)

Chapter 9   Classification Systems and Reimbursement

The expanded number of characters available in the ICD-10-CM/PCS code sets makes it possible to identify disease **etiology** (the cause of the disease or the condition), **anatomic site** (relating to the structure of the body), and the severity of the disease or the condition. Table 9.3 illustrates the ICD-10 code structure for a fractured right forearm.

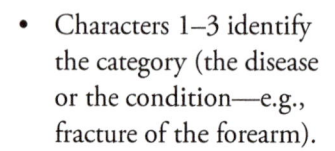

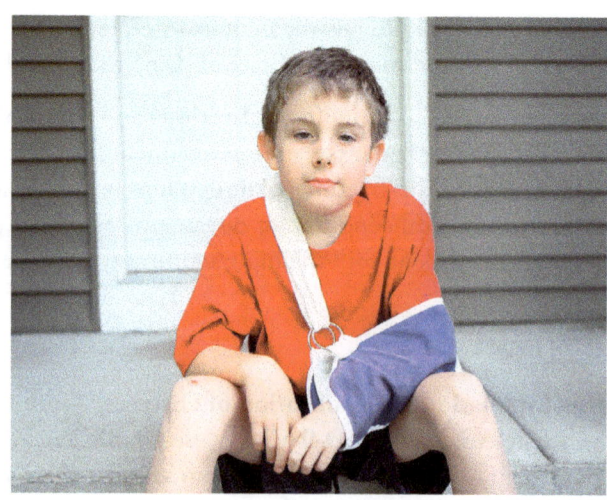

One of the benefits of the ICD-10 code set is that it allows for greater clinical detail, including a description of laterality, the side of the body where the affected area is located.

- Characters 1–3 identify the category (the disease or the condition—e.g., fracture of the forearm).

- Characters 4–6 identify the subcategory (fracture 5), anatomic site (torus fracture 2), and severity or other clinical detail (lower end of right radius, 1).

- Character 7 identifies the extension (the initial encounter for closed fracture).

Table 9.3 illustrates the ICD-10 codes for a fractured forearm.

Table 9.3 ICD-10 Codes for a Fractured Right Forearm

ICD-10 Code	Description	Code Part
S52	Fracture of the forearm	Category
S52.5	Fracture of the lower end of the radius	Identifies the anatomic site
S52.52	Torus fracture of the lower end of the radius (buckle fracture or incomplete fracture where there is a bulging of the cortex of the bone)	Provides additional clinical detail about the type of fracture
S52.521	Torus fracture of the lower end of the right radius	Defines *laterality* (the side of the body on which the fracture occurred)
S52.521A	Torus fracture of the lower end of the right radius; the initial encounter for closed fracture	Extension

In the ICD-10-PCS coding system, additional codes have been added to identify the body system, root operation, body part, approach, and device used. For example, the ICD-9-CM code for the suture of an artery is 39.31. The ICD-10-PCS code requires the coder to know the approach, whether the artery is right or left, and the part of the body where the artery is located (pulmonary, mammary, brachial, etc.).

For example, the ICD-10-PCS code for repairing a pulmonary trunk artery using an open approach is 02QP0ZZ. The code for repairing the same artery using a *percutaneous* (through the skin) approach is 02QP3ZZ.

Using a different example, the ICD-10-PCS code for a left knee replacement is 0SRD0JZ.

- 0 = Medical and Surgical Section (Name of Section)
- S = Lower Joints (Body System)
- R = Replacement (Root Operation)
- D = Knee Joint, Right (Body Part)
- 0 = Open (Approach)
- J = Synthetic Substitute (Device)
- Z = No Qualifier (Qualifier)

Due to its significantly more-detailed coding structure, the ICD-10 coding system provides a number of benefits. However, this level of complexity also requires coders to have a working knowledge of human anatomy and medical terminology and adequate training in the ICD-10 coding system.

International Classification of Diseases for Oncology, Third Edition

The **International Classification of Diseases for Oncology, Third Edition (ICD-O-3)** is the code set used primarily in tumor or cancer registry programs. The majority of the information used to identify the appropriate ICD-O-3 code is drawn from pathology reports. As Table 9.4 shows, ICD-O-3 is a 10-digit, multidimensional coding structure, identifying tumor **topography** (cancer site), **morphology** (cancer type), **behavior** (benign, malignant, or undetermined), and **grade** (differentiation).

For example, the ICD-O-3 code for ductal cell carcinoma in the body of the pancreas, stage 3, with metastasis to the lungs is C25.1 8500/3.3. Table 9.5 shows the code broken down into its component parts.

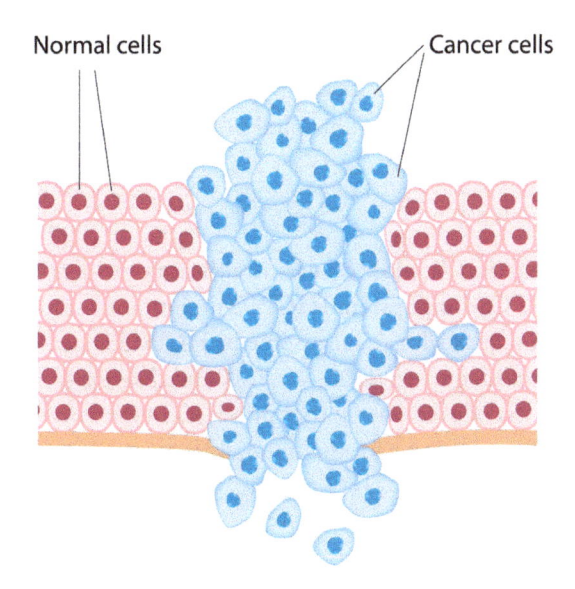

A tumor grade is based on how abnormal the tumor cells and the tumor tissues look under a microscope, and it is an indicator of how quickly a tumor is likely to grow and spread.

Table 9.4 ICD-O-3 Code Structure

Topography	Digits 1–4	Identify the cancer site
Morphology	Digits 5–8	Identify the specific histological term (type of cancer)
Behavior	Digit 9	Indicates whether the tumor is malignant, benign, in situ, or uncertain if benign or malignant
Grade (Differentiation)	Digit 10	Classifies tumors based on the abnormality of the cells (how different they look from normal cells)

Table 9.5 ICD-O-3 Sample Code for Ductal Cell Carcinoma

C25.1	Indicates carcinoma of the body of the pancreas with metastasis to the lungs (topography)
8500	Identifies ductal cell carcinoma (morphology)
3	Indicates that the tumor is malignant (behavior)
3	Indicates stage 3 (grade or differentiation); stage 1 cells look normal (slow growing, well differentiated), and stage 3 cells are abnormal (fast growing, poorly differentiated)

Current Procedural Terminology

Current Procedural Terminology (CPT) codes identify medical, surgical, and diagnostic procedures provided in an outpatient setting. CPT codes are used to submit reimbursement claims to insurance companies and other third-party payers. CPT codes consist of five-digit numeric codes that describe medical, surgical, radiology, laboratory, anesthesiology, and evaluation/management services provided by physicians, hospitals, and other healthcare providers. For example, the CPT code 99214 indicates an office visit; 90658 identifies a flu shot; and 12002 describes stitching a one-inch cut on a patient's arm. A two-digit modifier may be appended to the five-digit code when appropriate to clarify or modify the description of the procedure.

The American Medical Association (AMA) develops, maintains, and holds the copyright to the CPT codes, which are updated annually. The AMA publishes two versions of the CPT coding book. The most commonly used is the *CPT Physicians' Current Procedural Terminology*. A second version, the *CPT Physicians' Current Procedural Terminology: Specially Annotated for Hospitals: Hospital Outpatient Services*, contains all of the information in the original version and includes special Medicare guidelines and notations for identifying criteria applicable to outpatient hospital billing.

Healthcare Common Procedure Coding System

The Centers for Medicare & Medicaid Services (CMS) requires healthcare providers to use the **Healthcare Common Procedure Coding System (HCPCS)** (commonly pronounced "hick-picks") when submitting requests for reimbursement. HCPCS codes are based on the AMA's CPT code set and identify medical, surgical, and diagnostic services. CMS requires the use of HCPCS codes to ensure that providers in the same geographical region are reimbursed the same amount for the same procedure, such as a flu shot. Medicare reimbursement rates vary by region because the cost of providing care is higher or lower in certain areas of the country.

HCPCS codes are divided into two levels. HCPCS Level I codes are CPT codes. Level II codes identify services and supplies not included in Level I, such as an ambulance service or durable medical equipment. *Durable medical equipment* includes hospital beds, wheelchairs, oxygen equipment, and other physical supports used in home care.

Diagnostic and Statistical Manual of Mental Disorders, Fifth Edition

The *Diagnostic and Statistical Manual of Mental Disorders, Fifth Edition (DSM-5)* is the standard classification system for mental disorders. The *DSM-5* is used by physicians, psychologists, social workers, nurses, therapists (rehabilitation and occupational), and counselors across many different clinical settings. The *DSM-5* is also an important tool used for reporting public health statistics.

The DSM codes are divided into three major components:

- **Diagnostic classifications**   This is a list of DSM-recognized mental health disorders. The diagnostic codes for these disorders are derived from ICD codes.

- **Diagnostic criteria sets**   These are lists of conditions and symptoms that must or must not be present for each condition. Mental disorders can be difficult to diagnose. Signs and symptoms can vary depending on the disorder, the specific circumstance, and many other factors. Symptoms affect emotions, feelings, and actions, so diagnosing mental disorders can be much more subjective than diagnosing a medical disease or a condition for which a test can confirm the diagnosis (e.g., a chest X-ray showing the presence of pneumonia). Symptoms of mental disorders can include such things as feeling sad, an inability to concentrate, substance abuse, a major change in eating habits, hostility, and suicidal thoughts.

- **Descriptive text**   This is a systematic description of each disorder, including diagnostic features, supporting diagnoses, prevalence, and other features.

Comparing Nomenclature and Code Systems

The translation of words into numerical coding systems is difficult to understand. In coding systems, each number represents a term, an action, a concept, a timeframe, etc. Not all coding systems use the same translations. Coding classification systems may seem abstract to those with no training or actual experience in coding. The information presented in this chapter is intended as a brief introduction to the field of coding and to the coding systems in common use in the United States. However, HIM professionals will need to develop a deeper level of understanding and proficiency through additional coursework and practice.

Table 9.6 provides a quick reference guide for the nomenclatures and coding classification systems covered in this chapter, along with a sample code for each system.

Table 9.6 Nomenclatures and Code Systems

Coding System	Sample Code	Diagnosis/Condition Represented by the Sample Code	Focus of Code Assignment
SNOMED CT	25102003	acute type A viral hepatitis	Provides a standardized vocabulary for disease information
LOINC	2093-3	cholesterol, total	Facilitates the transmission of lab data electronically
ICD-9-CM	429.20	arteriosclerotic cardiovascular disease	Provides a code for diagnoses, descriptions of symptoms, and procedures
ICD-10-CM	572031A	displaced, midcervical fracture, right femur, initial encounter for a closed fracture	Codes for morbidity (disease or symptoms)
ICD-10-PCS	0DQ1022	repair the upper esophagus, open approach	Procedural codes that specify etiology, anatomic site, severity, and laterality
CPT	96360	IV infusion	Identify medical, surgical, and diagnostic tasks and procedures
ICD-O-3	188.5	malignant neoplasm of the bladder neck	Identify the site and the histology of neoplasms
HCPCS	95115	patient visit for allergy injection	Billing codes required by Medicare
DSM-V	290.11	dementia of Alzheimer's with delirium	Standard classification of mental disorders

Indices

Once a patient chart has been coded and abstracted, the information in the chart flows to the billing system so that the hospital or other healthcare facility can process the claim and send out a bill. The coded information in the chart also flows to the organization's data repository system where it resides as a part of an index. In general, an index is an organized set of data that operates somewhat like a road map in that it shows how information is organized and where information is located. For example, if you wanted to know more about coding, you could go to the back of this book in the alphabetical index, which lists all of the page numbers in the book where coding is mentioned or discussed.

Coding manuals have an alphabetic index that tells the coder where to find the correct code for a diagnosis or a procedure. Hospitals maintain several types of electronic indices, including the master patient index (MPI), diagnostic index, and operative (procedural) index. These indices allow healthcare organizations to locate, group, organize, and retrieve information. For example, if Good Health Hospital wanted to know "how many patients Dr. Berry admitted last month" or to drill down (look at something in depth) to see "how many of the patients Dr. Berry admitted who had a total knee replacement also developed a postoperative infection," the hospital could write a query using the ICD codes, and the index (an electronic database) would sort out all of the patient records containing that specific group of codes.

Master Patient Index

As discussed in Chapter 7, the **master patient index (MPI)** is a database or a list maintained by a hospital or another healthcare facility that records the names and the medical record numbers of all patients admitted or treated at that facility.

Key components of the master patient index include:

- internal patient identification
- patient name
- date of birth
- gender
- race
- ethnicity
- address
- alias/previous name
- social security number
- facility identification
- universal patient identifier (if available)
- account number
- admission date
- discharge date
- service type
- patient disposition

Each patient in the MPI is assigned one medical record number (MRN) to ensure that the patient is represented only once across all of the software systems used within the organization and that the patient's demographic and registration data are consistent across all systems. The MPI makes it easy to cross-reference essential demographic and clinical information between the different areas within a system and facilitates the tracking of patients and services.

Disease and Operations Indices

A **disease index** is a listing of all of the diagnostic codes for all patients treated at a facility. This list can be sorted by other information collected from the patient record, such as the demographic information from the MPI, or from miscellaneous data that is abstracted by the coder, such as a newborn's birth weight. If a hospital wanted to know what the top 10 diagnoses for the last year were, it would generate a computerized request for a report, listing the ICD diagnostic codes that appeared most frequently during a specific period of time.

The **operations/procedures index** works in a similar fashion. Inpatient data is coded using ICD codes while outpatient data contains both ICD and CPT codes. These indices are important tools healthcare organizations use to make operational decisions, to track and review the quality of patient care, for physician credentialing, and for comparison to other organizations of like size and complexity.

Disease and operations/procedures indices generally include:

- diagnostic and procedural codes
- data for additional conditions present or treated
- patient name, hospital number, sex, age, and ethnicity
- name of attending physician and/or surgeon

- hospital service to which the patient was assigned
- dates of admission, date of discharge, and length of stay
- disposition of the patient on discharge (e.g., the patient was discharged to home, discharged to another facility, or died)

Information in the disease and operations indices is used for a variety of internal and external reporting purposes. These include the following:

- **To track diagnoses by demographic group or another factor**   A state cancer-registry program may request a list of the 20 cancers most commonly diagnosed at the facility by age, sex, and other conditions present.

- **To analyze treatment outcomes**   A physician or an audit committee may request a list of patients who underwent a new procedure or were administered a new drug during the previous six months along with data on patient age, ethnicity, length of stay, and attending physician.

- **To track the frequency of diagnoses and procedures**   The billing or compliance department may want to know the most common diagnoses and procedures for the previous year.

The disease and operations indices are usually maintained in a computerized database, even in facilities that are not yet using an EHR system. As more facilities adopt EHRs, these indices will become even more essential, allowing data to be queried, shifted, and organized in new ways.

Other Activities Related to the Coding Function

For a number of years, HIM professionals have relied on encoder software programs and reference books to make identifying the correct medical codes for diagnoses and procedures faster and easier. More recently, HIM departments have begun turning to computer-assisted coding programs to improve the efficiency of coding and billing.

Encoder Software

Encoder software helps coders to identify the most appropriate code for a specific diagnosis or procedure. Encoders can streamline the coding process because the program can access information directly from the EHR. A paper chart is used as the source document if the facility does not have an EHR system.

Many different encoder-software programs are available. Encoders are either logic based or dictionary driven. A **logic-based encoder** requires the coder to type in a keyword. The encoder then asks a series of questions to refine and identify a specific diagnostic or procedural code. For example, if a patient's final diagnosis was listed as pneumonia, the coder would type the keyword "pneumonia" into the encoder. The software would then generate a series of questions to refine the diagnosis, such as, "With influenza or lung abscess?" If the coder selects "lung abscess," the encoder may query, "What specific organism?" As each question is answered, the diagnostic code becomes more specific until the appropriate code is identified.

A **dictionary-driven encoder** also requires the coder to enter a keyword or a code. The encoder then responds with a list of likely codes, definitions, and explanatory information in a format that is similar to the information provided in a printed coding book. The coder can then select the appropriate code by cross-referencing the information on the screen with the information in the patient's health record. Dictionary-driven encoders can speed up the coding process by eliminating the time it would take the coder to look up the appropriate code in the printed manual.

Computer-Assisted Coding

Computer-assisted coding (CAC) is a new and growing trend in health care. CAC utilizes a software program integrated into the EHR system to analyze documentation and generates codes based on specific terms and phrases. CAC software can identify and code many routine diagnoses and procedures, although human input and judgment is still required to code the more complex cases. Human coders are also needed to audit CAC output and verify that the correct codes have been assigned. CAC has advantages and disadvantages. Advantages include:

- increased productivity and efficiency
- greater consistency in applying coding guidelines
- an audit trail showing how a code was assigned
- the ability to create data queries when needed

Disadvantages include:

- the additional expense of purchasing the software
- an increased potential for upcoding and downcoding errors
- that coders still need to review the output

Coding References

Coders and encoders rely on a variety of reference books and websites when searching for the correct code. Many encoders integrate references, such as those listed here, into the software program for convenient access online. The most common resources include:

- *AHA Coding Clinic*, published quarterly by the American Hospital Association (AHA), provides ICD coding guidelines and advice for determining proper coding.
- *CPT Assistant*, published monthly by the AMA, provides up-to-date information on codes and industry trends.
- *Clinical Pharmacology*, a reference for drug identification and information
- *Dorland's Illustrated Medical Dictionary*
- *Coding Clinic for HCPCS,* published by the AHA, covers both Level 1 and Level 2 codes.
- ICD-9 and ICD-10 coding handbooks, including current guidelines and coding exercises

Chapter 9 Classification Systems and Reimbursement

- *The Merck Manual of Diagnosis and Therapy*
- *Mosby's Diagnostic and Laboratory Test Reference*, an alphabetic index of diagnostic and research tests with descriptions, alternate names, and other information
- *Dr. Z's Interventional Radiology Coding Reference* provides in-depth information on complex radiological procedures and applicable rules for CPT or HCPCS coding.
- *DRG Definitions Manual*, published by the CMS, lists the diagnosis-related groups for coding and reimbursement purposes.

Payment Methodologies

To the patient, a hospital billing statement may look like a confusing list of numbers and charges, and the cost of services and procedures may seem excessive. The *whys* and *why nots* of insurance or other third-party payer reimbursement can be even more confusing.

In this system, the patient is considered the "first party"; the care provider or healthcare facility where care is provided is considered the "second party"; and the insurance company, the managed care plan, or the governmental entity the "third party." In most cases, the third party may pay all or a portion of the cost of medical care provided to a patient. The remaining cost of care not covered by the third-party payer will then be charged to the first party (the patient). If the patient cannot or does not pay the remaining bill, the second party (the care provider) will need to absorb the expense.

In the modern healthcare system, the third-party payer often determines the rate of a particular procedure or service. CMS sets reimbursement rates for Medicare and Medicaid patient services. Insurers set their own reimbursement rates and negotiate costs with facilities.

It hasn't always been this way, however. Before Medicare was enacted in 1965, most care was reimbursed on a **fee-for-service** basis in which providers charged for the actual cost of the service provided (the test, the office visit, the procedure, or per day for inpatient care).

When Medicare was introduced in 1965, the federal government adopted the **retrospective cost-based reimbursement** system used by private insurance companies. Under this system, Medicare made periodic payments to hospitals throughout the fiscal year. Each hospital then filed a cost report at the end of its fiscal year. The interim payments were reconciled with **allowable costs** (charges for services and supplies for which benefits are covered under a health insurance plan) that were defined in regulation and policy.

Under this system, the cost of Medicare ballooned dramatically; between 1967 and 1983, Medicare payments rose from $3 billion to $37 billion annually. Three factors were blamed for driving the increase: the number of patients that were eligible for Medicare benefits and took advantage of the care provided; a payment system that paid providers based on services provided, which created an incentive for providers to provide more services; and the increased use of costly medical technology.

To curb the rising cost of Medicare, the federal government instituted a new **prospective payment system (PPS)** in 1983. In this system, inpatient admissions are classified into **diagnosis-related groups (DRGs)** based on final diagnoses. Providers are reimbursed for the cost of care based on the DRG rather than actual cost of providing care. Because Medicare pays hospitals a flat rate per case for inpatient hospital care, efficient hospitals are rewarded for their efficiency and inefficient hospitals have an incentive to become more efficient. Although it has been updated many times, the Medicare PPS system remains in place today.

Diagnosis-Related Groups

CMS categorizes similar treatments and procedures into approximately 500 DRGs. The DRG reimbursement rate reflects the level of services provided to an average patient in each DRG category. For example, when a hospital bills Medicare for a patient treated for hypertension, the hospital must either code the diagnosis as DRG 304 (hypertension with major complications and comorbidities), or as DRG 305 (hypertension without major complications and comorbidities). DRG 304 is a more complicated diagnosis, and the patient would likely require more care; therefore, the Medicare reimbursement rate for cases with that classification code is higher than for DRG 305. However, the amount of reimbursement would be nearly the same for all of the patients in each DRG classification, regardless of whether one patient was hospitalized for three days and another for five days, or whether one patient had different diagnostic tests and treatment than another.

DRGs focus primarily on resource intensity and not on the severity of illness. For that reason, in 2007, CMS adopted the use of Medicare Severity Diagnosis Related Groups (MS-DRGs) to shift the focus from facility characteristics to patient characteristics in order to capture the severity of illness. The MS-DRGs allow CMS to increase reimbursement to hospitals that treat more-severely ill patients. Even so, the DRG payment rate does not always cover the total cost of care, which is why facilities closely monitor reimbursement and the case mix index (discussed later in this chapter).

Individual Medicare claims may be adjusted for what are referred to as **outliers**, those patients for whom the cost of providing care (the value) is much higher or much lower than most others in the DRG. Identifying an accurate disposition on discharge is important for the DRG reimbursement to be split between facilities.

Because DRG assignment is based on ICD codes, an encoder can be used to identify the appropriate DRG number.

Ambulatory Payment Classifications

DRGs are used for inpatient services. The Medicare reimbursement classification system for hospital outpatient services is the Hospital Outpatient Prospective Payment System (OPPS). Similar to the PPS, the OPPS groups services into ambulatory payment classifications that set reimbursement rates for similar clinical services. Fees are based primarily on HCPCS codes.

EXPAND YOUR KNOWLEDGE

CMS has developed General Equivalency Mappings (GEMs) to help providers match the new ICD-10-CM/PCS codes to the correct DRGs. For more information, go to http://IntroHIM.ParadigmCollege.net/GEMs.

Ambulatory payment classifications (APCs) apply to outpatient surgery, outpatient clinics, emergency department services, and observational services. APC payments also apply to outpatient testing (such as radiology and nuclear medicine imaging) and therapies (such as certain drugs, intravenous infusion therapies, and blood products).

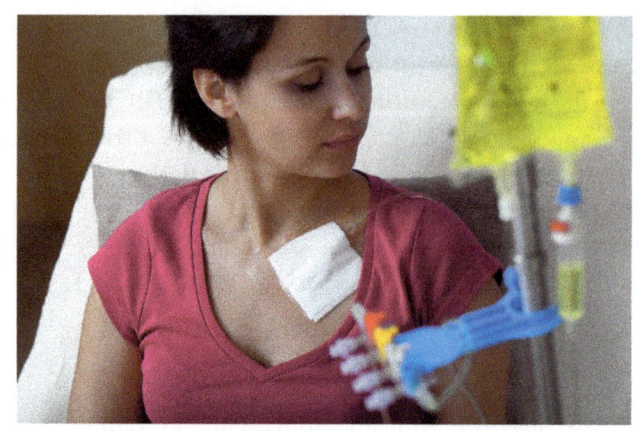

Increasingly, more medical services are provided on an outpatient basis.

Health Insurance Prospective Payment System/Resource Utilization Groups

CMS uses separate prospective payment systems to set reimbursement rates for acute inpatient hospitals, home health agencies, hospices, hospital outpatient facilities, inpatient psychiatric facilities, inpatient rehabilitation facilities, long-term care hospitals, and skilled nursing facilities.

The **Health Insurance Prospective Payment System (HIPPS)** was originally designed as a reimbursement system for skilled nursing facilities, but it has evolved to include home health agencies and inpatient rehabilitation facilities.

HIPPS works by creating tiers of payment levels, referred to as **resource utilization group (RUG)** levels, based on the level of nursing care required, room considerations (including isolation), and minutes of therapy provided. There are 66 RUGs. RUGs are determined periodically, and facilities are paid these set rates prospectively throughout a patient's stay.

Present on Admission

In response to a growing concern about the number of patients contracting preventable illnesses in the hospital, the federal Deficit Reduction Act of 2005 mandated a new reporting requirement for inpatient hospitals titled the "Hospital-Acquired Conditions and Present on Admission Indicator Reporting."

Effective for discharges after October 1, 2007, all inpatient hospitals submitting Medicare claims are required to include a **Present on Admission (POA)** indicator. POA refers to the conditions that are present at the time the patient is admitted to the hospital. This indicator is used to differentiate between conditions that the patient had at the time of admission and conditions that developed during the hospital stay, called **hospital-acquired conditions**. Conditions that develop during an outpatient encounter, during outpatient surgery, in the emergency department, or in observation are considered POA.

POA indicators provide an opportunity to monitor a hospital's quality of care and are an important part of CMS's efforts to link payment to quality. MS-DRG payments to hospitals may be reduced for specific conditions that were not present on admission (hospital-acquired conditions) and that could have reasonably been prevented through the application of evidence-based medicine. CMS annually updates the list of conditions determined to be reasonably preventable.

A POA indicator is assigned to the principal and secondary diagnosis and the external cause of injury code. Table 9.7 lists the five POA indicators.

Table 9.7 Present on Admission Indicators

Indicator	Definition
Y	Present at the time the patient was admitted to the hospital
N	Not present at the time of the inpatient admission
U	Unknown (documentation is insufficient to determine if the condition was present at the time of admission)
W	Clinically undetermined (the provider is unable to clinically determine whether the condition was present on admission)
Blank	Exempt from POA reporting

Case Mix Index

Case mix describes a group made up of patients with common traits such as age, insurance provider, diagnosis, or other criteria. A hospital's **case mix index (CMI)**, a number calculated by averaging the relative weights of the hospital's DRGs, has a significant impact on reimbursement. Medicare assigns each DRG a numerical weight (relative weight) that reflects the average amount of resources it takes for that hospital to treat a patient in that DRG. A high case-mix-index number indicates that the hospital treats more acutely ill patients and performs more-complex surgeries, which require more hospital resources. The higher a hospital's case-mix-index number, the more money the hospital receives per patient.

Case mix is related to coding since codes determine the DRG. Table 9.8 shows two different MS-DRGs, the corresponding diagnosis/procedural area and the relative weight.

Table 9.8 DRG Relative Weights

MS-DRG 1	MS-DRG 195
Heart transplant or implant of heart assist system with MCC	Simple pneumonia and pleurisy w/o CC/MCC (complication or comorbidity/major complication or comorbidity)
Weight 26.0295	Weight 0.7078

The patient with MS-DRG 1 is much sicker. More hospital time and resources will be required to treat that patient, so the relative weight of the DRG for heart transplant is much higher than the DRG for simple pneumonia.

To calculate the case index for an individual facility, follow these steps.

1. Determine the time period for the calculation to be done. (Commonly calculated for a specific period of time such as a month or year).

2. Identify the number of DRGs billed/submitted during that period.

3. Calculate the total relative weights for all DRGs billed/submitted for the period by adding the relative weights of each of the DRGs billed/submitted for the period. (DRG relative weights are available on the CMS website.)

4. Divide the total relative weights (from the calculation in step 3) by the number of DRGs billed/siubmitted (from calculation in step 2).

The product of the calculation in step 4 is the CMS (Case Mix Index) for the period.

TAKE THE CHALLENGE

Northstar Medical Center billed 100 DRG claims during a one-month period. The relative weight of the DRG claims for that month equaled 120. Calculate the hospital's case mix index for that month.

Hospitals use the CMI to estimate future reimbursement and to monitor it closely. Hospitals try to adjust costs to stay within the reimbursement amount by monitoring patient days in the hospital and decreasing the number of days, where possible, and by making sure that tests and diagnostic procedures are medically justified. Finance departments consider CMI when determining the hospital's budget. If the hospital's actual CMI is less than what the finance department predicted, the hospital loses revenue. Even seemingly small changes in the CMI have a large effect on the hospital's bottom line.

Billing Processes and Procedures

The billing processes and the procedures that support the billing processes are very important parts of the financial health of every healthcare facility. Billing is how the facility gets paid. An accurate record of patient identification and insurance information is essential to expediting the processing and the payment of claims. The billing process is supported by software used to prepare an electronic submission of claims.

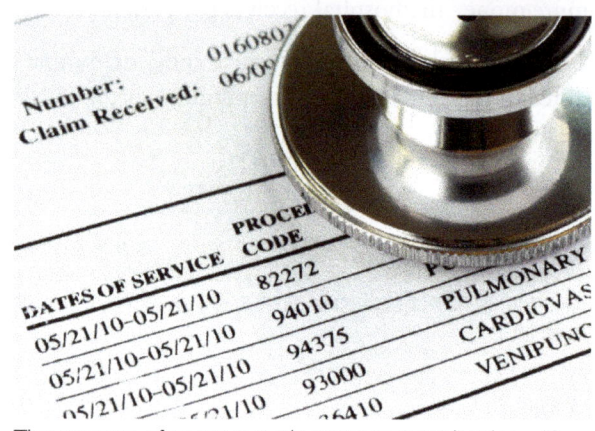

The process of revenue cycle management begins with patient scheduling and ends with payment appeals and the collection of unpaid bills.

The processes and procedures in billing can vary from facility to facility but should include these steps:

- At the time the patient is registered, the admissions office collects patient demographic and insurance information to determine who will be financially responsible for the cost of care (the patient, the insurance company, Medicare, etc.).

- If the patient has insurance, the admissions staff identifies the insurer, plan coverage, and guidelines, such as preapproval for care, that are required for reimbursement.

- The admissions, billing, or financial department determines the patient's financial obligation.

- After the patient is discharged but before billing, the patient record is coded, including the final diagnosis (identification of a disease or a condition) and all tests and procedures performed.

- The billing department takes the coded data, prepares a bill, and submits the bill to the payer.

- Responsibility for monitoring payments, resubmitting claims, and appealing denied or partially paid claims varies by facility but is often shared by the HIM and billing departments.

- The billing department generates patient billing statements for balances outstanding after the insurer's contribution.

Revenue Cycle Management

The Healthcare Financial Management Association (HFMA) defines **revenue cycle management** as "all administrative and clinical functions that contribute to the capture, management, and collection of patient service revenue."

As shown in Figure 9.1, the revenue cycle begins with patient scheduling and ends with payment appeals and collections. Each process in the cycle flows into and impacts the next.

To fully understand revenue cycle management, it is important to become familiar with each step of the process.

Scheduling and preregistration refers to the collection of patient registration information before the patient's arrival for inpatient or outpatient services, including eligibility, benefits, and authorizations.

Point of service registration counseling is the collection of a comprehensive set of data elements that is required to establish a medical record number and satisfy regulatory, financial, and clinical requirements.

Collections begins at the time of registration when any copayment or coinsurance payment is collected.

Encounter utilization review and case management is the process of evaluating the necessity, appropriateness, and efficiency of medical care provided by a facility for each patient against established medical standards, including regular reviews of admissions,

Figure 9.1 The Revenue Cycle

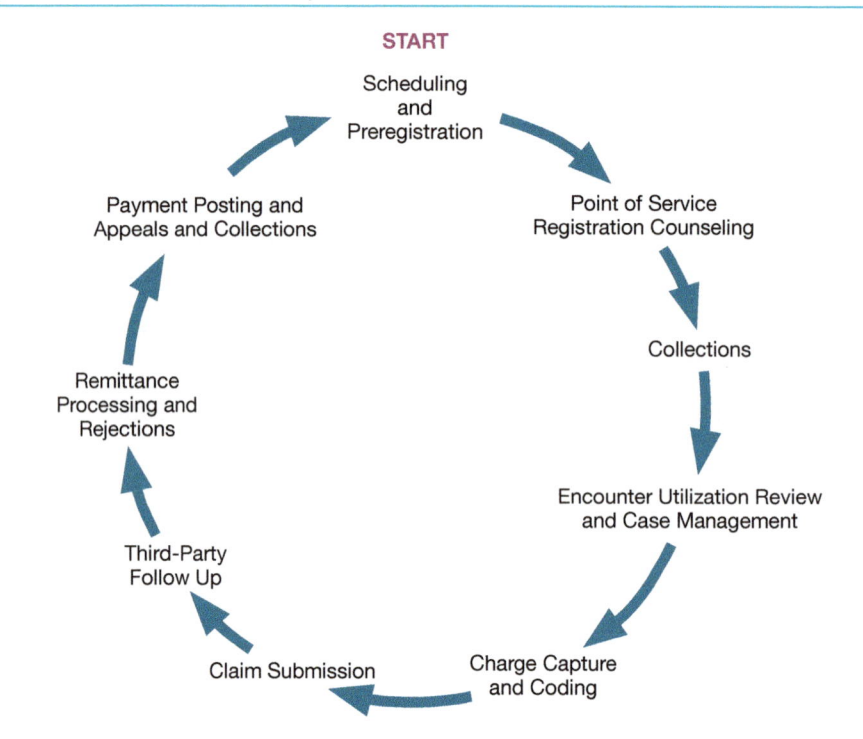

START

Scheduling and Preregistration → Point of Service Registration Counseling → Collections → Encounter Utilization Review and Case Management → Charge Capture and Coding → Claim Submission → Third-Party Follow Up → Remittance Processing and Rejections → Payment Posting and Appeals and Collections → (back to Scheduling and Preregistration)

lengths of stay, services performed, and referrals. This is done to ensure that the proposed hospitalization and care meet the criteria for reimbursement.

Charge capture and coding is the process of *capturing* (identifying) and coding all services provided to a patient for the purposes of billing and reimbursement. Medical billing is based on the codes assigned for services.

Claim submission is the process of submitting a universal claim form documenting all billable fees to the third-party payer for reimbursement.

Third-party follow-up involves collecting payments from insurers after the initial claim has been filed.

Remittance processing and rejections is the posting or the applying of payments or payment adjustments, including denied claims, to the appropriate accounts.

Payment posting and appeals and collections involves collecting medical fees not covered by insurance from patients and may include setting up payment plans.

Compliance

The term **compliance** refers to acting in accordance with established rules and guidelines. In relation to clinical coding, compliance is the practice of ensuring that diagnostic and procedural coding conforms to federal, state, and third-party payer regulations and guidelines, and that good coding practices protect against fraud and abuse in billing and reimbursement.

Coding inconsistencies can result in claims submitted for more reimbursement than is justified by the documentation in the patient record. This is known as **upcoding**. Upcoding may be the result of the coder's lack of coding experience or knowledge, or it may be an attempt to maximize reimbursement by assuming certain things that are not supported by documentation. Some healthcare organizations have used upcoding to intentionally increase reimbursement. Knowingly assigning incorrect codes to increase revenue is illegal and considered **fraud**, defined as wrongful or criminal deception intended to result in financial or personal gain. Payment of claims in which upcoding is present may be denied or reduced significantly. Penalties for fraud may include fines, imprisonment, restitution, and exclusion from participation in government healthcare programs.

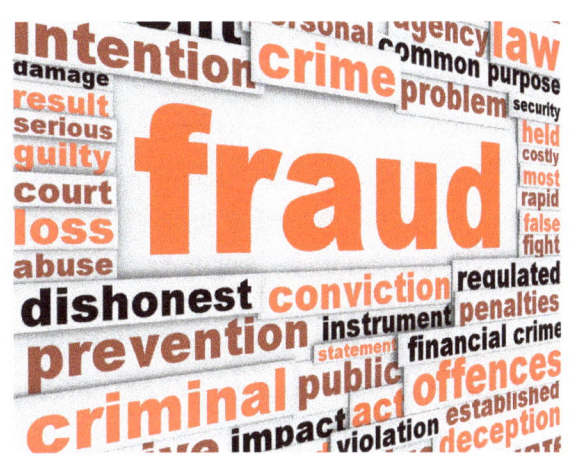

The Health Insurance Portability and Accountability Act of 1996 (HIPAA) established a comprehensive program to combat fraud committed against public and private health plans. In fiscal year 2013, the Department of Justice opened 1,013 new criminal healthcare-fraud investigations.

In some instances, coding does not sufficiently capture the severity of a patient's condition or the intensity of services provided to the patient. This is referred to as **downcoding** and may result in the provider or the facility not receiving full payment for the services provided. Downcoding usually stems from the coder's lack of knowledge of coding systems or fear of submitting an incorrect claim. Missing or incomplete documentation can also result in downcoding.

Healthcare organizations have implemented coding compliance programs to reduce the potential for fraud. The Patient Protection and Affordable Care Act provides coding compliance guidelines for healthcare organizations seeking reimbursement from federal programs.

These federal guidelines recommend that compliance programs include:

- a code of conduct that establishes the provider's commitment to accurate and ethical coding

- written policies and procedures for the provider's coding and billing procedures that cover:
    - documentation requirements
    - **medical necessity**, or justification that the care provided is reasonable, necessary, and/or appropriate based on evidence-based clinical standards of care
    - the **chargemaster**, or the comprehensive listing of all items billable to a patient or an insurance provider, including each medication, specific diagnostic test, minutes of anesthesia, etc.

- educational/training programs for physicians and staff, including the establishment of minimum qualifications and experience for coding positions and continued educational and training programs focused on proper documentation practices and guidelines

Think Ethics!

Upcoding can impact patient health if future care is based on incorrectly coded information in the medical record. Good documentation practices help to ensure that patients receive appropriate care.

Chapter 9   Classification Systems and Reimbursement

- a program to effectively communicate all coding changes to the appropriate staff and a requirement for staff to acknowledge the changes
- a means to ensure that staff are aware of the fraud-reporting process
- procedures for evaluating, auditing, and monitoring coding practices to ensure accuracy and consistency with the rules and the guidelines
- monitoring of trend-analysis data (e.g., an increase or decrease in denied claims, specific codes that lack documentation, or difficulty in code assignment, etc.) and the evaluation of claims denials (why they were denied)
- disciplinary and corrective procedures to support the coding function

Fraud

Do an Internet search for "Medicare" and "fraud," and dozens of entries are likely to pop up. Every year, criminal scams and fraudulent claims cost taxpayers and the federal government billions of dollars. Fraud involves making false statements or presenting false information for personal or financial gain. It is getting something of value by misrepresentation or concealment of factual information. Fraudulent acts can be committed by an individual, an institution, or a group.

Common examples of Medicare fraud include:

- knowingly billing for services that were not furnished and/or supplies not provided, including billing Medicare for appointments that the patient failed to keep
- knowingly altering claim forms and/or receipts to receive a higher payment amount

Several federal laws address Medicare fraud and abuse, including the False Claims Act, Anti-Kickback Statute, Physician Self-Referral Law (Stark Law), Social Security Act, and US Criminal Code. It is a crime to defraud the federal government or its programs. Punishment may include imprisonment, significant monetary fines, or both. Convictions may also result in exclusion from Medicare participation for a specified length of time. Medicare fraud may also result in civil liability.

TAKE THE CHALLENGE

Conduct an Internet search using the terms "Medicare" and "fraud," and then select three cases from the previous year in which different methods were used to defraud the federal government. Write a brief paragraph outlining each case. For each case, identify at least two other individuals or groups, in addition to Medicare, and explain how each group might have been victimized by the fraudulent activity.

False Claims Act

Under the federal **False Claims Act**, any person who submits a claim to the federal government that he or she knows (or should have known) is false is liable for monetary damages and penalties. For example, a practitioner who submits a bill to Medicare for payment for services that were not provided or who submits a bill in which services have been upcoded to increase reimbursement is committing fraud.

Whistle-Blower

A **whistle-blower** is someone who informs on a person or an organization that is engaged in illegal activity. There are many examples of hospital employees acting as whistle-blowers to report possible fraudulent activity. Whistle-blower cases have included illegal kickbacks (a partial return of money paid for a good or a service as part of a confidential and illegal agreement), cost-reporting fraud (inflating the cost of noncovered services and costs not related to patient care), illegal marketing practices, the sale of defective medical equipment, upcoding, and the submission of fraudulent claims.

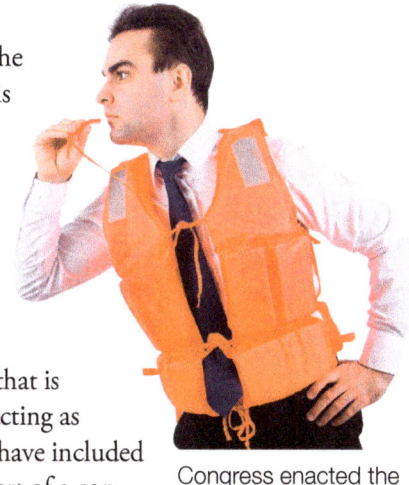

Congress enacted the False Claims Act during the Civil War in response to concerns that suppliers were defrauding the Union Army.

Whistle-blowers serve the public interest by reporting fraud and the illegal use of public resources. However, acting as a whistle-blower can carry significant risks, putting an individual's employment status, personal assets, and economic security in jeopardy. Therefore, there are some legal protections for individuals who inform on fraudulent or unethical business activity. For example, the federal False Claims Act includes protections for whistle-blowers as do some state laws.

Unbundling and Upcoding

Unbundling and upcoding are illegal billing practices used by medical practitioners or facilities to defraud the government. Unbundling is the practice of submitting multiple medical claims for services provided to a patient rather than a single claim in which all services provided are bundled together, as required by Medicare regulations. If a provider bills for each individual service, the provider can maximize reimbursement for those services. This is most often seen in billing for laboratory services—the most common example is in billing for blood tests. In this case, a provider orders a panel of tests, such as a blood chemistry profile, which tests many blood components. A blood chemistry profile may include fasting glucose, uric acid, BUN (blood urea nitrogen), sodium, a lipid profile (five different tests), and a CBC (complete blood count), which may require more than 10 separate tests. All of these tests should be bundled together under the description "chemical profile." However, if a facility submits individual claims for each test, it is likely to increase the amount of reimbursement it receives. Unbundling is fraud, and it is illegal.

WHAT WOULD YOU DO?

You are working as a coder in a small rural hospital. Your supervisor has told you to code and bill for each item in a patient's blood chemistry profile separately instead of using the single code for chemical profile, a practice known as *unbundling*. You know that unbundling is a violation of the law. What would you do?

Chapter 9 Classification Systems and Reimbursement

Clinical Documentation Improvement

Most healthcare facilities have a work group or a committee assigned to **clinical documentation improvement (CDI)**, a program to improve the quality of documentation to ensure that it is complete, legible, timely, concise, clear, patient centered, and accurate. The quality of documentation is important to patient care, and it also affects the facility's reimbursement. Facilities must be able to document services provided when billing insurers or other third-party payers for reimbursement. Improving the quality of documentation allows the coders to assign more-specific codes that more-accurately capture all of the care provided to the patient. Coding appropriately also reduces the number of claims denied. Monitoring clinical documentation is an important aspect of CDI because incorrect coding that results from a lack of documentation could be considered fraud.

CDI program goals generally include:

- identifying and clarifying missing, conflicting, or nonspecific physician documentation related to diagnoses and procedures
- supporting accurate diagnostic and procedural coding, severity of illness, and expected risk of mortality, leading to appropriate reimbursement
- promoting health record completion during the patient's course of care
- improving communication between physicians and other members of the healthcare team
- educating providers on appropriate documentation
- improving coders' understanding of the disease process, so they can identify the appropriate information and code as specifically and accurately as possible

Chapter Summary

The healthcare industry relies on nomenclature and classification systems that group together similar diseases and conditions in order to sort and organize healthcare data for the purposes of providing patient care, obtaining reimbursement, and conducting research.

A nomenclature is a system of naming things within a particular group. In science and medicine, nomenclatures are used to categorize and classify plants, animals, biological organisms, diseases, and surgical procedures, among other things. The two primary medical nomenclatures currently in use are the Systematized Nomenclature of Medicine—Clinical Terms and the Logical Observation Identifiers, Names, and Codes.

A classification system organizes groups or terms into categories. Medical coding classification systems group together diseases and procedures using corresponding numeric or alphanumeric codes. The most commonly used medical classification systems are the International Classification of Diseases, Current Procedural Terminology, and Healthcare Common Procedure Coding System.

The billing processes and the procedures that support billing processes are important parts of the financial health of every healthcare facility. Billing is how healthcare organizations generate revenue. Billing is just one part of the revenue cycle management process, which begins with patient scheduling and ends with payment appeals and collections.

In medical coding, compliance is the practice of ensuring that diagnostic and procedural coding conforms to federal, state, and third-party payer regulations and guidelines, and that good coding practices protect against fraud and abuse in billing and reimbursement.

Under the federal False Claims Act, any person who submits to the federal government a false claim or a claim that he or she should have known is false for the purpose of monetary gain is committing fraud. Upcoding and unbundling are examples of fraudulent billing practices. Several federal laws address Medicare fraud and abuse, including the False Claims Act, Anti-Kickback Statute, Physician Self-Referral Law (Stark Law), Social Security Act, and US Criminal Code. It is a crime to defraud the federal government or its programs. Punishment may include imprisonment, significant monetary fines, or both. Convictions also may result in exclusion from Medicare participation for a specified length of time.

HIM Review

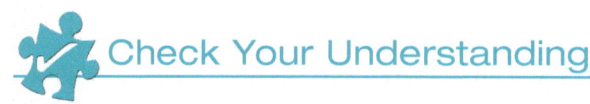

Check Your Understanding

Test your understanding of the material covered in this chapter by completing the following multiple-choice questions. For each question, select the best answer from the choices provided.

1. _____ is a method of arranging related disease entities in groups for reporting statistical data, and it usually includes all potential terms.

    a. A nomenclature

    b. Terminology

    c. A coding system

    d. A classification system

2. Submitting claims for more reimbursement than is justified by the documentation in the patient record is _____

    a. allowable if the coder believes it is the appropriate code.

    b. upcoding.

    c. downcoding.

    d. claim denial.

3. SNOMED CT is _____

    a. used for reimbursement purposes.

    b. a nomenclature of clinical terms and multilingual health terminology.

    c. a classification system.

    d. no longer used.

4. A disease index is _____

    a. used to find the names and the definitions of diseases.

    b. part of the reference software available to coders.

    c. used to identify patients with a certain condition.

    d. None of the choices are correct.

5. ICD-O-3 is used to code _____

    a. cancer.

    b. orthopedics.

    c. ophthalmology.

    d. operations/procedures.

6. _____ is software integrated into the EHR system to analyze patient documentation and to generate codes based on specific terms and phrases.

    a. Encoder
    b. CAC
    c. ICD-9-CM
    d. ICD-10

7. _____ is a tool used by coders to aid in assigning the most appropriate code.

    a. An encoder
    b. CAC
    c. ICD-9-CM
    d. ICD-10

8. Implementing the Medicare DRG system was an attempt to _____

    a. organize how claims are submitted.
    b. track additional information on charges.
    c. pay for only certain diseases.
    d. control the high cost of treating patients.

9. _____ is built into most encoders.

    a. CAC
    b. Reference software
    c. ICD-9 codes
    d. The ability to query physicians

10. The significance of POA is that _____

    a. the patient might not be justified for hospitalization.
    b. it puts the patient in a different payment category.
    c. payment may not be made for a portion of the claim if the condition arises during the hospital stay and was not present on admission.
    d. it is only captured for statistical purposes.

Think Critically

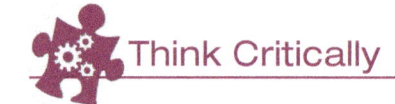

Consider the following real-world scenario and draft a response.

Review the ICD-9 codes in the first column, and compare them to the ICD-10 codes in the second column. Identify what documentation you would have to find in the patient record to code with ICD-10 that was not required for ICD-9; also indicate where you think you would find that information (by type of report). Be specific, and list all information needed to support the assignment of the ICD-10 code. Submit in a table with columns for the ICD-9 codes, one for the ICD-10 codes, and a third column where you identify the needed information as shown below. Use a medical dictionary if you need the definition of a term.

ICD-9 Codes	ICD-10 Codes	Additional Documentation Required
943.31 Full thickness skin loss due to burn (third degree NOS (not otherwise specified) of forearm	T22.311A Burn of third degree of right forearm, initial encounter	
453.41 Venous embolism and thrombosis of deep vessels of proximal lower extremity	I82.411 Embolism and thrombosis of right femoral vein	
813.45 Torus fracture of radius alone	S52.521A Torus fracture of lower end of right radius, initial encounter for closed fracture	

Sharpen Your Comprehension

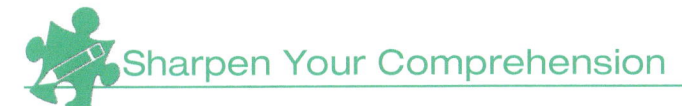

Complete the following matching exercise by selecting, from the list provided, the answer that best matches each of the numbered statements. For each statement, only one answer is correct.

a. case mix
b. chargemaster
c. clinical medical terminology
d. compliance
e. etiology
f. fraud
g. LOINC
h. nomenclature
i. unbundling
j. whistle-blower

1. _____ Standard medical language

2. _____ System for naming things within a particular group

3. _____ System for tests, measurements, and observations

4. _____ Cause of a disease or a condition

5. _____ Acting in accordance with established guidelines

6. _____ Listing of all potential billable items

7. _____ Type of patients treated by a hospital

8. _____ Making false statements to obtain benefits

9. _____ Informs on a person or an organization engaged in illegal actions

10. _____ Billing multiple, individual items when services are grouped together as one

Connect Theory to Practice

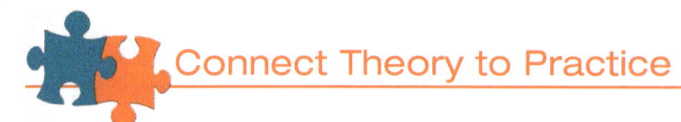

To help translate the concepts presented in this chapter to the workplace, complete the following exercise.

Research the requirements for a physician office medical coding compliance plan. List both the mandatory and optional items, if any. Explain each item and how it is used to support good coding practices.

Student eResources

*To enhance your comprehension of the chapter material, go to **Navigator+** and complete the additional practice items as advised by your instructor.*

Chapter Terms

allowable costs
ambulatory payment classifications (APCs)
anatomic site
behavior
case mix
case mix index (CMI)
charge capture and coding
chargemaster
claim submission
classification system
clinical documentation improvement (CDI)
clinical (medical) terminology
collections
comorbidities
compliance
complications
computer-assisted coding (CAC)
Current Procedural Terminology (CPT)
diagnosis-related group (DRG)
dictionary-driven encoder
disease index

downcoding
encoder software
encounter utilization review and case management
etiology
False Claims Act
fee-for-service
fraud
grade
Health Insurance Prospective Payment System (HIPPS)
Healthcare Common Procedure Coding System (HCPCS)
hospital-acquired conditions
index
International Classification of Diseases for Oncology, Third Edition (ICD-O-3)
International Classification of Diseases, Ninth Revision, Clinical Modification (ICD-9-CM)
International Classification of Diseases, Tenth Revision, Clinical Modification (ICD-10-CM)

International Classification of Diseases, Tenth Revision, Procedure Coding System (ICD-10-PCS)
logic-based encoder
Logical Observation Identifiers, Names, and Codes (LOINC)
master patient index (MPI)
medical necessity
morbidity
morphology
mortality
nomenclature
operations/procedures index
outliers
payment posting and appeals and collections
point of care
point of service registration counseling
present on admission (POA)
prospective payment system (PPS)
remittance processing and rejections
resource utilization group (RUG)
retrospective cost-based reimbursement
revenue cycle management
scheduling and preregistration
Systematized Nomenclature of Medicine—Clinical Terms (SNOMED CT)
third-party follow-up
topography
unbundling
upcoding
whistle-blower

> "Statistics: the only science that enables different experts using the same figures to draw different conclusions."
>
> —Evan Esar, American humorist

Think Ethics!

Using predictive analytics, researchers can now crunch data from millions of patients to determine, for example, which patients might respond best to certain therapies. However, the use of predictive modeling in health care raises ethical concerns as well. What if the analytical model suggests that a patient shouldn't receive treatment? And what about privacy? Should data crunchers have access to patient information without patient consent? Ethical questions like these often don't have easy answers.

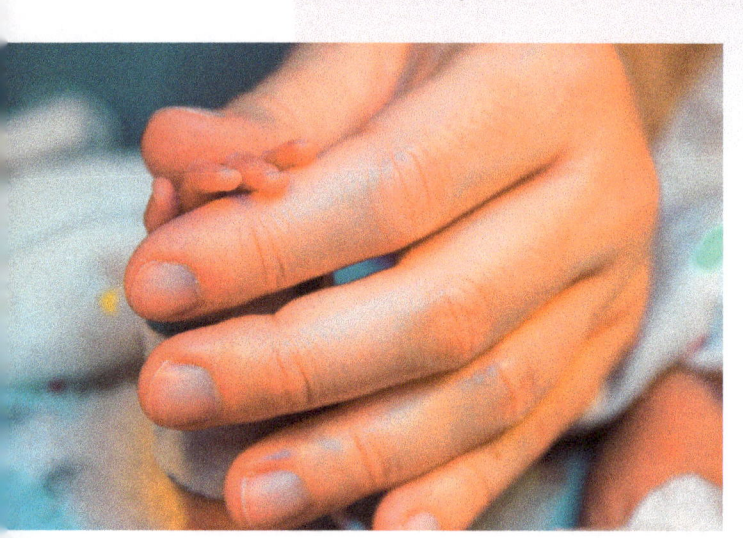

Future Trends: Big Data

With the adoption of the electronic health record, health information stored for decades is becoming useable, searchable, and actionable. Researchers are mining data to determine the most effective treatments and to identify patterns that can reduce hospital readmissions or drug side effects, and data-driven, clinical decision support systems put the best medical research at providers' fingertips.

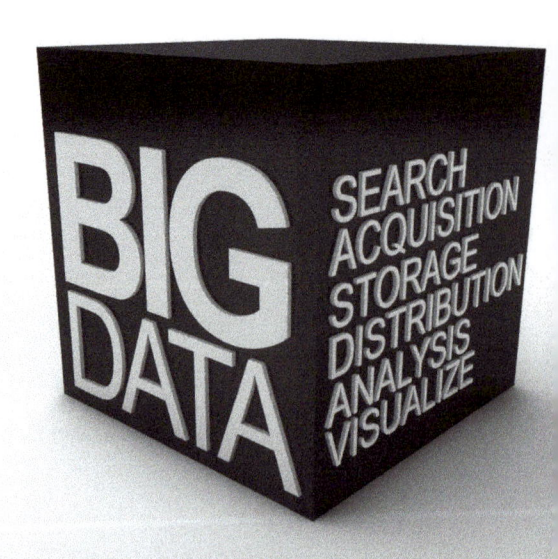

Chapter 10

Healthcare Statistics

> "Statistics is the science of learning from data, and of measuring, controlling, and communicating uncertainty."
>
> —Marie Davidian and Thomas A. Louis, "Why Statistics?" *Science*

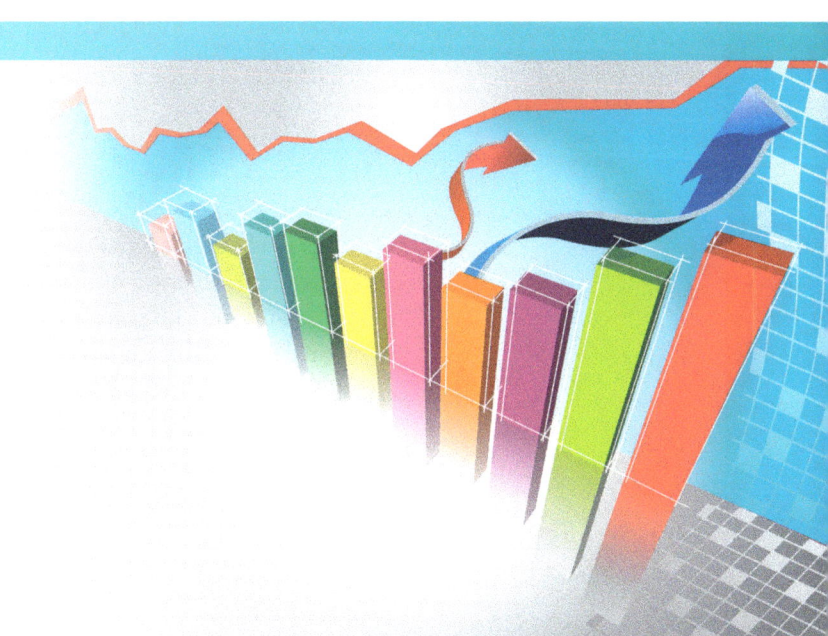

Fast Facts

The Indiana Health Information Exchange connects more than 90 hospitals, long-term care facilities, rehabilitation centers, community health clinics, and other healthcare providers across the state using a secure, standardized electronic format. This health information "superhighway" allows health information to follow the patient, and it gives the state's 25,000 providers access to the health information of millions of patients.

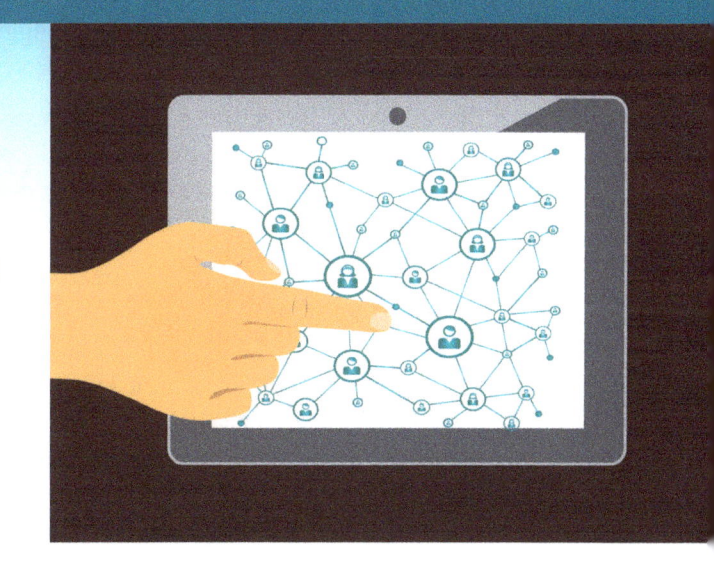

Learning Objectives

- Understand how statistics are used in health care.
- Explain the sources of data for compiling healthcare statistics.
- Understand basic statistical terms and commonly calculated statistics.
- Apply formulas for computing commonly used healthcare statistics.
- Know the appropriate methods of data display.
- Recognize how data is analyzed and used to support decision making.
- Explain vital statistics using examples.
- Understand the role of HIM professionals in healthcare research.

Statistics is a branch of mathematics that focuses on the collection, analysis, interpretation, and presentation of data. In general, statistics is a method of organizing large amounts of factual information (**data**) so that it can be more easily interpreted or compared. Health care is a data-driven field, and statistics hold the answers to many questions. Some questions are very broad. For example, data extrapolated from birth certificates can answer questions such as, *How many people were born in the United States last year?* (3,952,841 in 2012) or, *Is the number of teen births in the United States increasing or decreasing?* (decreasing).

Statistical Applications in Health Care

Statistics can be used to answer more detailed questions as well, such as determining the number and the success rate of procedures performed by an individual physician or a hospital, for example, or identifying what percentage of a hospital's patients are on Medicare and what percentage have private insurance.

Statistics can also be used to describe things. Compiling and analyzing information on people diagnosed with coronary heart disease, for example, can help to identify who is at greatest risk for the disease (in this case, smokers, individuals with high blood pressure and/or high cholesterol, and those who are overweight or obese).

Statistical information is also used as a basis for clinical and administrative decision making. If a hospital board of directors wants to know whether to recruit physicians with certain specialist credentials, such as neurosurgery or neonatology, they may look at data on the number of patients treated with these conditions, whether that number is increasing or decreasing, and the length of the trend to determine if the number of patients justifies recruiting the specialist to the area. If a physician wants to know if a specific treatment (e.g., laparoscopic surgery versus large surgical incisions) is more effective for one type of patient than another, she or he would likely look at the data on the length of stay for each patient group, incidence of infection, and complications related to both types of procedures. Physicians rely on statistical data to compare treatments and outcomes and to identify trends, such as an increase in the number of **nosocomial** (hospital-acquired) infections.

Reliability and Validity

Statistics are used in many ways, but not all statistics are equally reliable or valid. Therefore, it is important not to accept statistics at face value. Understanding how statistics are calculated is essential to recognizing whether statistical information is reliable and valid. Statistical measures are considered **reliable** when the same result is achieved on successive calculations. Statistics are **valid** if there is a sound basis in logic and if the statistics are accurate and relevant to the purpose for which they are used.

When evaluating statistical data, it is important to know where the data comes from, what information has been included and excluded, and how the statistics have been calculated and analyzed in order to recognize whether the data presented is "reasonable." Is the conclusion presented realistic in the context in which it is presented? Consider, for example, a statistic showing a community hospital having a mortality rate of 45 percent. Would you consider such a statistic reasonable? What about a hospital reporting a 2 percent occupancy rate, or a physician practice reporting two hours as the length of an average office visit? None of these statistics pass the test of reason. Death rates in hospitals are quite low (less than 4 percent); hospital occupancy needs to be between 64 and 75 percent for the facility to break even, and, depending on the type of physician, multiple studies indicate that the average face-to-face encounter between patient and physician lasts 15–20 minutes.

In health care, statistics help to determine methods of treatment, monitor care provided, and establish the need for services and other aspects of care.

Common Healthcare Statistics

Morbidity (incidence of disease) and **mortality** (death rates) are the most commonly computed healthcare statistics. Other common healthcare statistics include calculations of healthcare costs and the distribution of disease by demographic criteria (geographic area, ethnicity, gender, or socioeconomic status). **Vital statistics** are collected for births and deaths and provide information on population trends.

Individual practitioners or physician offices may also report healthcare statistics. Individual practitioners may report the number of patients seen per day, amount of time spent with patients, and patients' conditions reported by diagnostic code or payment source. Physician office reports may include patients sorted by diagnostic code, payment source, or age; the number of patients seen; or the number of return visits within a specific timeframe for the same condition. Every healthcare facility reports statistical information on practitioner-related events (e.g., acquired infections, complications, or length of stay for inpatients), outcomes (e.g., conditions improving or worsening, transfers to another facility for continued care, or complications), and services provided (e.g., surgeries, transfusions, or physical therapy).

Governmental and regulatory agencies compile statistical reports based on data from providers, hospitals, and other healthcare facilities. These reports are used to identify trends and compare outcomes. For example, statistical data is used to compare the average length of stay for a specific diagnosis at similar facilities or the types of services provided to patients with a specific diagnosis (e.g., the number of chest X-rays performed on patients with pneumonia). Governmental agencies gather statistical data on Medicare patients, which is used to set reimbursement rates and criteria for treatment based on such things as geographic area, cost of living, etc. The Joint Commission uses hospital performance data from accreditation activities to develop and support changes in performance standards to reflect current best practices.

Basic Statistical Terms and Calculations

To understand how data is used to create statistics it is necessary to become familiar with the terms that define the various statistical calculations. Some of the most commonly used terms are explained below.

Measures of Central Tendency

As the name implies, *measures of central tendency* are the methods used to determine the center of a group or a set of data in relation to the whole data group. The most common measures of central tendency are the mean, median, and mode. Each measure provides a different way of looking at the middle value in a range of data.

The **mean** of a group of numbers represents the mathematical average of that group. It is calculated by adding up all of the numbers in the group and then dividing that number by the quantity of numbers in the group. Calculating the mean is a useful and easy way to arrive at one number that is representative of the group as a whole. For example, if a hospital wanted to calculate the mean hospital stay for patients with pneumonia during the previous month, it would first run a computer query to abstract the data on the number of inpatient days for all patients with the diagnostic code for pneumonia. The list might look something like this:

Patient 1	7 days
Patient 2	5 days
Patient 3	8 days
Patient 4	2 days
Patient 5	4 days
Patient 6	6 days
Patient 7	7 days
Patient 8	25 days
Patient 9	7 days
Patient 10	6 days

To calculate the mean number of days in the hospital, add the inpatient days, and then divide the number by the number of patients.

$$\frac{77 \text{ days}}{10 \text{ patients}} = 7.7$$

The mean length of stay for this group of pneumonia patients is 7.7 days. The mean (average) is representative of the group.

The **median** is the number that falls in the middle of a set of numbers when the set is arranged in ascending or descending order. If the dataset contains an even number of items, the median is the middle point between the two middle numbers. To calculate the median from the list of inpatient stay days above, first organize the list of numbers in ascending order.

2 days

4 days

5 days

6 days

6 days

7 days

7 days

7 days

8 days

25 days

Because the list contains an even number of data points, the median falls in the middle of the two middle numbers: 6 and 7. Therefore, the median is 6.5.

Calculating the median is meaningful when there is an extremely deviating number (also referred to as an *outlier*), such as the 25-day length of stay in this list, which may **skew** (distort from a true mean value) the data when calculating the mean. In the case of the inpatient hospital stays presented here, the median is more representative of the group than the mean.

Mode is the value that occurs most frequently in a set of data. Looking at the lengths of stay data presented above, the mode is 7 because this is the number that appears most frequently in the dataset. The mode is useful when the most common item, characteristic, or value of a dataset is required.

Measures of Frequency

Many routine hospital statistics are reported as percentages. A **percentage** is the number of parts of 100. For example, a quarter is 25 percent of a dollar because a quarter equals 25 parts (cents) of a dollar (100 cents). Percentages can also be expressed as decimals or fractions (e.g., 25% = 0.25 = 25/100). Percentages are commonly calculated from a fraction. For example, if 12 of 25 patients in a hospital study on cancer are female, the number of female patients in the study expressed as a fraction is 12/25. To express this as a percentage, divide 12 by 25 and multiply by 100.

$$\frac{12}{25} = 0.48 \times 100 = 48\%$$

Hospital statistics expressed as percentages include death rates, infection rates, and percentage of occupancy.

Ratios provide a comparison between two numbers or quantities. A ratio is commonly displayed as two numbers separated by a colon. For example, if there are five credentialed coders and two noncredentialed coders in a health information management (HIM) department, the ratio of credentialed coders to noncredentialed coders is 5:2, which is read as "five to two."

Rate is a ratio that compares two quantities of different units of measure. Rate is often used to measure events over time. If the emergency department (ED) saw 250 patients a week and 40 of those patients were admitted to the hospital, the rate of ED admissions would be 40 patients per 250, or 40:250 when represented as a ratio. It is very common for percentages to be used in reporting healthcare statistics, so you need to be able to express a ratio as a percentage. One easy way to remember the formula for a rate expressed as a percentage is:

$$\frac{\text{the number of times something happened}}{\text{the number of times that it could have happened}} \times 100$$

Using the numbers from above,

$$\frac{40}{250} = 0.16$$

$$0.16 \times 100 = 16$$

The rate of ED patients admitted to the hospital is 16 percent.

Measures of Variation

Variability refers to the difference between a single value and every other value in a dataset. **Measures of variation** show the extent to which data points differ from each other or the spread of a group of numbers. The variation in a group of numbers may provide insight into why certain calculations resulted in certain numbers. One measure of variation is the **range**, which is the difference between the largest and the smallest values in a set of values. The range is an unrefined measure of spread. The range is most useful when there are extreme figures in the dataset.

Variation can also be seen on a **bell curve**, a symmetrical, bell-shaped line curve that represents a distribution of values, frequencies, or probabilities of a dataset. The mean value on a bell curve is the central point at the top of the curve. The sloping sides reflect the distribution of values above and below the mean. Aggregate data drawn from a large dataset tends to fall in the shape of the bell curve.

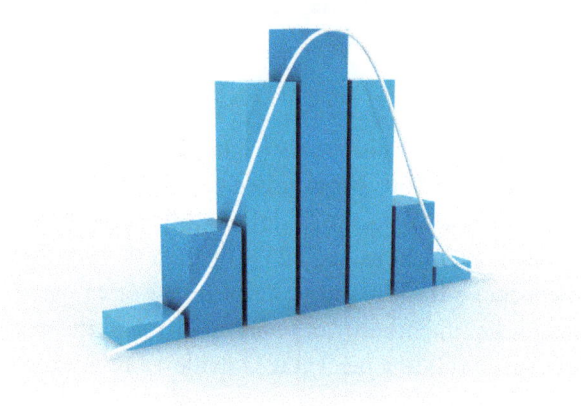

This bell curve provides a graphic representation of the distribution of data points in a set.

Standard deviation indicates how closely the data points (values) in a set of data are grouped around the mean. Standard deviation can be illustrated with a bell curve. In Example 10.1, the values of the blue line are clustered together, and the bell-shaped curve is steep. This indicates that the standard deviation is small. When the values are more spread apart, as depicted by the red line, the bell curve is flatter, and the standard deviation is greater. The standard deviation is useful when comparing values from different datasets to determine how diverse they are from one another.

Example 10.1 Standard Deviation

When the sides of the bell curve are steep, the standard deviation is smaller. When the curve is flatter, the standard deviation is greater.

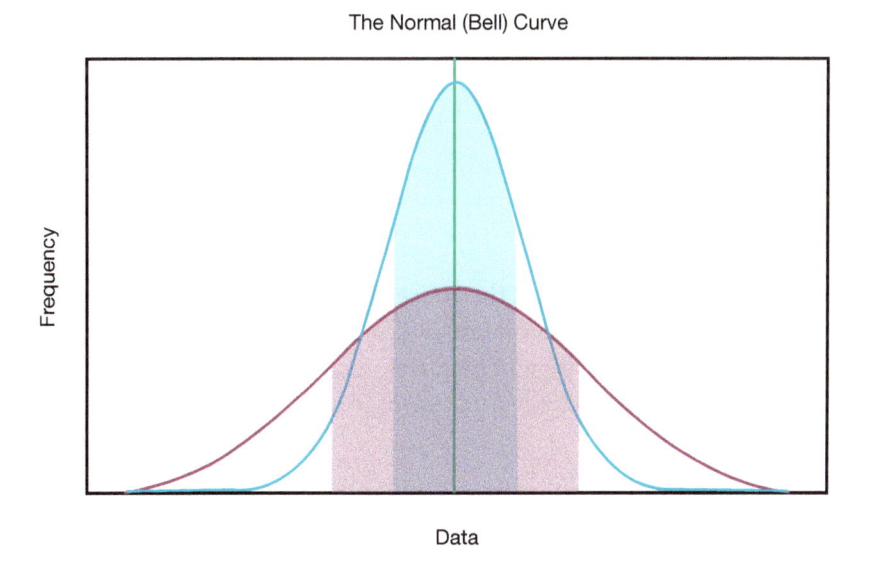

The Normal (Bell) Curve

Calculating Healthcare Statistics

The HIM department plays an important role in collecting, managing, analyzing, and disseminating healthcare data. An HIM professional needs to have a basic understanding of statistical principles and terminology and know how to identify and abstract the best available data. It is also important to understand how statistics are calculated and presented and be familiar with the routine statistical reports produced by a hospital or another healthcare facility. While there are many different computations that can be performed using patient data, some calculations are presented in monthly and yearly statistical reports.

Length of Stay

Length of stay (LOS) is the number of calendar days from the date of admission to the date of discharge. LOS is an important administrative statistic used to assess and manage facility resources, such as staffing for nursing care, housekeeping, and supplies. The data for this calculation comes from the **admission, discharge, and transfer (ADT) system**.

The **total length of stay**, also referred to as **discharge days**, is the sum of the lengths of stay for a group of inpatients discharged during a specific time period. The total lengths of stay may be compiled for all patients discharged, or it may be compiled for other identified groups—for example, by payment source (e.g., Medicare, Medicaid, private insurance, or self-pay), age group, final diagnosis, or physician.

To calculate the length of stay, subtract the date of admission from the date of discharge if both dates occur within the same month. Appropriate adjustments must be made when the stay extends past the end of a month. A one-day length of stay is assigned for a patient admitted and discharged within the same day, regardless of how long the patient was in the facility. A partial-day length of stay is never assigned.

For example, if a patient was admitted on May 28 and discharged on May 31, the LOS is three days (31 − 28 = 3). If the patient was admitted on May 28 and discharged on June 3, the LOS is six days (31 − 28 for the 3 days in May + the 3 days in June = 6 days). If the patient was admitted and discharged on May 28, a one-day length of stay is assigned.

> **! BE AWARE**
>
> When calculating length of stay, remember to make adjustments when a stay carries over from one month to another. Never assign a partial-day length of stay.

Average Length of Stay

The **average length of stay (ALOS)** is the average length of stay for all inpatients discharged during a specified period of time (e.g., a month or a year). Hospitals monitor the ALOS to assess the utilization of resources, such as beds, equipment, staff, and ancillary departments (emergency department, respiratory care, physical therapy, laboratory, etc.).

The ALOS is also one characteristic used to identify the patient population served. A facility's ALOS depends on the type of patients treated. In a hospital where a large percentage of the patient population is made up of mothers and newborns (NBs), the ALOS is probably fairly short—from one to three days. The majority of obstetric and NB patients do not stay in the hospital for very long. At a Level 1 trauma center that treats critically injured patients or at a hospital that provides psychiatric care, the ALOS would be much longer.

The ALOS is typically reported using two separate calculations: one for adult and child (A&C) patients and one for NB patients. These are very different patient types with different LOS. Calculating LOS for both groups together could distort the calculation.

Example 10.2 shows a sample ALOS calculation for adults and children. Example 10.3 shows a sample calculation of ALOS for newborns. In both cases, the number of total discharges includes deaths since death is a type of discharge.

To calculate the ALOS, divide the total patient discharge days by the number of patients discharged. Record the answer in days.

$$\frac{\text{discharge days}}{\text{total discharges (including deaths)}} = \text{ALOS}$$

Example 10.2 Adult and Children ALOS

A&C	9,588 discharges
	23,970 discharge days
	23,970/9,588 = 2.5

The ALOS for adults and children is 2.5 days.

Example 10.3 Newborn ALOS

NB (Live Births)	995 discharges
	1,895 discharge days
	1,895/995 = 1.9

The ALOS for newborns is 1.9 days.

Inpatient Census

The **inpatient census** is the number of inpatients present in the hospital at any one time. The inpatient census is also referred to as an *inpatient day*, *census day*, and *bed occupancy day*.

The inpatient census is monitored closely by hospital administration. When the census is very high, most of the hospital's beds are occupied, and there may be a concern that the hospital will not be able to accommodate new patients, especially intensive care or emergency surgery patients. In such circumstances, the hospital may need to move patients around or discharge patients who are healthy enough to go home or move to another type of care facility. When the census is low, especially if the census falls below the facility's financial break-even point, the hospital may have to temporarily reduce staffing levels.

To calculate the inpatient census, take the number of patients in the facility at the time the census was taken (at the end of the previous day), add the number of patients admitted during the census period, and then subtract the number of patients discharged during the census period. The result is the number of patients in the facility at the end of the day. This calculation is the first step in a series of calculations and is not included in statistical reports.

      number of patients in the facility at the beginning of the census period

+   number of patients admitted during the census period

−   number of patients discharged at the end of the census period

=   census at the end of the census period

Daily Inpatient Census

The **daily inpatient census** is the number of inpatients present in the facility at the time the census is taken, plus any inpatients who were admitted and discharged the same day but are not present when the census is taken. It is important to conduct the census at the same time each day. Most facilities conduct the census at 12 a.m. because it is the beginning and the end of the calendar day and is also a less active time in the facility when fewer patients are admitted or discharged. (The nursing staff sometimes performs a physical "head count" of each unit. The patient count is reported to the designated department so that any adjustments in admissions and discharges can be added or deleted to the ADT system and included in the census report.)

It is essential that the daily census provides an accurate patient count so that the HIM department can identify discharged patient records in the ADT system. When a patient is discharged, the patient's chart is processed and checked to see if all documentation is there, all signatures completed, etc. If the record is incomplete, it is flagged, and the person responsible for the missing document or documentation is notified that the record is incomplete. Transcribed reports and diagnostic test results continue to be generated after the patient is discharged and need to be incorporated into the chart at a later date.

To calculate the daily inpatient census, take the number of patients from the previous daily census, add the number of patients admitted during the previous 24 hours, and then subtract the number of patients discharged during the same one-day period. Finally, add the number of patients admitted and discharged within the 24-hour period. The step of adding the number of patients both admitted and discharged within the same day is necessary to capture their presence in the hospital since these patients are not present during the census-taking time period.

To calculate the daily inpatient census:

> number of patients in the facility at the beginning of the one-day period
- \+ number of patients admitted during the one-day period
- − number of patients discharged at the end of the one-day period
- \+ number of patients admitted and discharged within one day
- = daily inpatient census at the end of the one-day period

Remember, the inpatient census counts the number of inpatients at a given time and is conducted at the same time each day; the daily inpatient census includes the inpatient census plus all patients admitted and discharged within the 24-hour period.

Inpatient Service Day

An **inpatient service day** is a measure of the services provided to one patient in one 24-hour period—from census-taking time to census-taking time. The inpatient service day is also referred to as an *inpatient day, census day,* and *bed occupancy day*. **Total inpatient service days** refers to the sum of all inpatient service days during a select period.

The number of inpatient service days is equal to the daily inpatient census. There is no calculation for determining the inpatient service days. The rationale behind having these two separate numbers is that one indicates the number of patients (census) and the other number indicates the days of service provided (inpatient service days). As shown in Example 10.4, for every patient counted in the daily inpatient census, the hospital counts a day of service.

Example 10.4 Inpatient Days of Service

318 A&C daily inpatient census (patients) = 318 A&C inpatient days of service

59 NB daily inpatient census = 59 NB inpatient days of service

It is important to remember that the daily inpatient census must be used when a patient is both admitted and discharged within the same census day but not present at the census-taking hour to account for the service provided to that patient.

Average Daily Census

The **average daily census (ADC)** reflects the average number of inpatients present each day during specified periods of time (e.g., a month or a year). To calculate the average daily census, divide the total number of inpatient service days for the selected period by the total number of days in that period.

$$\frac{\text{total inpatient service days for a specified period}}{\text{total number of days in the period}} = \text{ADC}$$

For the ADC calculation to be meaningful, you must know the number of beds licensed in the facility. If a report indicates that a hospital's ADC is 243, there is no way to know if that number is high or low without knowing the total number of available beds. If the ADC is 243 and the hospital has 275 beds, it shows the ADC is relatively high given the size of the facility.

When calculating the ADC, remember to record the answer in terms of patients. Example 10.5, shows the calculations for the average daily census at Good Health Hospital during a one-year period. Remember, the ADCs for adults and children and for newborn patients are generally reported separately.

Example 10.5 Average Daily Census

There are 200 beds and 30 newborn beds in this facility.
The calculation is for one year (365 days).

Adults and Children $\dfrac{67{,}106 \text{ days}}{365} = 184$

Newborn $\dfrac{4{,}478 \text{ days}}{365} = 12$

The Average Daily Census is 184 A&C patients and 12 NB patients.

Percentage of Occupancy

Percentage of occupancy calculates what percentage of the facility's inpatient beds are occupied. Percentage of occupancy is based on the average daily census but presents the information in an easy-to-understand format that does not require the user to know the total number of beds in the facility. The percentage of occupancy is primarily an administrative statistic used to monitor bed utilization.

To calculate the percentage of occupancy, multiply the total inpatient days for the period by 100 (to convert to a percentage), and then divide by the total inpatient bed-count days for the period.

$$\frac{\text{total inpatient days for a period} \times 100}{\text{total inpatient bed count days for the time period}}$$

To calculate the number of bed count days, multiply the number of beds in the facility by the number of days in the specified time period. The number of bed count days reflects the facility's total capacity during the time period if each bed was filled. It should be noted that the bed capacity can change up or down during the time period. This will impact calculation of the occupancy rate. Example 10.6 shows how to calculate the percentage of occupancy for a 200-bed hospital during a one-year period.

Example 10.6 Percentage of Occupancy

Calculate the number of bed count days for the year.

total number of beds (200 beds) × 365 days = the total bed count days for adults and children (73,000)

Calculate the percentage of occupancy.

$$\frac{67{,}100 \text{ inpatient days for the period} \times 100}{73{,}000 \text{ bed count days for the period}}$$

$$\frac{6{,}710{,}000}{73{,}000} = 91.9\%$$

The percentage of occupancy is 92 percent.

TAKE THE CHALLENGE

As discussed previously, measuring variability is helpful in explaining statistics when the dataset contains extremely deviating values that can affect the statistical outcome. Table 10.1 displays lengths of stay for a group of patients at Good Health Hospital.

A hospital's ALOS is used as a **benchmark**, a standard or a reference point for comparison or assessment. Private insurers and the Centers for Medicare & Medicaid Services (CMS) monitor these numbers and may question a hospital with longer lengths of stay. If the LOS for a patient is too far outside the norm, the payer may refuse to reimburse the cost of care. Internally, hospitals monitor and evaluate ALOS numbers to identify trends: stays that are longer for certain diagnoses or for patients of specific providers. If the ALOS is shorter than other facilities, the hospital may be sending patients home too soon. In that case, the hospital may review readmission rates for the same diagnosis. Table 10.1 illustrates the LOS data for a group of patients. In the example, the first line shows 10 patients and each had a one-day LOS, and the total length of stay (10 days) for this group of 10 patients.

Table 10.1 Length of Stay Data for a Group of Patients

Length of Stay in the Hospital	Number of Patients with This LOS	Total Length of Stay for LOS and Number of Patients
1 day	10	10
2 days	16	32
3 days	15	45
4 days	22	88
5 days	15	75
6 days	3	18
10 days	5	50
234 days	1	234
	87 total patients	552 total days for all patients

Notice that the last entry on the chart indicates one patient stay of 234 days. While these situations do not happen frequently, they do occur. A patient may be too acutely ill to be in a long-term care or other type of extended stay environment (e.g., a patient waiting for an organ transplant, an infant born significantly prematurely, or a patient with extensive traumatic injuries from an accident).

For this challenge, it is your job as the HIM data analyst to calculate the ALOS and be able to explain the statistics to the hospital's board of directors.

First, calculate the ALOS for this group of patients.

Next, calculate the ALOS when the outlier is removed from the equation.

Finally, explain why the hospital should calculate the ALOS first by including the total LOS and then by leaving out the deviating figure.

Death Rates

Death is one outcome of care, and hospitals expect that some patients will die. A hospital's medical staff and quality of care committees review the number of and the causes of inpatient deaths to look for trends and unexplained increases (e.g., a spike in deaths among patients with a specific diagnosis or undergoing a particular procedure). If warranted, a death may undergo additional review to determine if the patient received the appropriate care and whether there is a need to improve care.

Gross Death Rate

To calculate the **gross death rate** (rate of discharges as a result of a death) multiply the number of inpatient deaths by 100, and then divide that number by the total number of discharges during the period (including deaths). The gross death rate is expressed as a percentage. As shown in Example 10.7, death rates for NBs and A&C are calculated together. The number of discharges includes deaths.

$$\frac{\text{number of deaths of inpatients in a period} \times 100}{\text{number of discharges (including deaths)}}$$

Example 10.7   Gross Death Rate

100 A&C deaths + 25 NB deaths for the year × 100 = 12,500

9,588 A&C discharges + 995 NB discharges = 10,583

$$\frac{12{,}500}{10{,}583} = 1.18$$

The gross death rate is 1 percent.

Net Death Rate

Facilities calculate the **net death rate** to determine the number of patient deaths that occur more than 48 hours after admission. If a patient dies within the first 48 hours, the cause of death is more likely to be a severe illness or condition and not the result of care provided. Hospital committees also monitor the net death rate.

To calculate the net death rate, first subtract the number of patient deaths occurring within the first 48 hours of hospitalization from the total number of inpatient deaths during the select period. Multiply the result by 100. Next, subtract the number of deaths occurring within the first 48 hours from the number of discharges (including deaths). Finally, divide the top number by the bottom number. As shown in Example 10.8, express the answer as a percentage.

$$\frac{\text{number of deaths of inpatients} - \text{deaths within the first 48 hours} \times 100}{\text{number of discharges (including deaths)} - \text{deaths within the first 48 hours}}$$

Example 10.8   Net Death Rate

$$100 \text{ A\&C deaths} + 25 \text{ NB deaths} - 26 \text{ deaths within 48 hours} \times 100 = 9{,}900$$

$$9{,}588 \text{ A\&C discharges} + 995 \text{ NB discharges} - 26 \text{ deaths within 48 hours} = 10{,}557$$

$$\frac{9{,}900}{10{,}557} = 0.9$$

The net death rate is 1 percent.

Remember to subtract deaths occurring within the first 48 hours from both the numerator and the denominator.

Fetal Death Rate

A *fetal death* is the spontaneous intrauterine death of a fetus at any time during pregnancy. The **fetal death rate** is calculated to determine the percentage of all births that result in fetal death.

Intermediate and late fetal deaths (20 weeks or more of gestation) are most commonly used for this calculation. State laws require hospitals to report fetal deaths, and federal law mandates the national collection of fetal death data.

To calculate the fetal death rate, first multiply the number of fetal deaths by 100. Then, add together the total number of live births and the number of fetal deaths. Divide the number of fetal deaths by the combined number. As shown in Example 10.9, the answer is expressed as a percentage.

$$\frac{\text{intermediate and late fetal deaths} \times 100}{\text{total live births} + \text{intermediate and late fetal deaths}}$$

Example 10.9   Fetal Death Rate

$$31 \text{ intermediate and late fetal deaths} \times 100 = 3{,}100$$

$$1{,}000 \text{ live births} + 31 \text{ fetal deaths} = 1{,}031$$

$$\frac{3{,}100}{1{,}031} = 3$$

The fetal death rate is 3 percent.

For this calculation, it is important to remember to add the number of fetal deaths to the number of live births to get the total number of births. A fetal death is not a live birth so it is not reflected in that number.

Maternal Death Rate

A **maternal death** is a death of the mother directly linked to or exacerbated by pregnancy. Direct maternal deaths result from complications during pregnancy, labor, or the *puerperium* (within six weeks of delivery). The maternal death-rate statistic is calculated to review the outcome of care. Maternal death rates are generally very low—less than 1 percent when there are any at all. The study of maternal deaths may help to identify the causes of maternal death. Tracking maternal deaths also provides information on other issues that may impact patient health, such as the prevalent age when maternal deaths occur, the presence or the absence of prenatal care, and other factors that could be addressed to reduce the number of maternal deaths.

To calculate the **maternal death rate**, multiply the number of maternal deaths by 100, and then add the number of obstetric discharges including the number of maternal deaths. Divide the first number by the second. As Example 10.10 shows, the answer is expressed as a percentage.

$$\frac{\text{total direct maternal deaths} \times 100}{\text{the total number of obstetric (OB) discharges} + \text{maternal deaths}}$$

Example 10.10 Maternal Death Rate

$$1 \text{ direct maternal death} \times 100 = 100$$

$$1{,}050 \text{ OB discharges} + 1 \text{ maternal death} = 1{,}051$$

$$\frac{100}{1{,}051} = 0.09$$

The maternal death rate is 0.09 percent.

Only direct maternal deaths are included in the statistical calculation. Deaths due to accidents or other medical conditions during pregnancy are not included in the maternal death rate.

Anesthesia Death Rate

Hospitals evaluate patients before surgery to determine if the use of anesthesia could put the patient at risk and if steps should be taken to mitigate that risk. The **anesthesia death rate** shows the number of deaths directly attributable to anesthesia. Hospitals generally have very few, if any, anesthesia-related deaths.

To calculate the anesthesia death rate, multiply the number of anesthesia deaths by 100, and then divide by the number of times anesthesia was administered. Express the rate as a percentage (see Example 10.11).

$$\frac{\text{number of anesthesia deaths} \times 100}{\text{number of anesthesia administrations}}$$

Example 10.11 Anesthesia Death Rate

$$\frac{1 \text{ anesthesia death} \times 100}{4{,}873 \text{ anesthesia administrations}} = 100$$

$$\frac{100}{4{,}873} = 0.02$$

The anesthesia death rate is 0.02 percent.

It is important to remember to calculate the rate using the number of anesthesia administrations, not the number of patients who received anesthesia because some patients receive anesthesia more than once.

Postoperative Death Rate

The **postoperative death rate** refers to deaths that occur after a surgical procedure and within 10 days of the procedure. Deaths occurring more than 10 days after a surgical procedure are not included in the calculation because other factors may have contributed to the death.

To calculate the postoperative death rate, multiply the number of deaths occurring within 10 days of surgery by 100, and then divide the total by the number of operations performed. The postoperative death rate is expressed as a percentage (see Example 10.12).

$$\frac{\text{number of deaths within 10 days of surgery} \times 100}{\text{number of operations performed}}$$

Example 10.12 Postoperative Death Rate

$$\frac{12 \text{ postoperative deaths} \times 100}{5{,}620 \text{ operations performed}} = 1{,}200$$

$$\frac{1{,}200}{5{,}620} = 0.21$$

The postoperative death rate is 0.2 percent.

Be sure to calculate the rate using the number of surgical procedures performed, not the number of patients operated on.

> **BE AWARE**
>
> Always check statistical calculations for accuracy by recalculating some statistics or by having someone else spot-check your calculations. It is also a good idea to compare statistics against the norm (death rates are low, percentage of occupancy is high, etc.). If your calculation is far from the norm, double-check the math.

Autopsy Rates

An *autopsy* is a postmortem (after death) medical examination of a body. Hospitals conduct autopsies on patients who died in the hospital for a number of reasons: to determine the cause of death for the family, the death certificate, and the patient record; for educational purposes; and for research. Autopsies are performed in a hospital if facilities are available for that purpose. If not, the autopsy may be done by a hospital's pathologist at a funeral home or at another hospital. Teaching hospitals generally have a higher autopsy rate because autopsies are an important instructional tool. In a nonteaching hospital, the autopsy rate is generally less than 10 percent. In an academic medical center, the rate may be 25–40 percent.

Autopsy rates are calculated in a number of ways, depending on whether the person who died was treated as an inpatient or an outpatient and whether the autopsy was conducted by a member of the hospital medical staff or as a part of a law enforcement investigation. All calculations are comparisons of deaths occurring within the same timeframe.

Gross Autopsy Rate

The **gross autopsy rate** is used to compare the number of autopsies conducted by hospital medical staff to the number of inpatient deaths. To calculate the gross autopsy rate, multiply the number of inpatient autopsies by 100. Divide the total by the number of inpatient deaths. As shown in Example 10.13, the answer is expressed as a percentage.

$$\frac{\text{number of inpatient autopsies} \times 100}{\text{number of inpatient deaths}}$$

Example 10.13   Gross Autopsy Rate

$$31 \text{ inpatient autopsies performed} \times 100 = 3{,}100$$

$$\text{inpatient deaths} = 125$$

$$\frac{3{,}100}{125} = 24.8$$

The gross autopsy rate is 25 percent.

Net Autopsy Rate

There are times when a coroner or a medical examiner performs the autopsy of a deceased hospital inpatient—most often if the cause of death is suspicious or if the death could be the result of a criminal act. In these cases, a law enforcement official, (a coroner or a medical examiner) conducts the autopsy to determine the cause of death and to identify and preserve potential *forensic evidence* (physical evidence related to the crime). When an autopsy is conducted by a county coroner or a medical examiner (ME), that body is not available for the hospital staff to autopsy and is not counted in the hospital's net autopsy rate.

To calculate the **net autopsy rate**, multiply the number of inpatient autopsies conducted during the time period by 100. Then, subtract the number of autopsies conducted by a coroner or a medical examiner from the total number of inpatient deaths. Divide the first number by the second. As Example 10.14 shows, the answer is expressed as a percentage.

$$\frac{\text{the number of inpatient autopsies for the time period} \times 100}{\text{the number of inpatient deaths} - \text{coroner/ME autopsies (bodies available for autopsy)}}$$

Example 10.14 Net Autopsy Rate

$$31 \text{ inpatient autopsies} \times 100 = 3{,}100$$

$$125 \text{ inpatient deaths} - 5 \text{ coroner/ME autopsies} = 120$$

$$\frac{3{,}100}{120} = 25.83$$

The net autopsy rate is 26 percent.

Notice that the net autopsy rate is higher than the gross autopsy rate. Subtracting the number of autopsies conducted by the coroner and the medical examiner better reflects the activity of the hospital personnel.

Hospital Autopsy Rate

A hospital pathologist or a medical staff member performs an autopsy of patients who died during a hospital stay. However, hospital staff may also autopsy former patients who died outside of the hospital and whose bodies are made available for autopsy. The **hospital autopsy rate** calculates the total number of autopsies done by hospital staff.

To calculate the hospital autopsy rate, multiply the total number of inpatient (IP) and outpatient (OP) autopsies by 100. Divide the result by the total number of IP and OP bodies available for autopsy during the same period. Calculate the number of OP bodies available for autopsy by adding the number of IP deaths and the number of OP deaths and subtracting the number of autopsies conducted by the coroner/ME. As shown in Example 10.15, the answer is expressed as a percentage.

$$\frac{\text{number of hospital (IP and OP) autopsies} \times 100}{\text{total number of bodies available for autopsy}}$$

Example 10.15 Hospital Autopsy Rate

$$31 \text{ IP} + 3 \text{ OP autopsies} \times 100 = 3{,}400$$

$$125 \text{ IP deaths} + 3 \text{ OP deaths} - 5 \text{ coroner/ME cases} = 123$$

$$\frac{3{,}400}{123} = 27.64$$

The hospital autopsy rate is 28 percent.

The hospital autopsy rate is higher than the autopsy rates in previous calculations. This higher number is the true reflection of the number of autopsies performed by the hospital pathologist and the medical staff. Remember that autopsy rates reflect physician activity in the performance of autopsies. A higher number is considered positive. Teaching facilities must be able to provide this educational experience for medical students.

Other Statistical Calculations

There are many statistics derived from information contained in the patient record. The calculations explained in this chapter are the most common statistics hospitals calculate on a monthly or yearly basis. Statistical reports are distributed internally to hospital administration, medical staff, and department leaders for review and for use in planning, monitoring care, and understanding the facility. Some statistical measures are reported to licensing and accrediting entities, educational organizations, third-party payers, and governmental entities.

Internal and external groups (hospital administration, medical staff, accrediting organizations, third-party payers, etc.) may sometimes request additional statistical analysis on an as-needed basis. For example, a regional health-planning agency may ask for a report of patients by county of residence. A state birth registry may request data on congenital anomalies present at birth. A hospital administrator may want to review lengths of stay for common operative procedures or information on patient morbidity, including the nosocomial infections by type of infection, final diagnosis, and location in the hospital. Review of data on morbidity, the state of disease of patients in a healthcare facility, is an important component of quality management.

> **BE AWARE**
>
> As reported in the *Journal of Patient Safety*, the third leading cause of death in the United States is death from preventable medical errors. As many as 440,000 such deaths are reported each year. A number of healthcare agencies, including the Centers for Disease Control and Prevention (CDC), have made reducing the number of HAIs a top priority.

Nosocomial Infection Rate

Many patients are admitted to the hospital with existing infections. However, some patients develop an infection in the hospital. The **nosocomial infection rate** indicates the number of patients who acquired an infection while in the hospital compared to the total patient population. Knowing the nosocomial infection rate is essential to providing high-quality care.

To calculate the nosocomial infection rate, multiply the number of hospital-acquired infections (HAIs) during the specified period by 100, and then divide that number by the total number of hospital discharges during the same period. As Example 10.16 shows, the rate is expressed as a percentage.

$$\frac{\text{number of nosocomial infections} \times 100}{\text{total number of patients discharged}}$$

Example 10.16 Nosocomial Infection Rates

$$\frac{19 \text{ nosocomial infections} \times 100}{799 \text{ A\&C discharges}} = 1{,}900$$

$$\frac{1{,}900}{799} = 2.38$$

The hospital's nosocomial infection rate is 2.4 percent.

It is important to remember that only nosocomial infections are counted in this rate. Nosocomial infections occur in all hospitals, but the rate of HAIs should be below 10 percent of the patients discharged. The World Health Organization (WHO) reports that the nosocomial, or hospital-acquired, infection rate is 7 percent in developed countries and 10 percent in developing countries.

Consultation Rate

During an inpatient hospital stay, the attending physician may ask another physician to examine the patient health record and the patient and provide an opinion or a treatment recommendation in a written report. This is referred to as a **consultation**. Consultations can be valuable, but the practice may also be abused. The overuse of physician consultations increases the cost of care, so knowing the facility's consultation rate is an important factor in controlling costs. The use of consultants depends on the facility, patient population, conditions treated at the facility, and types of physicians available to consult.

To calculate the **consultation rate**, multiply the number of patients who received consultation by 100. Divide that number by the number of patients discharged. The consultation rate is given as a percentage (see Example 10.17).

$$\frac{\text{number of patients receiving consultation} \times 100}{\text{number of patients discharged}}$$

Example 10.17 Consultation Rate

646 patients receiving consultation for the year × 100 = 64,600

A&C discharges for the year = 9,588

$$\frac{64,600}{9,588} = 6.74$$

The hospital's consultation rate is 6.7 percent.

When calculating the consultation rate, it is important to use the number of patients who received consultations, not the number of individual consults performed (as one patient may have multiple consultations).

Data Display and Presentation

Translating data into graphs and charts is one way to make statistics more meaningful and easier to understand. However, not all graphic tools are equal. Tables, bar charts, pie charts, histograms, and line graphs are best used for presenting specific types of data. The most commonly used methods for displaying data are discussed here along with recommendations on the best use for each.

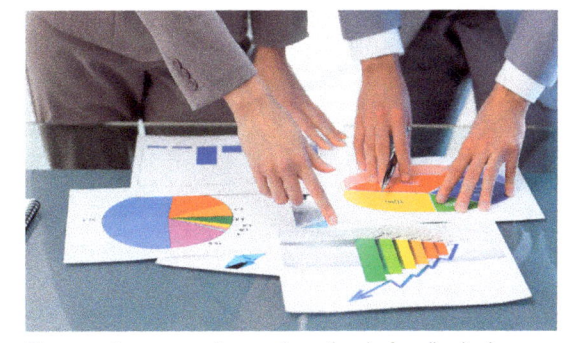

The most commonly used methods for displaying data include tables, bar charts, pie charts, histograms, and line graphs.

Chapter 10 Healthcare Statistics

293

Data Table

A *table* is used to visually display numbers and/or words organized on a grid. A table is most appropriate for presenting exact numbers, comparisons, or correlations in rows and columns. As Table 10.2 shows, a **frequency distribution table** may be used to show numerical ranges rather than individual numbers.

Table 10.2 A Bar Graph Displays Data on a Grid

Patient Age	Number of Inpatients
Under 16	98
16–34	34
35–49	107
50–64	238
65 and over	393
Total	**870**

By displaying patients by age range, it is easy to see in which age group the largest number of patients falls. Almost half of the 870 patients are age 65 and older. Certain illnesses are common among this group, such as pneumonia, congestive heart failure, and complications of chronic and comorbid conditions. Knowing how many patients are in this group helps the hospital administration and medical staff plan for the most beneficial utilization of hospital beds, staffing, and other needed services.

Bar Chart

Data is either **discrete data**, meaning it has finite values such as the number of days or the number of tests, or it is **continuous data**, meaning it is measured on a continuous scale with an indefinite number of points along a continuum. Examples of continuous data include height and weight. Different types of data display should be used when displaying discrete and continuous data.

A *bar chart*, also called a *bar graph*, displays data as horizontal or vertical bars. Bar charts are used to present categories of discrete data. Example 10.18 shows how a bar chart can be used to show, by diagnosis, the number of patients who had a breast mass surgically removed.

Example 10.18 A Bar Chart Presents Discrete Data

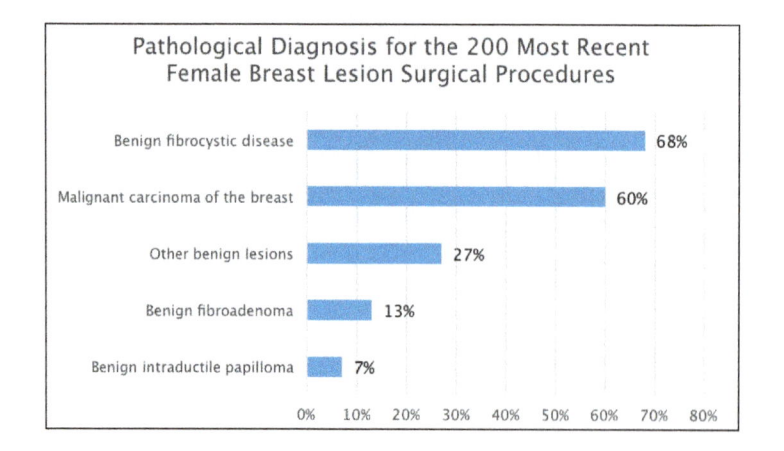

Pathological Diagnosis for the 200 Most Recent Female Breast Lesion Surgical Procedures

Diagnosis	Percentage
Benign fibrocystic disease	68%
Malignant carcinoma of the breast	60%
Other benign lesions	27%
Benign fibroadenoma	13%
Benign intraductile papilloma	7%

This type of graph is useful for comparing data so that the frequency of something—in this case, breast lesion surgical procedures—is easily observable and the actual number of occurrences can be easily read.

Histogram

A *histogram* is a way to represent a frequency distribution of continuous data. Although Example 10.19 displays the percentage of occupancy by month for a single year, the graph could be expanded to show the same data continuously over several years. A histogram often shows the bars touching to reflect the continuous nature of the data.

Example 10.19   A Histogram Displays Continuous Data

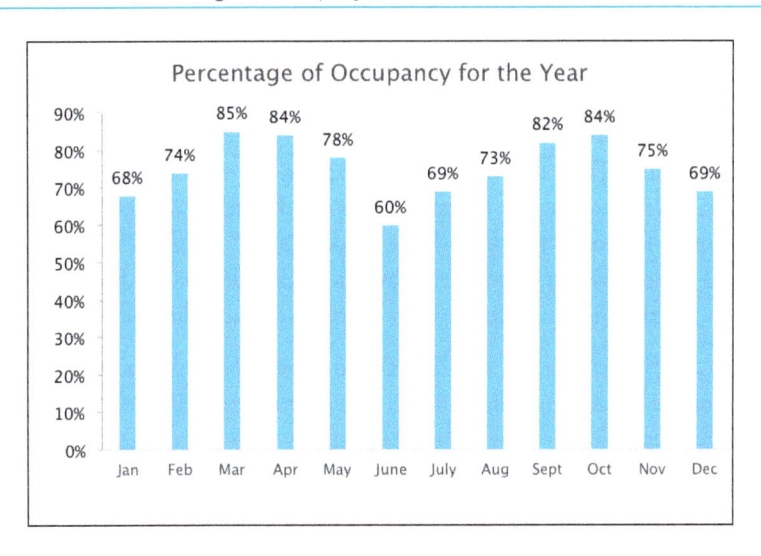

Percentage of Occupancy for the Year

Month	%
Jan	68%
Feb	74%
Mar	85%
Apr	84%
May	78%
June	60%
July	69%
Aug	73%
Sept	82%
Oct	84%
Nov	75%
Dec	69%

In reviewing this data, hospital administrators might question why the patient census is lower in June and whether the June numbers are just an anomaly or if June typically has a low census due to fewer seasonal illnesses or some other issue.

Line Graph

A *line graph* presents data points plotted over time, most often connected by a straight line. This type of data display is effective for showing similar data over time. Example 10.20 compares nosocomial infection rates at the same hospital in 2015 and 2016. The data points represent monthly infection rates.

The use of a line graph makes it easy to compare similar data over the same time period. This example, which shows infection rates for each month, makes it easy to compare data month to month and to identify trends, such as the spike in infection rates in February of both years.

Example 10.20 A Line Graph Displays Similar Data Over Time

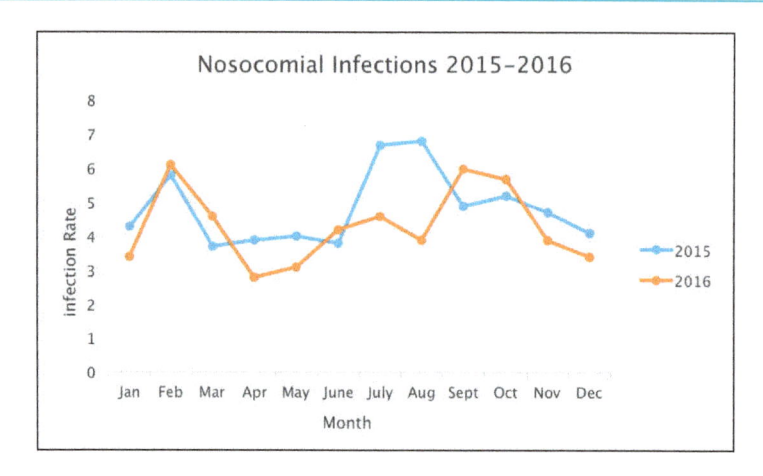

Nosocomial Infections 2015–2016 (line graph showing infection rate by month for 2015 and 2016)

Pie Chart

A pie chart looks just like it sounds—like a pie divided into slices. In a *pie chart*, data is displayed in a way that shows the relationship of different segments of data to the whole. Data must be percentages. Each "piece of the pie" illustrates a percentage of the whole (100 percent). The pie chart shown in Example 10.21 identifies hospital patients by payment source. Note the clear labeling of each slice of the pie.

A pie chart is an effective way to display data to show relationships and to emphasize one or more of the values. In this example, it is easy to see that Medicare is the payment source for nearly half of the hospital's patients. This information could have an impact on hospital budgeting because the Medicare prospective payment system caps reimbursement for medical care.

By drilling down into the data, the hospital administrator could review the data on the most common diagnoses for this group of patients and look at the average number of patients for each diagnosis. Such information would help the hospital to develop income projections from this group of patients for budgeting purposes. The same review could be done for privately insured patients, the next largest patient group.

Example 10.21 A Pie Chart Shows the Relationship of Segments to the Whole

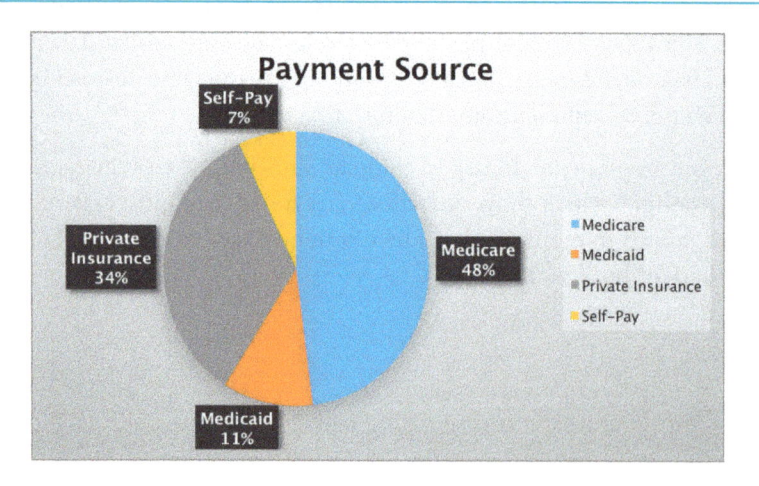

Payment Source pie chart: Medicare 48%, Private Insurance 34%, Medicaid 11%, Self-Pay 7%

Analytics and Decision Support

Analytics is defined as the systematic analysis of data or statistics and as the identification and communication of significant patterns in data. A **decision support system (DSS)** is an interactive computer application that generates data to facilitate decision making. The use of DSSs is relatively new, and management of these systems falls largely under the jurisdiction of the informatics department in facilities that have such a department.

The HIM department typically interacts with the DSS to make sure the appropriate data (real time and retrospective) is available to meet the information needs of the facility. As HIM experts, the HIM department has a comprehensive and thorough understanding of the statistical needs of the facility, where the information comes from, and how the statistics are calculated.

Information commonly generated by DSS software includes:

- comparative utilization data (e.g., the number of patients in the hospital or the number of services provided by day or week)

- business projections (e.g., revenue projections based on LOS data)

- evaluations of treatment options based on clinical data (e.g., recovery times for invasive surgery versus laparoscopic surgery)

- comparison data before and after process change (e.g., the impact of changing ED staffing patterns on wait times)

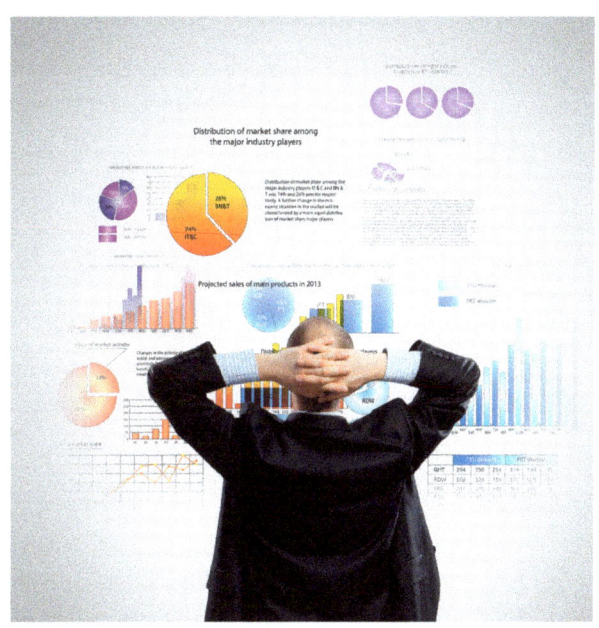

Calculating and displaying statistics can be informative, but the next and most important step is to analyze what the statistics mean for your healthcare facility.

Trend Analysis

Trend analysis is the process of collecting and analyzing data to identify patterns or trends over time. Trend analysis can be applied to historical data to predict future outcomes by comparing the same data—for example, data on the utilization of hospital outpatient services—over several years to identify patterns or relationships between variables. A trend analysis may show how new treatment technologies or changing patient-population demographics could increase or decrease the future utilization of hospital outpatient services. Trend data can be presented in graphic format as a trend line (a line chart) that displays the general pattern of the projected change.

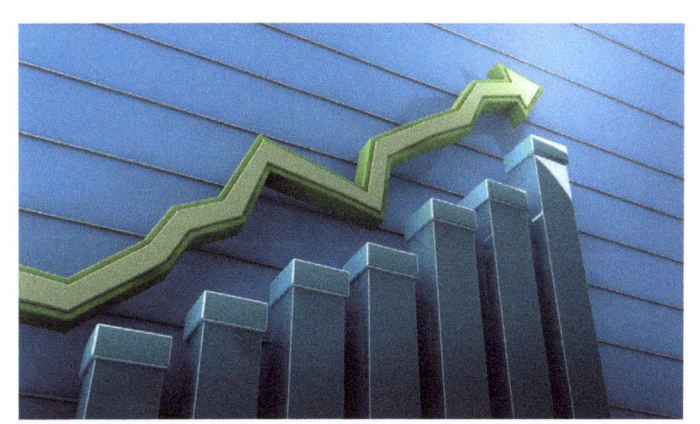

When a trend or a pattern is identified, trend analysis can be used to determine what factors are driving the trend, if the trend will continue, and what impact the trend may have on the organization.

Chapter 10 Healthcare Statistics

One example of a current trend impacting hospitals is the increase in freestanding treatment centers that provide care and services, such as outpatient surgery and long-term acute care, which were at one time only available in hospital settings. Advances in medical technologies and equipment are making it possible to provide even more services on an outpatient basis, and, eventually, reimbursement may no longer cover some services provided in an inpatient setting.

Some areas in health care where trend analysis will become very important include reimbursement, electronic health record (EHR) adoption, preventive care, and new and evolving patient-provider relationships.

- Reimbursement is beginning to move from a fee-for-service model (payment for each service provided) to models that pay for quality and efficiency.
- EHRs are integrating patient care across healthcare providers and organizations and allowing for better information sharing between providers, practitioners, and the population as a whole.
- There is a growing emphasis on patient-provider collaboration on preventive care to improve health outcomes.
- Developing new ways to strengthen patient-practitioner relationships is becoming increasingly vital to the financial success of the practitioner.

Vital Statistics

In health care, vital statistics refers to the critical life events of birth and death. Healthcare facilities are responsible for facilitating the completion of birth, death, and fetal death certificates. Some of the information required for birth certificates is available in the patient record and the HIM department is responsible many times for providing information for the completion of the birth and death certificates. The statistics clerk may also interview a new mother to obtain additional information. In most states, a physician signature is required to authenticate all birth and death certificates. Once completed, birth and death certificates must be filed with the local registrar or the county or state agency. This varies by state, but there is commonly a city or county office for vital records. These agencies are then responsible for reporting required vital statistics data.

The actual birth or death certificate does not become a part of the patient record; rather, a worksheet with the required information is routinely filed in the record in case questions arise in the future. To obtain an official copy of a birth or death certificate, individuals request one from the state agency responsible for the official recording of the birth or the death. This varies by state but often is the state's department of health or office of vital statistics.

County, state, and local registrars report vital statistics data to the **National Vital Statistics System (NVSS)**, which is a part of the **Centers for Disease Control and Prevention (CDC)**. The CDC's National Center for Health Statistics uses data reported to the NVSS to publish statistical and trend analysis in the National Vital Statistics Reports. Example 10.22 shows how information reported to the NVSS is used to track infant mortality data.

Example 10.22 Infant Mortality Trend Reported by the National Vital Statistics System

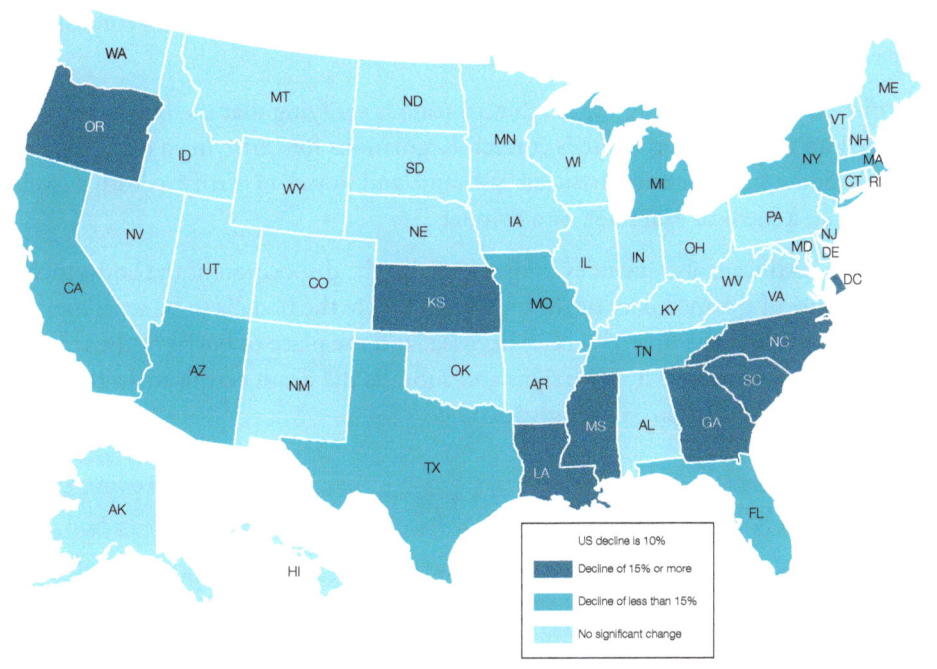

Percent change in infant morality rate, by state: United States, 2005–2010
Source: CDC/NCHS, National Vital Statistics System

> ## TAKE THE CHALLENGE
>
> Turn to Appendix D and review copies of the standard birth and death certificates. Both documents capture a lot of information that does not become a part of the legal health record. Some of the information captured is de-identified and reported in aggregate form, becoming the source of many population statistics published in news reports.
>
> For this challenge:
>
> 1. Identify what portion of each document becomes a part of the legal certificate.
> 2. List three pieces of information on each form that appear in publically reported health statistics.

The HIM department is less involved in the completion of death certificates. The patient chart may provide some of the required demographic information for these documents. A family member or a legal representative will be needed to provide information not included in the health record. The person(s) qualified to pronounce death varies widely by state. In some states, a medical student is allowed to pronounce death in a teaching hospital. In nonteaching hospitals, it is most often a physician or a nurse. In the case of a hospice patient who dies at home or in the hospital, a hospice nurse commonly pronounces the death. Some states explicitly require a physician, a medical examiner, or a coroner to pronounce death.

It should be noted that there is a difference between pronouncing a death and certifying a death. *Pronouncing a death* is declaring the death, time, and date. The physician or the person who pronounces the death is responsible for recording the time and the immediate cause of death in the patient record as well as any underlying conditions that might have led to the cause of death.

Certifying a death by signing the death certificate is verifying that the information recorded on the death certificate is correct. Regulations for certifying a death also vary by state. Some states permit physician assistants and nurses to certify a death as well as a physician, a medical examiner, or a coroner.

The death certificate also includes information on the disposition of the body, including the name of the mortuary or the crematory where the body is to be sent, the funeral facility and the funeral service licensee, and the place of burial or the release of ashes. The funeral service licensee signs and submits the death certificate to the designated city, county, or state vital statistics office.

Research

EXPAND YOUR KNOWLEDGE
Learn about FDA regulations for conducting clinical trials at http://IntroHIM.ParadigmCollege.net/FDAClinicalTrials.

Healthcare research covers a wide variety of issues and is conducted in many different locations, including patient care facilities, teaching hospitals, university and government laboratories, and private research facilities.

Medical research involves the study of diseases and conditions and the development of new drugs, treatments, and equipment to improve health and prolong life. Many healthcare facilities also conduct *administrative research* to improve the quality and the efficiency of care and to reduce the cost of providing care. *Population-based research* looks at the broader effects of disease and the allocation of healthcare resources on specific population groups, such as the poor, the elderly, or people living in one geographical region. The potential topics for healthcare research are almost limitless.

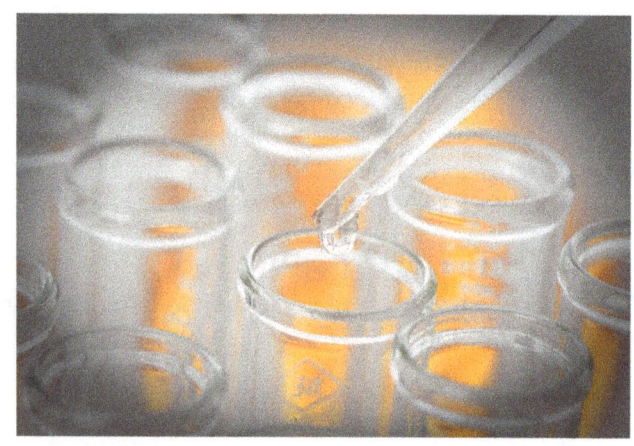

Research relies on data and valid statistical analysis to be able to draw conclusions and make good decisions. Healthcare research directly impacts the health and the well-being of patients' lives.

HIM's Role in Research

The wealth of data captured in the patient record serves as a basis for research, and as the EHR is increasingly integrated into all healthcare settings, that data becomes more accessible to researchers. The HIM department plays a role in research through its data management functions—the coding, processing, and analysis of data from the patient record. HIM also plays a key role in maintaining the privacy and the security of protected health information when information from the patient records is being used in research. In addition, HIM serves in a support role to an organization's Institutional Review Board, discussed later in this chapter.

Research methodology (how research is conducted) varies greatly based on the type of facility (teaching versus nonteaching) and the type of research (grant- or contract-funded or independent research conducted by one or more physicians).

A **clinical trial** is a type of research study conducted to test the effectiveness of a new drug or treatments on human subjects. During development of a new drug, the US Food and Drug Administration (FDA) requires researchers to conduct a series of clinical trials to determine if the drug is effective and to identify potential side effects.

In order to be valid, research must conform to accepted scientific practices and protocols. The US Department of Health and Human Services' Office for Human Research Subjects Protection (OHRP) provides guidelines, training materials, and federal regulatory oversight of biomedical research. The FDA requires researchers to comply with its guidelines for good clinical practice (GCP), which include human subject protection (HSP), a universally recognized critical requisite for any research that involves human subjects.

The Health Insurance Portability and Accountability Act of 1996 (HIPAA) also regulates the use of protected health information in research. The HIPAA Privacy Rule defines research as "a systematic investigation, including research development, testing, and evaluation, designed to develop or contribute to generalizable knowledge."

Under the HIPAA Privacy Rule, covered entities may use or disclose de-identified health information for research purposes. Covered entities may disclose protected health information with individual authorization or without individual authorization in limited circumstances as identified in the rule. The Privacy Rule also spells out how covered entities must inform patients of any use or disclosure of their information for research.

HIM professionals may find career opportunities in the areas of medical and administrative research. Graduates of health information technology (HIT) programs have the skills and the knowledge needed for entry-level positions, such as data entry clerk, data or research assistant, data collection clerk, and data analyst. Senior positions, such as data manager, compliance officer, database administrator, and statistician may require additional education or certification within the HIM field. More advanced positions, such as research coordinator, research project manager, and investigator/researcher may be held by HIM professionals with the appropriate education and experience.

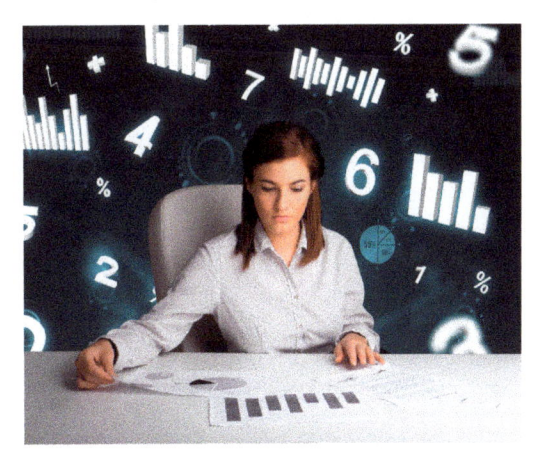

Research positions involve working with a great deal of data and require a thorough understanding of statistics, data analytics, graphing, and data presentation as well as good written communication skills.

EXPAND YOUR KNOWLEDGE

Information on HIPAA regulations governing the use of patient information in research is available from the US Department of Health and Human Services. To learn more, go to http://IntroHIM.ParadigmCollege.net/ResearchGuidelines.

As previously discussed, the patient record is a valuable source of primary data used for research. However, patient information contained in indices (disease and operation) or logs (surgery, blood administration, etc.) also provides useful data for research. Furthermore, new information may be compiled from databases created specifically for the purpose of a study.

Basic Steps in the Research Process

There are many different types of research and many different ways to design and conduct a research study. However, all research studies follow these same basic steps.

Develop a Hypothesis

The first thing a researcher or a research team does is to develop a hypothesis, or a problem statement or topic. A **hypothesis** is a tentative assumption established for the purpose of giving direction to a study. This may actually be one of the more difficult steps—determining what the problem is, not just the symptom that is presenting.

In this hypothetical example, Our Town Hospital's HIM department is conducting research for process improvement to address frequent backlogs in the coding department. Most research studies are done on a much larger scale and deal with more-complex issues, but this simplified example follows the same steps.

To address the coding backlog, the hospital's HIM department has requested that the hospital hire additional coders. In order to research the problem (the coding backlog), the HIM manager might first form a hypothesis that states that the coding backlog is the result of understaffing.

But is that really the problem? The backlog could be caused by a lack of coders, but the problem could also be caused by poor workflow, poor training, or assigning coders other tasks that take them away from the more important coding function.

To thoroughly investigate the issue, the research hypothesis may have to be broader in scope. A broader hypothesis might state, "The workflow of patient information from discharge through completion of the coding process is not adequate to support the coding function."

Review the Literature

Once a hypothesis has been established, the next step is to review the available literature. Before designing and undertaking a study, a researcher must become as knowledgeable about the subject of the research as possible. In this case, the manager would look to see if other similar studies had been done on coding workflow. He or she would consider the question, What is the standard number of charts a coder should be able to code in a set period? By reviewing the available literature, including other studies on the topic, the manager will be able to further refine the problem statement and the study design, identify what data needs to be gathered, and determine the method(s) to be used to gather the data.

Conduct the Research

Data collection is the actual process of gathering the data for a study. This is finding new knowledge about a topic. *Methodology* is the general strategy or approach used to gather data and conduct the research. Two commonly used methodologies for gathering data are the qualitative method and the quantitative method.

Qualitative research is descriptive. It refers to meanings, definitions, concepts, characteristics, and descriptions of things, including non-numerical data. Qualitative research involves collecting, analyzing, and interpreting data based on observations. Qualitative research can be subjective, and data collection often includes interviews and focus groups with a small number of participants. Compared to quantitative research, qualitative research is more exploratory and open-ended.

Quantitative research relies on numbers, counting, and measuring. The data must be objective, *quantitative* (expressed in terms of quantity), and *statistically valid* (the sample size must be large enough to produce a valid conclusion).

Once the data has been gathered, the researcher(s) interprets the data using statistical techniques and draws conclusions based on information known before the study, information in the literature, and the study findings.

Review the Data and Submit It for Publication

After the study is completed, the researcher(s) should go back and review the study process to identify any factors that may have affected the outcome of the study. Study limitations could include such things as poor study design, a low participation rate, or some other unforeseen problem with the data collection or analysis.

Before publishing the findings, the completed study should include a pertinent, current bibliography that demonstrates that a thorough review of the available literature was conducted in developing the research project.

The final step is the dissemination of the study findings through presentations at professional meetings, in industry publications, and in peer-reviewed journals. This is a very important part of the process.

Institutional Review Board and Compliance

An **institutional review board (IRB)** is a formally appointed group within each facility where research is conducted. The purpose of the IRB is to review and monitor **biomedical research** (applications of the sciences to study diseases) involving **human subjects**. The role of the IRB is to protect the rights and welfare of human research subjects, consistent with regulatory guidelines and ethical principles. HIM professionals may serve as advisors to the IRB with respect to health information privacy protection. The HIM director or privacy officer may sit on the board.

Many universities and healthcare organizations that conduct research have an office or an individual to monitor compliance. This office or individual works with the IRB. *Compliance monitoring* ensures that all research is conducted in compliance with federal, state, and local laws and regulations and in accordance with the sponsor and/or funding agency guidelines and internal policies and procedures.

Think Ethics!

The National Commission for the Protection of Human Subjects of Biomedical and Behavioral Research was created in 1974 to identify basic ethical principles and develop guidelines governing the conduct of research involving human subjects. Learn more about this important aspect of healthcare research in the Belmont Report at http://IntroHIM.ParadigmCollege.net/BelmontReport.

Ethical Issues

Ethics are rules of behavior based on societal views of morality and what are considered the right things to do. Healthcare organizations confront a number of ethical issues in the delivery of health care. Medical research also raises many ethical questions; sometimes, even just asking the question may raise ethical issues.

Institutional review boards are charged with the protection of human subjects participating in medical research, but a number of other mechanisms have been put into place over the years to promote ethical research practices. These include special protections for **vulnerable subjects**—individuals and population groups who may be susceptible to coercion or undue influence, including the mentally or physically infirm, those who are illiterate, children, prisoners, addicts, and students of the instructor conducting research. When vulnerable subjects are to be included in a study, the researcher should implement additional safeguards to protect their well-being.

A number of guidelines have been adopted over the years to address the protection of human research subjects and to ensure that ethical principles are adhered to throughout the research process—one such example is the Nuremberg Code. The **Nuremberg Code** is a set of ethical principles for research involving human experimentation. The code was developed as a result of the Nuremberg trials that took place at the end of World War II to address the inhumane treatment of prisoners of war in research studies. The **Declaration of Helsinki**, developed by the World Medical Association, outlines a similar standard regarding the treatment of human subjects in experiments and has become widely accepted as the ethical foundation for the treatment of human subjects. Researchers working with human subjects are required to obtain a written informed consent from all study participants. This informed consent ensures that the study participants have agreed to participate in research and that they have a full understanding of its possible consequences along with a full knowledge of its risks and benefits.

A **conflict of interest** is a situation or circumstance in which financial or other personal considerations have the potential to compromise or bias an individual's professional judgment and objectivity. Conflicts of interest are inherent in research. Conflicts of interest often arise in medical research and can influence the conduct of a study or the reporting of study findings. Conflicts of interest also arise in the day-to-day operations of healthcare facilities. A hospital may want to promote statistics that are beneficial and obscure statistics that reflect poor or substandard performance for financial benefit, to win recognition, to secure accreditation, or to bolster its ability to recruit top professionals. With so much at stake, there is a temptation to make the statistics reflect positively on the facility. However, such actions may violate ethical standards and can, when taken to extremes, even violate the law.

EXPAND YOUR KNOWLEDGE

The National Institutes of Health provides extensive resources on the ethical use of and protections for human subjects in research as well as information on current guidelines and standards. Learn more about this important topic at http://IntroHIM.ParadigmCollege.net/NIHEthics.

WHAT WOULD YOU DO?

Pharmaceutical drug trials and research studies are highly regulated because drug studies can be influenced in a variety of ways. The financial rewards are great for the pharmaceutical company if a drug is approved for use, but the potential side effects of a drug that has not been adequately tested can have debilitating and even fatal effects on the participants. The reliability of the data in drug research can be compromised by including or excluding certain types of study participants, eliminating data on some participants, using flawed methodology to analyze the data, etc.

Go to http://IntroHIM.ParadigmCollege.net/DrugTrialChallenge. Read the descriptions of the four phases of clinical trials. For each phase of a clinical trial, first read the statement, and then rewrite the statement in your own words to reflect what it means to you. Second, for each phase, identify at least one potential ethical issue that might arise, and describe what safeguards you, as a researcher, could put into place to protect the subjects of the trial and the ethical integrity of the study. Your answers may address issues related to participant protections, study design, and other potential situations.

Chapter Summary

Health information is a primary resource for patient care, but the data in patient records has many other uses as well. Statistics calculated from health records data provide the basis for administrative and healthcare delivery decisions and for reports submitted to governmental and accrediting agencies. The health record serves as a legal document and is used to substantiate claims for reimbursement for care provided.

Healthcare organizations use statistics to aid in the collection, analysis, interpretation, and presentation of healthcare data. Statistics represent facts about the data in a succinct manner that allows them to be easily interpreted and compared. Graphic displays, such as bar charts, line graphs, and data tables provide a means for displaying and comparing statistical information in a visual format. Familiarity with these displays and understanding how best to use them is an important aspect of working with patient information.

The HIM department routinely calculates statistics for monthly and annual reports. It is important to understand where the data for these calculations comes from, the type of information present, and whether the statistics presented are reliable and valid. To be reliable, the same data when calculated the same way should achieve the same result. Statistics should have a sound basis in logic to be relevant to the purpose for which they are used.

It is essential for HIM employees to be familiar with common statistical measures and how to apply them. These measures include standard deviation; measures of central tendency, frequency, and variance; and the formulas used to calculate routine healthcare statistics. Commonly calculated statistics include the hospital length of stay; the daily inpatient census; and birth, death, autopsy, and infection rates. When using charts, graphs, and other visual methods to display statistics, choose the type of visual display best suited to represent the data.

Vital statistics, which include birth and death information, are compiled nationally. The statistics are used for monitoring aspects of illness and care for large populations. HIM's role in vital statistics is to provide information via that which is contained on the birth and death certificates.

Statistical analysis can be used to identify trends to support clinical and business decisions. Trend analysis also plays a key role in *medical research*, the study of diseases and conditions and the development of new drugs, treatments, and equipment to improve health and prolong life.

The research arena provides many opportunities suitable for individuals with HIM education and experience. HIT graduates may be suited to entry-level positions related to data management, coding, processing, and basic data analysis. HIM professionals should be familiar with the importance of ethics and the role of an IRB within an organization conducting human subjects research.

HIM Review

Check Your Understanding

Test your understanding of the material covered in this chapter by completing the following multiple-choice questions. For each question, select the best answer from the choices provided.

1. Administrative statistics are _____
    a. used to monitor the utilization of services.
    b. used to monitor financial reports such as those for the payment and the nonpayment of claims.
    c. used to determine the need for new services.
    d. All of the choices are correct.

2. Study participants who might be subject to coercion or undue influence in research are _____
    a. those who receive payment for their participation.
    b. vulnerable subjects.
    c. known to have a condition that could benefit from the approval of the study drug.
    d. those who have not signed the informed consent.

4. Good Health Hospital treated 535 patients in March; 358 patients did not have surgery, and 182 patients had a surgical procedure. What is the ratio of patients who had surgery to those who did not?
    a. 182:540
    b. 182:358
    c. 358:182
    d. 358:540

5. Using the data presented in the previous question, select the correct formula to calculate the hospital's surgery rate for the month of March.
    a. 182/358
    b. 182 x 100/358
    c. 358 x 100/182
    d. 182 x 100/540

Chapter 10 Healthcare Statistics

307

6. Which of the following statements is not a realistic statistical calculation?

    a. 57% hospital infection rate

    b. 6% hospital death rate

    c. 38% autopsy rate

    d. 0.4% fetal death rate

7. A _____ measure shows the extent that data points differ from each other.

    a. rate

    b. ratio

    c. mode

    d. variability

8. _____ is a research study using human subjects for the purpose of improving treatment.

    a. Performance data

    b. A quantitative study

    c. A clinical trial

    d. A qualitative study

9. An institutional review board (IRB) _____

    a. is found in every facility where research is conducted.

    b. reviews the participation of human subjects in research.

    c. is a compliance program for medical research.

    d. reviews the results of individual research studies.

10. Vital statistics _____

    a. use quantitative data.

    b. are reported on specified population groups.

    c. use data legally required for reporting vital events.

    d. All of the choices are correct.

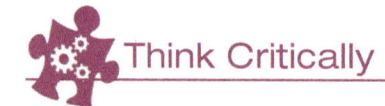

Think Critically

Consider the following real-world scenario and draft a response.

In May, the City Medical Center reported 50 inpatient deaths. Of those, four deaths were coroner's cases; two deaths were former patients who died in hospice and who were autopsied by the hospital pathologist; and the hospital pathologist performed the 44 remaining inpatient autopsies. Use this data to calculate the following rates. Round your answer to one decimal point.

1. The gross autopsy rate for the month
2. The net autopsy rate for the month
3. The hospital autopsy rate for the month

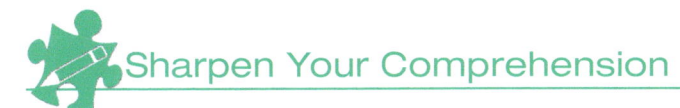

Sharpen Your Comprehension

Complete the following matching exercise by selecting, from the list provided, the answer that best matches each of the numbered statements. For each statement, only one answer is correct.

a. data
b. discrete data
c. inpatient census
d. nosocomial
e. rate
f. ratio
g. reliable
h. skew
i. valid
j. vital statistics

1. _____ When the same results are achieved on successive tests

2. _____ A count of the hospital's patients at a given time

3. _____ Relevant and meaningful for the purpose they are used for

4. _____ Facts or statistics gathered for analysis retrieval

5. _____ Compares two quantities of different units of measure

6. _____ Based on quantitative data of specified population groups

7. _____ Hospital acquired

8. _____ To distort

9. _____ Categorized into a classification and based on counts

10. _____ Provides a comparison between two numbers or quantities

Chapter 10   Healthcare Statistics

Connect Theory to Practice

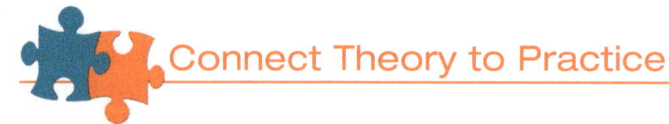

To help translate the concepts presented in this chapter to the workplace, complete the following exercise.

Access the guidelines for obtaining an official copy of a birth certificate for the state where you reside. Prepare a handout for new parents with instructions on how to obtain an official copy of their baby's birth certificate.

Student eResources

To enhance your comprehension of the chapter material, go to **Navigator+** and complete the additional practice items as advised by your instructor.

Chapter Terms

admission, discharge, and transfer (ADT) system
analytics
anesthesia death rate
average daily census (ADC)
average length of stay (ALOS)
bell curve
benchmark
biomedical research
Centers for Disease Control and Prevention (CDC)
clinical trial
conflict of interest
consultation
consultation rate
continuous data
daily inpatient census
data
data collection
decision support system (DSS)

Declaration of Helsinki
discharge days
discrete data
ethics
fetal death rate
frequency distribution table
gross autopsy rate
gross death rate
hospital autopsy rate
human subjects
hypothesis
inpatient census
inpatient service day
institutional review board (IRB)
length of stay (LOS)
maternal death
maternal death rate
mean
measures of variation

median
mode
morbidity
mortality
National Vital Statistics System (NVSS)
net autopsy rate
net death rate
nosocomial
nosocomial infection rate
Nuremberg Code
percentage
percentage of occupancy
postoperative death rate
qualitative research

quantitative research
range
rate
ratio
reliable
skew
standard deviation
total inpatient service days
total length of stay
trend analysis
valid
variability
vital statistics
vulnerable subjects

Professionalism Tip

Healthcare professionals who recognize or report on quality and patient safety outcomes have been pressured, harassed, and threatened with serious legal and licensure repercussions. New financial models that tie quality outcomes to payment are likely to increase the stakes associated with quality results.

In 2012, the National Association for Healthcare Quality, an organization dedicated to improving healthcare quality and safety, called on healthcare organizations to implement measures to ensure integrity in quality and safety evaluation and comprehensive, transparent, and accurate data collection, including:

- establishing accountability for the integrity of quality and safety systems
- protecting those who report quality and safety findings
- reporting quality and safety data accurately
- responding to quality and safety concerns with robust improvement

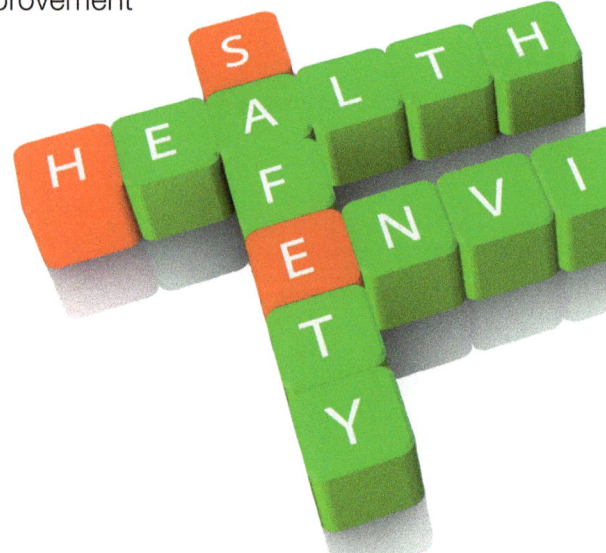

Think Ethics!

The idea that ethics are integral to quality is a central tenet of IntegratedEthics, a care model developed by the National Center for Ethics in Health Care at the Department of Veterans Affairs (VA). The model suggests that in health care, ethics and quality cannot be separated. A healthcare provider who fails to meet established ethical standards is not delivering high-quality health care. Conversely, care that fails to meet minimum quality standards raises ethical concerns.

Chapter 11

Quality Management and Data Collection

Fast Facts

More people die each year from nosocomial or hospital-acquired infections (HAIs) than breast cancer and automobile accidents combined. However, national efforts over the past several years to reduce HAIs are paying off. In 2012, the Centers for Disease Control and Prevention reported:

- a 44 percent decrease in central line-associated bloodstream infections (2008–2012)
- a 20 percent decrease in surgical-site infections for 10 procedures tracked (2008–2012)
- a 4 percent decrease in hospital-onset methicillin-resistant Staphylococcus aureus (MRSA) staph infections (2011–2012)
- a 2 percent decrease in hospital-onset Clostridium difficile infections (2011–2012)
- a 3 percent increase in catheter-associated urinary tract infections (2009–2012)

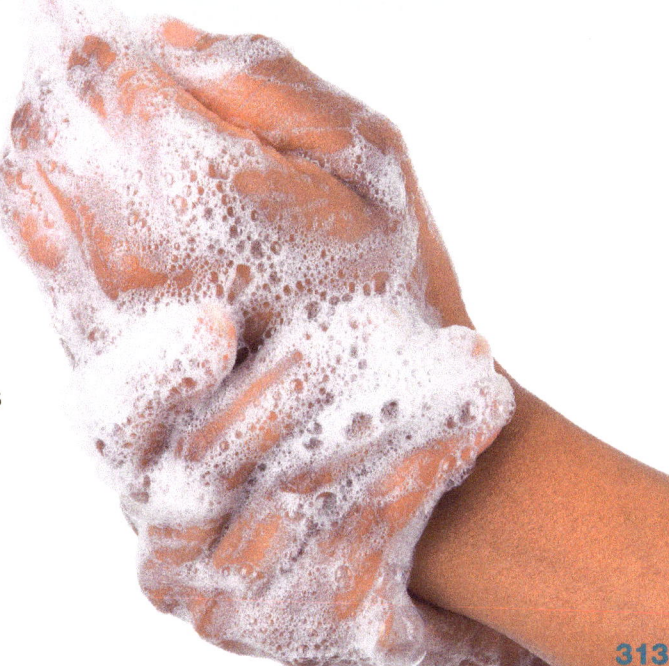

> ## Learning Objectives
>
> - Explain the steps involved in quality and process improvement.
> - Identify the organizations that monitor and regulate patient safety.
> - Recognize the accuracy and the integrity of health data.
> - Analyze data to identify trends.
> - Explain the functions of case management.
> - Describe the responsibilities of risk management.
> - Describe the data collected by the most common healthcare databases and registries.

Most of the people who work in health care do so because they want to help other people. Furthermore, most healthcare providers want to provide patients with the safest, most cost-efficient, and highest-quality care available. But how can providers and healthcare facilities know if the care they provide is the best, safest, and most cost-efficient? They can assess this concern by measuring and analyzing the data.

Health care is a data-driven field, particularly when it comes to evaluating the quality of care. Since the beginning of the 20th century, healthcare organizations and providers have been working to develop ways to measure and monitor the quality of care provided.

One way to measure and monitor quality of care is to evaluate information collected from patient health records against a variety of quality standards. These quality standards include industry best practices, licensure and accreditation standards, and internal organizational standards and goals.

As experts in data collection and the organization of clinical data, health information management professionals play a key role in quality management. These professionals define what data elements are collected as part of the health record and by working to improve documentation content and accuracy. This way, providers have the best information available, allowing them to provide the best-quality patient care.

In addition to ensuring high-quality patient care, healthcare organizations rely on timely, accurate, and complete data to make operational and financial decisions, such as setting staffing levels and deciding when to purchase new diagnostic equipment.

As discussed in Chapter 2, most hospitals have a quality/performance improvement committee. The committee reports to the hospital's board of directors on quality activities and oversees external reporting on quality issues to the Joint Commission, state health departments, and other regulatory entities. The committee recommends changes that will improve the quality and the safety of patient care. For example, if an organization's rate of **hospital-acquired infections (HAIs)** is significantly higher than the national average, the committee may order an investigation into the root cause (the reason[s] for the problem or the cause of the failure) and, depending on the result of that investigation, recommend policy changes, such as new hand-washing procedures, to reduce the HAI rate.

Quality Management

Quality is excellence as defined by the "customer" in meeting or exceeding desired outcomes. Or, as the Agency for Healthcare Research and Quality (AHRQ) states, "Quality health care means doing the right thing, at the right time, in the right way, for the right person—and having the best possible results."

In health care, the primary customer is the patient, but patients are not healthcare organizations' only customers. Healthcare organizations also serve employers, insurance providers, governmental agencies, patients' family members, and the general public. A healthcare organization must apply quality standards and employ quality controls to provide the best possible care and service to all of its customers.

Quality control refers to the operational techniques and activities that are used to regulate performance and prevent an undesirable change in a process. One example of quality control in health care is the monitoring and the recording of refrigerator temperature to ensure the safe storage of medication. If the temperature rises above or falls below a prescribed range—an undesirable change in process—the safety or the efficacy of the medication stored within may be compromised.

Quality improvement (QI) is a methodology that is used to identify and implement necessary changes to advance the efficiency, effectiveness, and reliability of a process or a procedure. In health care, the term **continuous quality improvement (CQI)**, also referred to as **process improvement (PI)**, is used daily to ensure care that is safe, effective, patient centered, timely, efficient, and equitable.

Each person who works in a healthcare facility has the opportunity and the obligation to improve a process at the time of an undesirable event. For example, if a biomedical engineer repairing a piece of biomedical equipment notices that the same type of equipment has failed in the same way throughout the facility, the engineer will follow the procedures to initiate quality improvement immediately. Initiating quality improvement may involve calling a hotline to report the problem, filling out a quality improvement report, and/or initiating contact with the equipment vendor.

A number of regulatory and accrediting bodies have established minimum requirements for quality patient care, including the Centers for Medicare & Medicaid Services (CMS), the Joint Commission, national medical societies, and state departments of health. Healthcare organizations may also have their own more rigorous standards for patient care.

The rate of hospital infections resulting from the placement of a urinary catheter is one example of a standard of patient care. Table 11.1 shows a comparison of three hospitals' infection rates to the national average for all hospitals.

Table 11.1 Infection Rate Data from a Urinary Catheter

Hospital	Infection Rate
Hospital A	0.465
Hospital B	0.324
Hospital C	0.080
National Average	0.316

> **TAKE THE CHALLENGE**
>
> Use the data from Table 11.1 to answer the following questions.
>
> 1. Which of the hospitals listed have met the minimum requirement for quality patient care? (Hint: Their rates are below the national average.)
> 2. Which of the hospitals listed need to implement continuous quality improvement to reduce the incidence of urinary catheter infections?
> 3. How can the hospitals collect data to monitor improvement in urinary catheter infection rates?

When a medical facility's performance falls outside or below the expected standard, it may choose to implement a continuous quality improvement (CQI) program to improve performance in that area. CQI is a multistep process. The steps include:

- Identify the problem. What is not working? Why is the facility failing to meet the minimum standard?
- Identify the steps or the process change(s) necessary to fix the problem.
- Train the staff on the new process.
- Once staff training is complete, implement the process.
- Monitor outcomes as the change(s) takes place, and tweak the process if necessary until the desired outcome is achieved (the standard is met).

Once the standard has been met, employees may think that the process is complete. However, as the word "continuous" implies, continuous quality improvement is an ongoing process. The goal of CQI is to continue to improve the process and to exceed rather than just meet expectations.

Health care is a dynamic environment. New diagnoses and procedures are being discovered all the time while new mandates and regulations are also being added. Healthcare providers are always trying to find ways to do things more efficiently and effectively while also improving the safety and the quality of patient care.

Safety and Regulatory Standards

Healthcare safety is regulated and monitored by a number of different agencies and organizations, including federal, state, and local governments; the Joint Commission; and consumer groups.

The Joint Commission

As described in Chapter 2, the **Joint Commission** is an independent, nonprofit organization that sets standards and evaluates the safety of thousands of healthcare organizations across the country through its voluntary accreditation process.

Hospitals accredited by the Joint Commission undergo an ongoing, rigorous evaluation process, including an unannounced on-site evaluation every three years, conducted by nurse, physician, and administrator surveyors. Hospital performance is measured against the evidence-based standards for quality and safety developed by the Joint Commission in consultation with healthcare experts, providers, and researchers. Hospitals that meet or exceed those standards are awarded Joint Commission accreditation. Medicare and many third-party insurers require Joint Commission accreditation.

The Joint Commission sets **National Patient Safety Goals** for hospitals, ambulatory and behavioral healthcare facilities, and home care. These goals are intended to protect patient safety and improve the quality of patient care. The goals address issues such as improving patient identification procedures to reduce "wrong patient" errors, improving medication safety through better labeling and storage practices, preventing infection, and reducing surgical errors by ensuring that the "correct surgery is done on the correct patient and at the correct place on the patient's body."

Hospital Performance Measures

ORYX for Hospitals is the Joint Commission's performance measurement and improvement initiative. Introduced in 1997, ORYX integrates performance measures into the accreditation process with the goal of improving patient outcomes and the quality of care. Hospitals are required to collect and submit outcomes data to the Joint Commission on a minimum of six performance measure sets both for individual patients and patient groups within specific diagnostic areas. ORYX core measures are divided into mandatory and discretionary measure sets, and each addresses a specific area of patient care. Acute care medical/surgical facilities must report outcomes on all five mandatory-performance measure sets and one discretionary measure set.

Examples of the current (as of publication) Joint Commission mandatory and discretionary measure sets for acute care medical/surgical facilities are listed in Table 11.2. Joint Commission measures are subject to frequent changes.

Table 11.2 Joint Commission ORYX Performance Measures

Mandatory Performance Measure Sets
• Heart attack care
• Pneumonia
• Surgical care improvement
• Heart failure
• Prenatal care (hospitals with more than 1,100 births per year)
Discretionary Performance Measure Sets
• Children's asthma care
• Tobacco treatment
• Immunizations
• Stroke
• Emergency department

EXPAND YOUR KNOWLEDGE

The Joint Commission provides a free online tool called the "Core Measure Solution Exchange," which reports success stories from accredited and critical access hospitals that have received an "excellent" status. View the report at http://IntroHIM.ParadigmCollege.net/JointCommission.

One example of a reportable measure in the area of heart attack care is "aspirin on arrival." If a heart attack patient is administered aspirin upon arrival at the hospital, the criterion is met. If a heart attack patient is not administered aspirin on arrival, it does not necessarily mean that the physician/facility provided suboptimal care. Further review of the medical record would be needed to fully assess the level of care provided. The record may show that the patient had aspirin "before" arrival in the ambulance, that the patient is allergic to aspirin, or, perhaps, that the patient was in a full code and unable to swallow aspirin upon arrival.

Complete, timely, and accurate documentation protects the patient during treatment and ensures that the information needed to review the quality of care is recorded.

TAKE THE CHALLENGE

The Joint Commission publishes an annual report, *Improving America's Hospitals: The Joint Commission's Annual Report on Quality and Safety*, that lists top-performing hospitals based on key quality measures. View or download the most recent report, and identify five hospitals in your state that have achieved a high ranking on at least three core quality measures. Next, identify five hospitals in your state that are not highly ranked on at least three core quality measures. (Hint: These hospitals will not be listed in the report.) Write a brief summary explaining which hospital(s) you would prefer to receive services from and why.

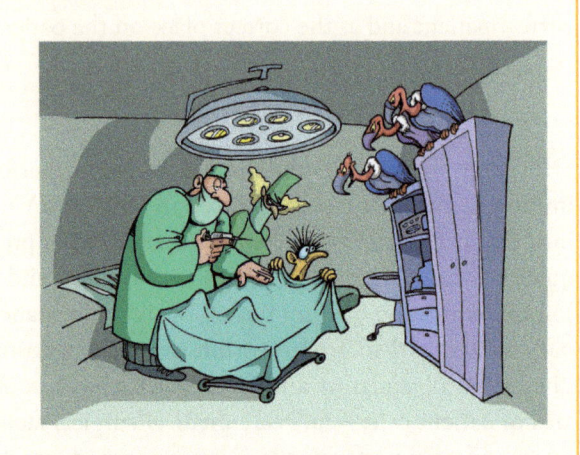

Sentinel Events

As a part of its efforts to improve the safety and the quality of health care and as a part of its accreditation process, the Joint Commission reviews healthcare providers' responses to sentinel events. A **sentinel event (SE)** is an unexpected occurrence that results in a patient's death or in serious physical or psychological injury. The occurrence is referred to as *sentinel* because it requires an immediate investigation and response. The Joint Commission automatically reviews certain sentinel events, including:

- medication errors that resulted in death, coma, or a major and permanent loss of function
- an operation conducted on the wrong side of a patient's body
- intrapartum (related to the birth process) maternal death
- the abduction of a patient from a hospital or another medical facility

- an assault, a homicide, a suicide, or another crime involving a patient
- a foreign body left in a patient after surgery

This is a partial list of sentinel events. To see a complete list of reviewable sentinel events, go to http://IntroHIM.ParadigmCollege.net/SentinelEvent.

IT REALLY HAPPENS

A hospital's newborn nursery is the area with the highest risk for patient abduction (a sentinel event). Hospitals must have a security system in place, including security cameras, to limit access to the nursery. Many facilities use colored name tags to identify obstetric nurses so that a new mother knows who is taking her baby. If an infant or a child is missing, a hospital will issue a special alert, such as "code pink" (similar to the "code blue" for cardiac arrest). The hospital is then locked down, meaning no one is allowed in or out of the facility. Employees are also positioned to guard all doors to the outside. There is always a collective sigh of relief when the infant or the child is found and the "all clear" is sounded.

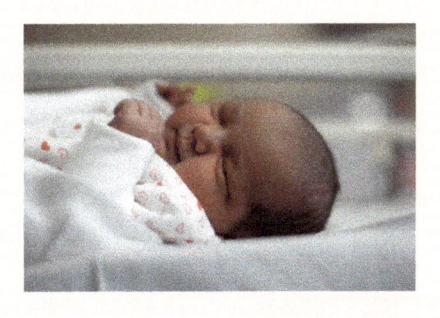

Federal Quality Standards

One example of the government's involvement in the regulation of quality is the **National Quality Strategy**, established as a part of the Patient Protection and Affordable Care Act (ACA) to serve as a catalyst for quality improvement efforts. The National Quality Strategy seeks to align the efforts of public- and private-sector stakeholders (individuals, family members, payers, providers, employers, and communities) to achieve better health and health care for all Americans. This voluntary strategy has three broad-based goals:

- **Better care** Improve the overall quality of health care by making it more patient centered, reliable, accessible, and safe.
- **Healthy people/healthy communities** Improve the health of the US population by supporting proven interventions to address behavioral, social, and environmental determinants of health in addition to delivering higher-quality care.
- **Affordable care** Reduce the cost of quality health care for individuals, families, employers, and government.

Consumer-Based Quality Measures

In addition to government standards, consumer-based organizations monitor and evaluate healthcare quality and performance. The **Healthcare Effectiveness Data and Information Set (HEDIS)** is a set of standardized performance measures developed by the National Committee for Quality Assurance (NCQA), a nonprofit organization

---

EXPAND YOUR KNOWLEDGE

Learn more about the National Quality Strategy online at http://IntroHIM.ParadigmCollege.net/Quality. Notice how the National Quality Strategy principles are in line with the meaningful use requirements covered in Chapter 7.

dedicated to improving health care quality. Healthcare consumers (e.g., employers, consultants, and patient advocates) use HEDIS data along with accreditation status to help identify the best-performing health plan to meet their needs. HEDIS data is often used as the basis for health plan "report cards" that appear in media newspapers and websites.

Increasingly, employers are negotiating health insurance contracts based on healthcare quality outcomes. This is called **value-based purchasing (VBP)**. VBP is a market-driven strategy that rewards healthcare providers who provide high-quality, efficient health care in a cost-effective way. VBP uses payment incentives to reward health plans, hospitals, physician groups, and individual healthcare practitioners that meet or exceed nationally approved measurements.

Under the ACA, CMS implemented a hospital VBP Program. Hospitals that provide care to Medicare patients are no longer paid based solely on the quantity of services but also on the quality of care provided: how closely the hospital follows best clinical practices and how well it enhances patients' experiences of care during hospital stays.

Documentation Quality

The quality of the documentation in the medical/health record is of utmost importance to the quality of patient care. Clinical documentation is the primary communication tool between providers. High-quality clinical documentation ensures that all providers are focused on the same patient goals and outcomes, and it provides the information needed to determine a patient's next course of treatment. High-quality clinical documentation also ensures greater accuracy in coding and reimbursement. Hospital admitting and utilization management departments and patient advocates use administrative documentation, which includes information on a patient's next of kin, his or her insurance carrier, and other nonclinical items, to move the patient through the healthcare system seamlessly. If any of this information is incomplete, inaccurate, or missing, it can delay patient care or result in denied reimbursement claims.

Documentation quality is monitored and evaluated by the hospital committee or the department that is responsible for overseeing a particular area of patient care. For example, an **infection-control committee** would review documentation related to HAIs, and the department of physical therapy would review documentation related to that area of patient care. If needed, these hospital committees and departments are also responsible for developing strategies to improve documentation quality.

Documentation review should be conducted concurrently, while a patient is hospitalized, and, when possible, by providers who document, such as physicians, nurses, or therapists while the patient is still in the facility. The advantage of **concurrent review** is that documentation gaps can be identified immediately and then resolved while a patient is still undergoing treatment. For example, every nursing unit conducts a daily chart check to verify that every physician order is initialed and dated by the patient care provider responsible for that patient's order, indicating that the order had been completed. If an order has not been initialed and dated (i.e., has not been documented), the nurse conducting the chart check is responsible for ascertaining whether the person executing the order forgot to document the care provided or if the order had not been fulfilled. Both scenarios require immediate corrective action.

If concurrent documentation review is not possible (as with a review of the components of a discharge summary, for example), a health information management (HIM) department employee may conduct a **retrospective review** of a patient's discharge summary, including discharge instructions and final diagnosis, after the patient has been discharged. The review findings are then compiled in a report and/or graph format and presented to the medical staff department, hospital department, or individual provider responsible for the documentation. If necessary, a documentation improvement plan will be developed.

Data integrity and reliability are the essential ingredients of high-quality documentation. The American Health Information Management Association (AHIMA) has developed a data quality management model to illustrate the challenges to producing high-quality data. Table 11.3 lists and defines the characteristics of data quality.

Table 11.3 Characteristics of Data Quality

Characteristic	Definition
Accuracy	Data is free of typographical or misprint errors.
Accessibility	Data items are readily available but well protected from unauthorized access.
Comprehensiveness	All required data items are included, the information is complete, and there are no missing documents or data elements.
Consistency	Data is reliable, and all providers have documented the same information throughout the record.
Currency	Data is updated to provide the most current information. Old information, such as an old lab result, is not used for current decision making.
Definition	The specific meaning of a healthcare-related data element, such as abbreviations, is clear and well documented.
Granularity	The level of detail is well defined; individual data elements cannot be subdivided. For example, the data element of the patient's middle name cannot be subdivided into another data element.
Precision	Data values, usually numbers, are exactly stated to support the purpose. For example, a medication dosage would be exact; it would never be rounded up.
Relevancy	Data is useful for the purposes for which it is collected.
Timeliness	Data is up-to-date and available within a useful timeframe, meeting or exceeding regulatory requirements.

Documentation Timeliness

The Joint Commission, CMS, and state departments of health all have requirements regarding the timely access to and the timely completion of documentation. As discussed in Chapter 4, many of the documents in the patient record must be completed within a specific timeframe. For example, nursing assessments must be completed within 24 hours. Additionally, providers need timely access to up-to-date information in the patient record to accurately diagnose and treat patients. A physician preparing for emergency surgery would not expect to wait 24 hours for the result of a radiology examination, for example.

The HIM department may coordinate a committee to assess timeliness data. Such reviews may be conducted by the HIM/medical record (MR) committee or by a specific hospital department (such as the department of nursing). The committee or the department reviews the graphs and spreadsheets to evaluate the timeliness of the data and decides if improvements and subsequent changes need to be made. Timeliness is an important factor in quality patient care. It should be monitored continuously and reported at least monthly to the HIM/MR committee or to the appropriate department.

Illegible Documentation and Abbreviation Use

Illegible documentation and the misuse or the misinterpretation of abbreviations in patient documentation can have serious consequences for patient health. These types of miscommunications between healthcare providers can lead to poor patient care, medication errors, and other mistakes that can result in patient injury or death.

Joint Commission standards require that all entries in the medical record be legible—that documentation can easily be read and understood. During an accreditation site visit, the Joint Commission survey team will review a sample of patient records for legibility. If the documentation in a record appears illegible in the surveyor's opinion, he or she will hand the record to a healthcare provider, such as a nurse, and ask that individual to read the documentation. If that person cannot read the documentation, the surveyor will ask another provider to read it. If neither provider can read what is written, the hospital will receive a low score for that standard. Problems with illegible documentation will impact a hospital's overall accreditation score.

Illegible documentation is becoming less of a problem, however, as healthcare facilities adopt the electronic health record (EHR). Because EHR documentation is typed, legibility is not as much of an issue. Not all healthcare facilities have fully transitioned to the EHR, however. As discussed in previous chapters, some facilities continue to work with hybrid medical records, which include both paper and electronic files.

Abbreviations are commonly used in healthcare settings to save time, but abbreviations can often be misused or misunderstood. Providers in one specialty may not recognize an abbreviation commonly used by providers in a different specialty, or they may use the same abbreviation but for a completely different term. For example, an orthopedic physician or a physical medicine physician would use the abbreviation ROM to mean "range of motion." An obstetric physician, however, may use the same abbreviation to mean "rupture of membranes." The use of ROM is globally accepted in both scenarios.

Abbreviation mistakes can have serious consequences for patient health, including errors in medication administration and miscommunication between providers.

In the past (and still published in some textbooks), the Joint Commission standard recommended that each abbreviation be limited to a single use. This proved to be unrealistic in today's healthcare environment, though, so the Joint Commission standard was changed. To ensure that all healthcare providers share a common understanding of medical abbreviations, each healthcare facility should compile and maintain a list of approved abbreviations, signs, and symbols. Signs document the presence of a specific characteristic observed during a medical examination. Historically, signs were named after the physician who first described the characteristic. For example the +

Babinski sign is named after neurologist Joseph Babinski. It demonstrates an abnormal plantar reflex. Commonly used symbols include:

♀ female sex

♂ male sex

↓ decrease

↑ increase

The most hazardous use of abbreviations in health care is in communicating medication orders; the most frequent error is the use of the abbreviation "U" for units.

IT REALLY HAPPENS

A physician prescribing 20 units of insulin for a patient wrote a medication order for 20 U of insulin. The nurse administering the medication mistook the U for zero. The patient was accidentally injected with 200 units of insulin and died of an insulin overdose.

Facilities must adopt a "do not use" list of abbreviations, acronyms, and symbols, including—at a minimum—the Joint Commission's official "do not use" list shown in Table 11.4.

Table 11.4 Joint Commission's "Do No Use" Abbreviations List

Do Not Use	Potential Problem	Use Instead
U, u (unit)	Mistaken for "0" (zero), the number "4" (four), or "cc"	Write "unit."
IU (international unit)	Mistaken for IV (intravenous) or the number 10 (ten)	Write "international unit."
Q.D., QD, q.d., qd (daily)	Can be mistaken for each other.	Write "daily."
Q.O.D., QOD, q.o.d, qod (every other day)	Period after the Q mistaken for "I" and the "O" mistaken for "I"	Write "every other day."
Trailing zero (X.0 mg)*	Decimal point is missed.	Write X mg.
Lack of leading zero (.X mg)		Write 0.X mg.
MS	Can mean morphine sulfate or magnesium sulfate	Write "morphine sulfate."
MSO4 and MgSO4	Can be confused with one another	Write "magnesium sulfate."

*Exception: A "trailing zero" may be used only where required to demonstrate the level of precision of the value being reported, such as for laboratory results, imaging studies that report size of lesions, or catheter/tube sizes. It may not be used in medication orders or other medication-related documentation.

© The Joint Commission, 2014. Reprinted with permission.

The Joint Commission, the US Food and Drug Administration (FDA), and the Institute for Safe Medication Practices (ISMP) have worked diligently to provide resources, recommendations, and education on potential dangerous abbreviations. While facilities are required to adopt the Joint Commission's official "do not use" list, the list is far from complete. To reduce adverse events and avoidable medical errors, each healthcare organization must carefully evaluate and provide written policies on the use of abbreviations while educating all patient care providers on abbreviation use and the "do not use" list.

EXPAND YOUR KNOWLEDGE

The Institute for Safe Medication Practices publishes a list of error-prone abbreviations, symbols, and dose designations. To view the list, go to http://IntroHIM.ParadigmCollege.net/Abbreviations.

Inconsistent Documentation

The HIM professional plays a major role in identifying and rectifying inconsistencies in documentation. For example, a surgical consent form may indicate that surgery is to be performed on a patient's right arm, but the operative report states that the surgery was performed on the patient's left arm. Problems with documentation consistency can also occur when more than one provider is treating or evaluating the same patient. One provider may document that a patient is short of breath; the other may document that the patient has no shortness of breath. Physicians may document differing diagnoses. Even basic descriptors are sometimes inconsistent, such as "patient is male" and "patient is female." Inconsistencies in documentation are often discovered during an HIM department analysis of the patient record. Documentation inconsistencies should be sent back to the author of the documentation for revision.

Incomplete Data Components for the Condition

Review of documentation should always be done concurrently (while a patient is still in the hospital) so that any changes and improvements in documentation can be made while the provider's memory is fresh.

Reviewing documentation to ensure high-quality patient care is sometimes referred to as *clinical pertinence*. The HIM department reviews the individual data components in the patient record to make sure that all required documentation is complete. Consider the example of postoperative pain assessment. Does the record show that the patient's postoperative pain level, assessed on a level of 1–10, was documented every 30 minutes? If the answer were "yes," then the HIM staff member reviewing the documentation would mark on a review sheet that the documentation standard had been met. If not, the reviewer would mark "no" to indicate that the requirement was not met.

Once the record review is completed, the HIM department tallies the yes and no responses on the checklist and then calculates the percentage of records that have met the documentation standard. To continue with the example above, for the month of March, the record review showed the documentation standard for postoperative pain assessment was met 74 percent of the time; 26 percent of the records reviewed failed to meet the standard. This information can also be broken down by nursing unit to allow for a more focused analysis of where the data was or was not captured, so the department of nursing can initiate an improvement plan.

Sometimes, information needed to assess a patient's health issue or disease process is missing from the documentation. For example, if a patient comes to a hospital with shortness of breath and the hospital physician is concerned that the patient may have congestive heart failure (CHF), then the physician's documentation of the initial physical exam should include all of the documentation requirements for congestive heart failure (see Table 11.5). An HIM professional will review a sample representative of CHF records. If the documentation is missing one or more data components, the patient record will be forwarded to a physician member of the HIM/MR committee for review. The committee representative will then make a determination as to whether the documentation is adequate.

Table 11.5 Documentation Requirements for Congestive Heart Failure

Measurement of vital signs including weight and blood pressure
Assessment of the abdomen for hepatojugular reflux
Assessment of the neck veins for jugular venous distention
Assessment of the extremities for • the presence of pitting edema • color (cyanosis of the nail beds)
Assessment of the lungs for • rales • rhonchi • decreased breath sounds
Auscultation (listening) to the heart for • murmurs • arrhythmias • gallop • extra heart sounds (e.g., clicks, ventricular filling gap)

Case Management

In hospitals and other types of healthcare facilities, the **case management department** plays a key role in ensuring that patients get the right care, at the right time, and in the appropriate setting. The case management department fulfills many roles, including utilization management, discharge planning, care coordination, and resource management.

Utilization management is the process of evaluating the appropriateness of a patient's level of care (e.g., inpatient versus observation) against objective criteria.

Transitional (discharge) planning is the coordination of services for a patient after discharge from a hospital. This process may begin as soon as a patient is admitted to a hospital, particularly in cases in which the patient will be discharged to a facility that has a waiting list (e.g., a long-term care facility).

Care coordination is done in conjunction with a patient's insurance provider to evaluate the patient's progress toward treatment goals. Care coordination begins during the *precertification process* (the insurance company's preauthorization for the provision of care at a certain level [acute inpatient versus rehabilitation], for a procedure, or for hospitalization) and continues during hospitalization and until the patient is discharged to an appropriate setting.

Resource management is the process of evaluating the cost and the efficiency of patient care services concurrently to control expenses (e.g., moving a patient from the intensive care unit [ICU] to a standard patient-care room once the patient is stable). Additional information is collected retrospectively, or after the patient is discharged (e.g., unnecessary or duplicate diagnostic testing), and the results are provided to the utilization review committee for trend analysis and process improvement opportunities.

A hospital's **case manager** evaluates the level of service provided to an individual patient to determine if the care meets the criteria for medical necessity. **Medical necessity** refers to care that is reasonable, necessary, and/or appropriate according to evidence-based clinical standards of care. Medical necessity also plays a key role in reimbursement. Insurers and other third-party payers will only reimburse care that is medically necessary. Claims for care deemed "not medically necessary" may be denied.

When a hospital or a physician signs a contract with CMS or a private insurance company, as a condition of payment the payer may require the provider to evaluate care decisions against evidence-based guidelines specified by the payer. CMS and many private insurers use guidelines provided by one of two firms: MCG and McKesson's InterQual.

For example, when a patient is treated in the emergency department (ED), the patient's physician with guidance from the patient's case manager, will review these guidelines to determine medical necessity: Does the patient's condition meet the criteria for admission, or should the patient be placed in observation? This determination is based on two factors, intensity of service and severity of illness.

Intensity of service (IS) challenges the case manager to justify via documentation in the medical record that the patient meets criteria or is "sick enough" to require acute inpatient hospitalization. Some questions the payer may ask the case manager include:

- Why did the patient come to the hospital?
- Which criteria are documented in the medical record to support acute inpatient hospitalization?
- Was outpatient treatment attempted, and did it fail?

Severity of illness (SI) requires that documentation in the medical record provide proof that care in an acute inpatient setting is medically necessary. Questions the payer may ask the case manager include:

- What is the care plan?
- Could care provided to the patient in the acute care setting be provided safely in an alternative level of care (ALC) setting, such as home health, or in a long-term care facility?

After the case manager contacts the payer and provides the information requested to justify an acute inpatient admission, the payer approves a specified number of inpatient hospital day(s). If the patient is not healthy enough to be discharged within the approved number of day(s), the case manager will again contact the payer and provide additional information explaining why the patient requires additional time in the hospital.

The payer will compare the information provided by the case manager against discharge criteria to determine if additional inpatient care is warranted or if the patient can be discharged to his or her home or to an alternate care setting. Examples of discharge criteria include:

- pain controlled with PO (by mouth) meds
- temperature between 97.0 and 99.8
- heart rate between 50 and 100 beats per minute
- PO fluids tolerated
- wound healing

If the patient meets the discharge criteria and has no other medical issues that require an acute care level of service, the payer will no longer pay the charges for any subsequent days or services.

One of the most common symptoms presented in a hospital emergency department is chest pain. Table 11.6 provides an example of documentation for two patients, both of whom presented to the ED with chest pain, and the patients' responses to initial treatment. Patient A will be placed in observation while Patient B meets the criteria for acute inpatient care. The highlighted areas provide enough information for the case manager to make this determination.

Table 11.6 Comparison of Admission Criteria for Chest Pain

Patient A	Patient B
Male, age 76	Male, age 54
Left-sided chest pain radiating to left arm	Left-sided chest pain radiating to left arm
Received aspirin, nitroglycerin SL, and morphine/1 with relief of pain	Nitroglycerin/3 SL and intravenous morphine/1 without relief of pain; titrated IV nitroglycerin started
O2 saturated @ 95% on room air	O2 saturated at 90%, requiring supplemental oxygen 3 L/min. per NC (nasal cannula)
Respiratory normal to auscultation and percussion	Bilateral basilar crackles without wheezes or rhonchi.
Chest X-ray normal	Chest X-ray shows mild heart failure.
Electrocardiogram (ECG) normal	ECG—ST elevation consistent with acute anterior MI (myocardial infarction)
Admit to observation for cardiac monitoring to R/O (rule out) MI.	Admit to inpatient status in the cardiac care unit (CCU) for MI protocol.

Both patients will continue to be closely monitored. Patient A will be observed for approximately 24 hours or less during which time a decision will be made to admit the patient as an acute inpatient or to discharge the patient.

Traditionally, the case manager position has been held by a registered nurse; however, HIM professionals are moving into these roles more often because of their expertise in pertinent and accurate clinical documentation. The HIM professional can help to educate physicians on how to write clear and precise documentation that will support the level of care a patient needs, for as long as it is needed. Table 11.7 illustrates the difference between supportive and vague documentation for intensity of service.

Table 11.7 Documentation Guidelines for Intensity of Service/Severity of Illness Criteria

Vague Documentation	What the Documentation Suggests	Clear Documentation to Support Patient Care
Patient stable	The patient is well enough to be discharged; lack of severity of illness.	Describe why the patient must remain in the hospital (severity of illness), and document acute care services provided (intensity of services).
Patient doing well; will discharge in the a.m.	The patient may go home immediately because he or she is no longer meeting severity of illness criteria. Last day of stay may be denied.	Patient may be discharged in the a.m. if tolerating his or her diet without vomiting for at least 12 hours.
Awaiting ICU bed transfer	The patient's condition is not severe enough to need an ICU level of care. The first day of ICU care may be denied.	Transferring to ICU bed soon; one-on-one nursing care in place until transfer. Demonstrates intensity of service need.
Patient ambulatory	The patient is able to walk and no longer meets severity of illness criteria required for acute care.	Patient ambulating five feet with slow and unsteady gait; requires assistance of two staff members. Demonstrates both severity of illness and intensity of service needed.

Risk Management

In every healthcare facility, large or small, **risk** (a situation involving exposure to danger, harm, or financial loss) is a concern. **Risk management** seeks to prevent or reduce accidents or injuries in a healthcare facility and limit the hospital's *liability* (legal responsibility) if an accident or an injury does occur. Large healthcare facilities have a risk management department. In smaller facilities, risk management may be handled by the quality management department. Risk management responsibilities involve identifying, tracking, and evaluating risk; implementing loss prevention and reduction (developing and implementing new policies for the removal of ice from a hospital's parking lot, for example); and resolving litigation stemming from risk events.

Although patient care is a primary area of focus for risk, the hospital risk management department works to prevent all types of risk. One common area of risk in a hospital is falls. A visitor, a vendor, a physician, an employee, or a patient could slip and fall on a freshly mopped floor, for example. The risk management department tracks injuries from falls and other events, identifies the cause of each incident, and implements preventive measures.

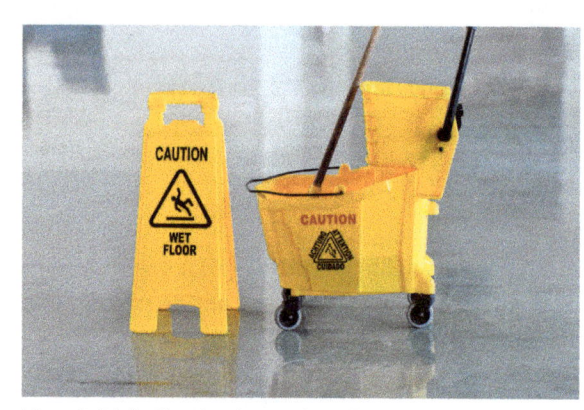

Hospital falls that lead to serious injury may be attributed to negligence. Hospitals need to take appropriate precautions to minimize falls, including displaying "caution" signs during floor cleaning.

The risk management department oversees the hospital's response to all medical malpractice and personal injury litigation brought against the healthcare facility. Potential legal issues are identified through the healthcare incident-reporting process and through coordination with the HIM department. The HIM department notifies the risk management department of any subpoena or record request pertaining to a medical malpractice investigation.

Databases for Reporting Purposes

In a healthcare setting, data from patient records is used in a variety of ways. Some uses are related to direct patient care, but many are not. The case management department collects data from patient records and uses the aggregated data to evaluate trends, track costs, support claims for reimbursement, and ensure patient safety. Risk management programs use healthcare data to identify risks, to defend the hospital from malpractice claims, and in loss prevention. The quality management department collects and analyzes data from patient records when looking at issues such as patient safety, infection control, and diseases or procedures in specific diagnostic areas (myocardial infarction or cesarean sections, for example).

As discussed in earlier chapters, once primary data is collected from the patient record, it can be used as **secondary data** in reporting to external registries (e.g., a cancer registry), in vital statistics reporting (birth and death certificates), for accreditation purposes, and for use by other healthcare databases.

Secondary data provides a big-picture view that is used within a healthcare organization to track trends and identify patterns to improve the quality of patient care, in budgeting, and for planning purposes. Secondary data is also used in research to evaluate and track the efficacy of treatment for diseases and procedures.

Recall that a **database** is a collection of related data stored on a computer system that is organized so that its contents can easily be accessed, managed, updated, and extracted. Databases are developed and used by researchers and state and federal governments and in the form of indexes within a healthcare facility. Data is grouped together by like items, such as diagnosis (e.g., diabetes, pneumonia), patient demographics (e.g., gender, age, race), or providers (e.g., physicians, hospitals).

Databases can be multifaceted. For example, the National (Nationwide) Inpatient Sample (NIS), the largest all-payer inpatient-care database in the United States, is a part of the Healthcare Cost and Utilization Project (HCUP), which is pronounced "H-CUP." HCUP is a national information resource for healthcare data. It brings together the data from federal and state databases and those operated by hospital associations and private data organizations to enable research on health policy issues. These issues include the cost and the quality of health services, patterns of medical practice, access to healthcare programs, and treatment outcomes. The NIS was created in 1988 and contains data on more than seven million hospital stays. Because of its large sample size, HCUP data is used to calculate *regional cost estimates* (how expensive it is to treat patients in a particular area of the country) and hospital-to-hospital cost comparisons. It is also used for analysis of common treatments and special populations. Much of the data accessible through HCUP is drawn from hospital billing systems

> **BE AWARE**
>
> To save time, some hospitals only report enough diagnostic and procedural codes to get the bill paid (get an accurate DRG). By not including *all* of the diagnostic and procedural codes that describe a patient's condition, information aggregated in databases like the NIS will be skewed. (In general, the patient will appear healthier.)

(coded and abstracted from patient records) and includes more than 100 clinical and nonclinical data elements for each hospital stay, including:

- primary and secondary diagnoses
- primary and secondary procedures
- admission and discharge status
- patient demographics (e.g., gender, age, race, median income for zip code)
- expected payment source
- total charges
- length of stay
- hospital characteristics (e.g., ownership, size, teaching status)

Hospitals contribute information to and use data from a number of publicly available data sets.

The national Centers for Disease Control and Prevention (CDC) compiled the National Hospital Discharge Survey (NHDS) annually from 1965 to 2010. This national probability survey was designed to track information on characteristics of inpatients discharged from nonfederal, short-stay hospitals in the United States. Data from the survey is used to examine important topics of interest in public health and for a variety of activities by governmental, scientific, academic, and commercial institutions. The NHDS was discontinued in 2010 and its data replaced with the National Hospital Care Survey.

The National Hospital Ambulatory Medical Care Survey (NHAMCS) collects data nationwide from the ED, outpatient department (OPD), and ambulatory surgery center (ASC).

The National Hospital Care Survey (NHCS) integrates inpatient data formerly collected in the NHDS with emergency department, outpatient, and ambulatory surgery center data. Integration of data from these two surveys along with the collection of personal identifiers (protected health information) make it possible to link care provided to an individual patient through the ED, OPD, ASC, and other inpatient departments. Survey data may also be linked to the National Death Index and to Medicaid and Medicare data to provide a more complete picture of patient care.

Registries

A **healthcare registry** is a collection of data elements that correlate to specific diseases, conditions, or procedures. Registry data is collected by healthcare workers, most often registered nurses, for internal use and to meet government reporting requirements. Some of the most common registries track trauma, birth defects, and immunizations. Cancer registry data is most often collected and maintained by certified tumor registrars (CTRs) who work as a part of the HIM department.

Trauma Registry

A **trauma registry** collects demographic and clinical information on all hospital trauma cases, such as injuries, falls, accidents, burns, and cuts. Registry reporting requirements are determined by individual states. Information collected in the trauma registry can impact public health. For example, trauma registry data prompted a product recall of baby walkers after data collected on infant trauma cases showed a high incidence of infants in walkers falling down stairs. A new federal safety regulation was thus implemented, requiring new walkers to stop at the edge of a step.

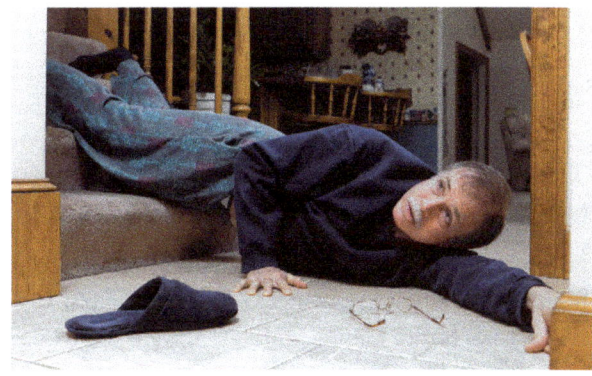

Each year, one in every three adults age 65 and older falls. Falls can cause moderate to severe injuries, such as hip fractures and head traumas, and can increase the risk of early death. Fortunately, falls are a public health problem that is largely preventable.

Birth Defects Registry

The emotional turmoil of having a newborn with a birth defect can be devastating and have lifelong effects for a family. **Birth defects registry** data provides information to monitor, investigate, and make changes to reduce or eliminate birth defects. According to the CDC, hospitalizations for birth defects cost the United States more than $2.6 billion annually. Registry information on birth defects is collected by the National Center on Birth Defects and Developmental Disabilities (NCBDDD), under the direction of the CDC, and birth defects registries that are regulated by individual-state reporting requirements.

Immunization Registry

The documentation and the tracking of immunizations and vaccines have been inconsistent in health care. Most states operate an **immunization registry** that can download data to the CDC's immunization information systems (IIS). Through the IIS, vaccination information is available regardless of where an individual lives or moves. The IIS is intended to increase the number of individuals vaccinated, make vaccination information easily accessible to providers and patients, and enable the CDC to send out reminder and recall notices.

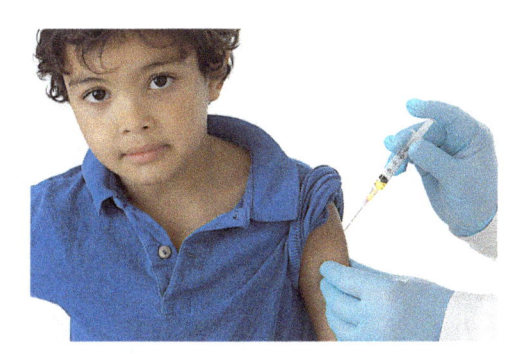

Routine childhood immunizations prevent 14 diseases: diphtheria, hepatitis A, hepatitis B, Hib, influenza (flu), measles, mumps, pertussis (whooping cough), pneumococcal disease, polio, rotavirus, rubella, tetanus, and varicella (chickenpox).

Chapter 11 Quality Management and Data Collection

Cancer Registry

A **cancer registry**, also referred to as **tumor registry**, collects, stores, manages, and analyzes data on people diagnosed with and treated for malignant cancer and people diagnosed with certain benign yet aggressive tumors. Healthcare facilities report cancer cases to a central or state cancer registry, which is a mandatory requirement for hospitals in all 50 states, the District of Columbia, Puerto Rico, and the US Pacific Island jurisdictions. The CDC's National Program of Cancer Registries (NPCR) collects data on cancer occurrence (including the type, extent, and location of the cancer) and the type of initial treatment. National registry data allows physicians and public health agencies to access up-to-date information on treatments and mortality data by cancer type.

Hospital cancer registries are maintained by a *cancer registrar*, often a member of the health information department. The cancer registrar's duties include case finding, abstracting, tumor coding and staging, and following up with reportable cancer patients.

Some smaller hospitals and hospitals not accredited by the American College of Surgeons may not maintain internal cancer registries. Instead, these institutions may hire a certified tumor registrar contractor to abstract and report the basic data required by state regulation.

Case Finding

Case finding is a process used to identify all reportable cancer diagnoses, inpatient or outpatient, which are diagnosed or treated at a facility. Two common methodologies used to identify cancer cases include reviewing pathology reports and reviewing all diagnostic codes within a certain range (for example, all codes for malignant and metastatic cancers listed during the previous month).

The cancer registrar determines which cases are reportable based upon the state list of reportable cancers and, for facilities accredited by the American College of Surgeons (ACS), the Commission on Cancer's (CoC) reportable list. The cancer registrar determines if the patient has been previously entered into the facility's registry. If not, the registrar assigns the patient a case number, a unique eight-digit number called an **accession number**. The first four digits of the case number designate the year the patient was first diagnosed or treated at the facility; the second four digits indicate when the patient was abstracted into the registry database.

For example, patient Mary Hancock is diagnosed with breast cancer in 2015. Her case is assigned accession number 20150189-00. The first four digits of the accession number, 2015, identify the year that her cancer was diagnosed. The numbers 0189 indicate the number of cases entered into the hospital's registry for the year so far. Therefore, Mary Hancock is the 189th patient added to the registry database in 2015.

Cancer registries count the number of primary cancers diagnosed rather than the number of patients with cancer. A **primary cancer** is the anatomical site where the cancer started, such as breast cancer. Once the breast cancer has spread to other locations, such as the liver or the brain, these cancers are not considered primary but rather *metastatic*, cancers that originated from the primary site. A patient diagnosed with a metastatic cancer would not be issued a separate accession number in the registry. Rarely, a patient may be diagnosed with an **unknown primary** in which metastatic cancer cells are found in the body, but the primary origin cannot be determined. In this case, a physician member of the hospital's cancer committee will review the patient's medical record and may even speak with the attending physician to ensure that the cancer is in fact an unknown primary before it is entered as such in the cancer registry system. On occasion, a cancer patient will develop more than one primary site, known as a **multiple malignancy**. Because the cancer registry counts primary cancers, the registrar will designate the additional primary with a sequence number indicating how many primary cancers an individual has. A patient with one primary would have a sequence number of 00, while a patient with three primaries would have a sequence number of 02.

IT REALLY HAPPENS

In 2003, a 65-year-old male patient was diagnosed with chronic lymphocytic leukemia (CLL). He was then treated with chemotherapy, which put the CLL into remission. In 2007, the patient was diagnosed with prostate cancer. In 2011, a routine CT scan to check on the patient's CLL status detected a shadow on his pancreas. The shadow turned out to be pancreatic cancer, a new primary cancer. The patient also had a few basal cell carcinoma lesions removed from the skin of his face and ears. Because he has multiple malignancies, three of which were diagnosed and/or treated at one facility, the facility's cancer registrar assigned the patient more than one accession number: 20030369-00 for the CLL, 20070087-01 for the prostate cancer, and 2011474-02 for the pancreatic cancer. Because the patient's skin cancer was diagnosed and treated at a different facility, that cancer was not accessioned in this facility's cancer registry.

Abstracting

After the cancer registrar has assigned an accession number and a sequence number, the registrar reviews all available patient information and abstracts select data elements, such as demographic and family information, social history, diagnostic studies, cancer stage, treatment, and follow up. This data is then entered into the cancer-registry computer system, or it's manually recorded on a paper form and submitted to the applicable state cancer registry. Hospitals accredited by the American College of Surgeons' Commission on Cancer (ACS/CoC) also report their registry information to the National Cancer Data Base (NCDB).

Coding and Staging

The cancer registrar uses a number of different books and manuals to identify and code the cancer location, type, and stage. Cancer staging reflects the extent to which the cancer has spread from the original site. The most common cancer references include:

The *International Classification of Diseases for Oncology (ICD-O)* is used to code tumor topography (the location or the site of cancer), histology (cell type), behavior (benign, in-situ, or malignant), and grade (how abnormal the tumor cells and the tumor tissue look under a microscope).

EXPAND YOUR KNOWLEDGE

A *tumor grade* indicates how quickly a cancer may grow and spread. Grading systems differ depending on the type of cancer. To learn more about tumor grades, check out the National Cancer Institute fact sheet at *http://IntroHIM .ParadigmCollege.net /TumorGrade*.

- The *Facility Oncology Registry Data Standards (FORDS)* defines what tumor types require data collection.
- The American Joint Committee on Cancer (AJCC) provides staging resources to help identify a tumor's extent and any node involvement and metastasis, also known as *TNM staging*.
- The *Surveillance, Epidemiology, and End Results (SEER) Summary Staging Manual* provides information to help determine the extension of tumors and the differentiation of blood and lymphoid neoplasms.

Cancer staging is based on universal standards. The **cancer stage** describes the severity of a patient's cancer based on tumor location, size, and histology, and how far the cancer has spread. Staging provides the healthcare professional with the information needed to determine a patient's prognosis and the best course of treatment.

TNM Staging System

The **TNM staging system** is one of the most commonly used cancer staging systems in use around the world. The TNM is accepted by the AJCC and the Union for International Cancer Control (UICC). It is a tool that enables physicians to stage different types of cancers based on standardized criteria.

The TNM staging system shown in Table 11.8 is used by most medical facilities. It classifies cancer based on the size or extent (reach) of the tumor (T), the spread to the lymph nodes (N), and the presence of metastasis (M).

Table 11.8 *TNM Staging System*

T describes the original (primary) tumor.
• TX: The primary tumor cannot be evaluated.
• T0: No evidence of primary tumor
• Tis: Carcinoma in situ (abnormal cells are present; not yet a cancer but may develop into one).
• T1, T2, T,3 or T4: The size and/or extent of the primary tumor
N describes whether the cancer has reached nearby lymph nodes.
• NX: Regional lymph nodes cannot be evaluated.
• N0: No regional lymph node involvement (no cancer found in the lymph nodes)
• N1, N2, N3: Involvement of regional lymph nodes (number and/or extent of spread)
M indicates whether there are distant *metastases* (the spread of cancer cells to other parts of the body).
• MX: Distant metastasis cannot be evaluated
• M0: No distant metastasis
• M1: Distant metastasis

For example, breast cancer classified as T3 N2 M0 indicates a large tumor that has spread outside the breast to nearby lymph nodes but no distant metastasis. Prostate cancer T2 N0 M0 indicates a tumor in the prostate but no spread of cancer cells to the lymph nodes or any other part of the body.

Once the T, N, and M are determined, the cancer is assigned an overall stage of 0, I, II, III, or IV. Criteria for cancer staging differs for different types of cancer. These stages may be subdivided as well, such as IIIA and IIIB. Stage I cancers are the least advanced and these patients often have a better prognosis. Stage IV cancers are the most advanced.

Follow Up

Hospital cancer registries that are accredited by the American College of Surgeons continue to collect data on all accessioned cancer cases in the registry throughout the patient's life. This process called **follow up** tracks disease status, including any recurrence of the cancer, any additional cancer treatment provided, and quality of life. Most importantly, the data collected is used to calculate survival rates by cancer site and stage.

TAKE THE CHALLENGE

Go online and locate your state's cancer registry and data reports. (If you are unable to find your state's cancer registry data, use the Texas Cancer Registry data at http://IntroHIM.ParadigmCollege.net/TexasCancerRegistry.)

Find the top 10 anatomical cancer sites for your chosen state for the most recent year or the accumulative years listed (e.g., 2010–2013). Then, create a bar graph showing the top 10 sites broken down by gender. Note which cancer sites appear on both lists. Submit the results to your instructor.

Chapter Summary

Everyone who works in health care does so with the desire to provide the highest quality of care. Quality management is the process of collecting, monitoring, and evaluating data to ensure high-quality care. Physicians, staff, and other hospital employees all play a role in quality management by identifying problems and areas where quality can be improved and by helping to implement the changes needed to advance the efficiency, effectiveness, and reliability of a process or a procedure. Continuous quality improvement is an ongoing process that involves identifying a problem, developing the steps needed for process change, training employees on the new process, and implementing and monitoring the change.

Many regulatory and accrediting bodies and consumer organizations are focused on ensuring safe, high-quality patient care. Joint Commission accreditation is the most recognized and sought after accreditation in health care. It sets standards for patient quality and safety.

Quality documentation is an essential component of safe, high-quality care and is also integral to quality assessment efforts. AHIMA has developed a data quality management model that outlines the characteristics of data quality: accuracy, accessibility, comprehensiveness, consistency, definition, granularity, precision, relevancy, and timeliness.

The case management department ensures that patients get the right care at the right time in the appropriate setting. Case management includes utilization management, transitional planning, care coordination, and resource management. Case managers review patient records for intensity of service and severity of illness criteria.

The risk management department is responsible for preventing and reducing accidents and injuries in a healthcare facility and for limiting the hospital's liability. The risk management department reviews all safety concerns for all persons who enter the facility; the number one area of concern is falls.

Information used by the HIM, case management, risk, and quality departments is collected as data and maintained in databases; it is then used for reporting and evaluation purposes. Data is also collected and maintained in a number of public healthcare databases. This information can be used to compare healthcare providers. Consumer groups often make this comparison data available in the form of healthcare report cards.

Secondary data, abstracted from the patient medical/health record, is collected in databases and by healthcare registries. Some of the most common healthcare registries collect data on trauma, birth defects, immunizations, and cancers. A hospital's cancer registry is usually managed by the HIM department and a certified tumor registrar. The American College of Surgeons has an accreditation process for hospitals with more-detailed cancer registry systems and processes.

HIM Review

Check Your Understanding

Test your understanding of the material covered in this chapter by completing the following multiple-choice questions. For each question, select the best answer from the choices provided.

1. Which of the following is not a component of case management?

    a. utilization review

    b. care coordination

    c. case finding

    d. transitional planning

2. _____ is a set of standardized measures developed to facilitate employer efforts to assess health plan performance.

    a. VBP

    b. ORYX

    c. HEDIS

    d. SE

3. _____ refers to the operational techniques and activities used to regulate performance and prevent undesirable changes in a process.

    a. Continuous quality improvement

    b. Resource management

    c. Process improvement

    d. Quality control

4. Once a problem is identified, it is important to investigate the _____, or the reason for the problem or the failure.

    a. trend

    b. root cause

    c. performance standard

    d. outcome

5. A risk management department _____

    a. files malpractice suits.

    b. develops a methodology for risk prevention or reduction.

    c. abstracts data for national databases.

    d. None of the choices are correct.

6. A cancer registrar _____
    a. collects data on malignant cancers.
    b. collects data on benign yet aggressive tumors.
    c. submits data to a state registry.
    d. All of the choices are correct.

7. Hospitals report core measures to _____
    a. CMS.
    b. the Joint Commission.
    c. the FDA.
    d. the US Department of Health and Human Services.

8. The National Quality Strategy areas of care do not include _____
    a. pneumonia.
    b. perceptions of patient care.
    c. hospital-acquired infections.
    d. cancer.

9. A _____ refers to an unexpected occurrence involving a patient death or a serious physical or psychological injury.
    a. sentinel event
    b. quality
    c. fall
    d. risk

10. Which of the following is not included in the National Quality Strategy's broad-based goals?
    a. affordable care
    b. healthy people/healthy communities
    c. durable care
    d. better care

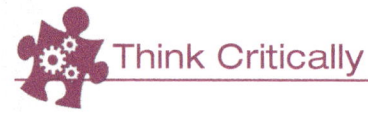

Think Critically

Consider the following real-world scenario and draft a response.

An HIM departmental review of physician progress notes determined that 90 percent of the physicians on staff use the phrase "patient improving" in progress note documentation. Write a short (two-page) paper from your perspective as an HIM professional describing why use of this phrase is a concern and listing the specific steps you would take to help the medical staff improve documentation practices. Explain how you would evaluate the results of your efforts to induce change.

Sharpen Your Comprehension

Complete the following matching exercise by selecting, from the list provided, the answer that best matches each of the numbered statements. For each statement, only one answer is correct.

a. accession number
b. quality control
c. intensity of service
d. medical necessity
e. risk management
f. case finding
g. utilization management
h. value-based purchasing
i. continuous quality improvement
j. cancer stage

1. _____ The process of evaluating the appropriateness of a patient's level of care

2. _____ Operational techniques and activities used to regulate performance and prevent an undesirable change in a process

3. _____ Describes the severity of a patient's cancer based on tumor location, size, and histology and how far the cancer has spread

4. _____ This department is responsible for all medical malpractice and personal injury litigation brought against a healthcare facility.

5. _____ A process used to identify all reportable cancer diagnoses, inpatient or outpatient, that are diagnosed or treated at a facility

6. _____ Refers to care that is reasonable, necessary, and/or appropriate with regard to evidence-based clinical standards of care

7. _____ A unique eight-digit identifier a cancer registrar assigns to each reportable cancer case

8. _____ A payment methodology that rewards quality of care through payment incentives

9. _____ Justification via documentation in the medical record that a patient meets criteria or is "sick enough" to require acute inpatient hospitalization

10. _____ Ensures care that is safe, effective, patient centered, timely, efficient, and equitable

Connect Theory to Practice

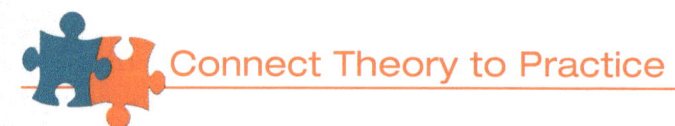

To help translate the concepts presented in this chapter to the workplace, complete the following exercise.

Create a database in Microsoft Access and populated it with enough data elements to be able to run a report to accomplish the tasks listed below.

- a list of patients who live in McClean County who are male and between the ages of 0 and 55 who have had a fractured femur

- a list of charts to review (Hint: You will need to have the medical record number.) for patients who are female and Hispanic with an advance directive on file

Next, do the following:

1. Name your database.

2. Provide a list of database elements.

3. Abstract at least 25 patients into your database.

4. Run the reports above (do not forget to name your reports), and submit the list of database elements and the reports to your instructor.

Student eResources

*To enhance your comprehension of the chapter material, go to **Navigator+** and complete the additional practice items as advised by your instructor.*

Chapter Terms

- accession number
- birth defects registry
- cancer registry/tumor registry
- cancer stage
- care coordination
- case finding
- case management department
- case manager
- concurrent review
- continuous quality improvement (CQI)
- database
- follow up
- Healthcare Effectiveness Data and Information Set (HEDIS)
- healthcare registry
- hospital-acquired infection (HAI)
- immunization registry
- infection-control committee
- intensity of service (IS)
- Joint Commission
- medical necessity
- multiple malignancy
- National Patient Safety Goals
- National Quality Strategy
- ORYX
- primary cancer
- process improvement (PI)
- quality
- quality control
- quality improvement (QI)
- resource management
- retrospective review
- risk
- risk management
- secondary data
- sentinel event (SE)
- severity of illness (SI)
- TNM staging system
- transitional (discharge) planning
- trauma registry
- unknown primary
- utilization management
- value-based purchasing (VBP)

> "Trust is the glue of life. It's the most essential ingredient in effective communication. It's the foundational principle that holds all relationships."
>
> — Stephen R. Covey, author, *The 7 Habits of Highly Effective People*

Professionalism Tip

Management by Walking Around

"Management by walking around" is an easy way for managers to keep in touch with those on the team. Dropping in on employees builds rapport, increases visibility, and allows the manager to have eyes on staff members, equipment, and the status of work.

Dos and Don'ts
- Do visit each employee.
- Do follow up on questions and concerns raised.
- Do not use this time to criticize or correct.

Fast Facts

Healthcare benefits are an important factor when taking a new job or staying with a current one. Approximately 25 percent of employed individuals choose employment based on better healthcare benefits.

(*Source: Kaiser Family Foundation*)

Chapter 12
Management

> "The leaders who work most effectively, it seems to me, never say 'I.' And that's not because they have trained themselves not to say 'I.' They don't think 'I.' They think 'we'; they think 'team.' They understand their job to be to make the team function. They accept responsibility and don't sidestep it, but 'we' gets the credit. This is what creates trust, what enables you to get the task done."
>
> — Peter Drucker, management consultant, author, educator

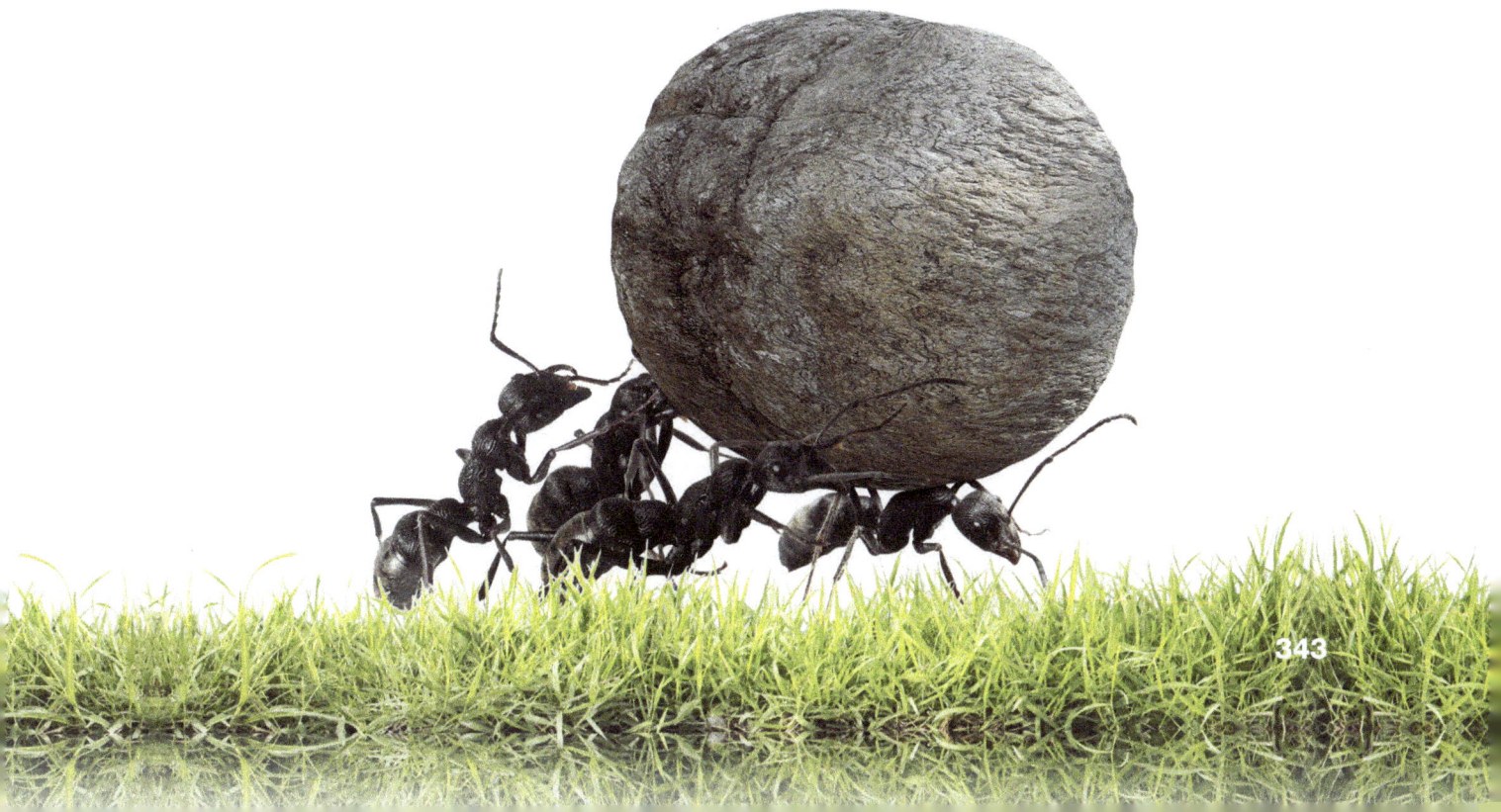

Learning Objectives

- Distinguish between management and leadership.
- Explain the steps used to build excellent teams.
- Evaluate workflow and improve efficiency.
- Explain the techniques used to evaluate and improve processes.
- Describe two types of projects and explain how they are different.
- Identify the steps in the project management process.
- Understand good communication techniques.
- Understand the manager's role in selecting, evaluating, and motivating employees.
- Be able to conduct employee orientation and training programs.
- Understand the use of staff productivity data.
- Know how to write policies and procedures.
- Demonstrate an understanding of the budget process.

Management and Leadership

There are many opportunities for health information management (HIM) professionals to pursue management and leadership roles within healthcare organizations. Some of those positions are discussed in Chapter 1. Titles such as director, manager, and supervisor all encompass varying levels of management responsibility.

What is the difference between a manager and a leader? A **manager** plans, organizes, and delegates tasks. He or she works with systems and procedures and supervises employees. Management is about processes. A **leader** inspires and motivates others. He or she works with people and has followers. Leadership is about behavior. These two approaches complement each other and both are necessary for success.

IT REALLY HAPPENS

When the hospital's HIM department was suddenly faced with unplanned staffing shortages, Salina, a transcription clerk, knew that something had to be done to ensure that important job duties were covered. She sought help from other employees and together they devised an immediate coverage plan and a plan to catch up any backlog that developed because of the staffing shortage. Salina presented the staff's recommendations to her manager and then "rallied the troops," inspiring everyone to work together.

In this example, Salina is acting as an **informal leader**. A leader does not need to be at the top of the organizational chart or have a formal title to lead. The most successful companies have leaders at all layers of the organization. In this case, Salina is perceived by her peers and by the organization as someone who is both experienced and knowledgeable. Informal leaders do not hold positions of authority or power, but they can influence the decisions and actions of those around them in both positive and negative ways. It is important for a manager to identify these individuals and then to develop clear expectations and parameters for them.

Manager

One of the responsibilities of a manager is to delegate tasks. **Delegating** is assigning responsibility and authority for a particular task or role to another person or group or, as in this case, to an employee. Delegating is not easy. It is not uncommon for a manager to think he or she can perform a particular task faster and more accurately than the employee. However, one of a manager's responsibilities is to train employees, set expectations, and then follow up to ensure those expectations are met. Managers who fail to delegate often become overwhelmed and may lose the respect of the employees they supervise.

A manager is also a decision maker. A **decision** is the act of choosing a course of action from among the available alternatives. A manager in the HIM department must make many decisions each day, from deciding which employee should conduct a deficiency system audit, to deciding how to discuss concerns about personal hygiene with an employee. To make the best decision, it is important for a manager to:

- know when he or she has gathered enough information to make a good decision
- understand the organization's priorities and evaluate each decision against the organization's other competing needs and priorities
- know whether the decision is supported by his or her personal ethics and values

TAKE THE CHALLENGE

You are the manager of the HIM department and have discovered that Dr. Houng, a popular staff physician, has shared his username and password with his office manager. The office manager is electronically signing Dr. Houng's verbal and telephone orders. The Joint Commission, the Centers for Medicare and Medicaid Services (CMS), and the US Department of Health and Human Services (HHS) all have standards that clearly state that *only* the physician may sign orders. Dr. Houng also signed a security statement before receiving his computer login in which he agreed not to share his username and password with anyone, a requirement of the Health Insurance Portability and Accountability Act of 1996 (HIPAA) regulations. When you approach the hospital administrator about your concern, she instructs you, "Leave him alone. He is one of the hospital's biggest admitters and is also on the board of directors. We do not want to upset him!"

Outline the issues. Describe in detail how you would handle this situation.

Leader

Leaders are often described as visionaries. They look beyond the day-to-day responsibilities and consider how an organization can grow and develop in the future. They encourage change and persuade people to accept change. Leaders are risk takers. A **risk taker** is someone who chooses an action that offers an opportunity for gain but also has potential risk. Risk taking is like gambling; you may win or you may lose. A leader evaluates risk to determine whether potential gain is worth the risk.

WHAT WOULD YOU DO?

As an HIM leader at a medium-sized metropolitan hospital, you have been asked to decide whether to outsource the hospital's transcription work overseas. By outsourcing, the hospital can reduce its need for staff and equipment, resulting in substantial cost savings, and recapture valuable space in the facility that can be repurposed to accommodate revenue-generating services. However, outsourcing has substantial risks. Transcription services located outside the United States are not regulated under HIPAA, and transcriptionists in other countries may not understand English slang, which may result in errors within the medical report.

Do you think outsourcing is worth the risk? Explain the reasoning behind your decision.

Leaders are excellent change agents. A **change agent** assists individuals, teams, and organizations in moving from the current state to a desired future state. Being an agent of change is an important aspect of leadership because change can be unsettling, and people naturally resist change. A change agent should:

- effectively communicate the reason for the change
- engage key stakeholders (people affected by the change)
- provide counseling and support to those affected by the change
- keep communication flowing throughout the change process
- measure, monitor, and tweak changes as necessary

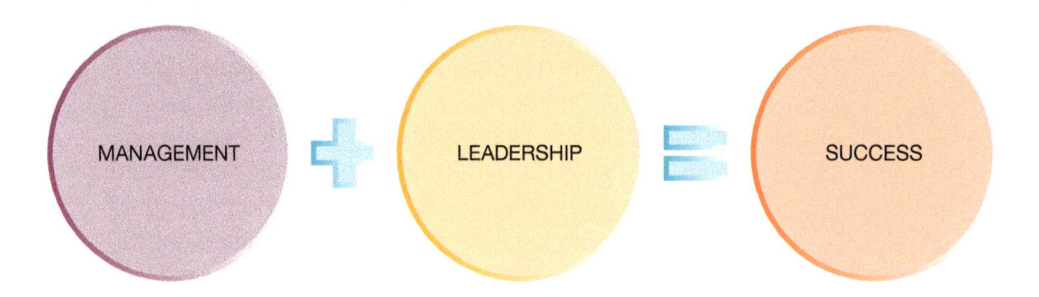

MANAGEMENT + LEADERSHIP = SUCCESS

Working in Teams

One of the most important responsibilities of a leader is forming and developing successful teams. In the current healthcare environment, it is essential that employees work together to provide high-quality, low-cost services. Consider how you would feel as a patient in a hospital. You would want every employee to work cooperatively and seamlessly to ensure you received the best care possible.

A team is a group of individuals organized to work together. **Teamwork** is the cooperative effort by a group or team to achieve a common goal. As a healthcare leader, you may be asked to develop a team to achieve certain goals. So, how do you get started?

First, it is important to define the team's goal. A **goal** is a desired result, an endpoint toward which effort is directed. For a team to succeed, a goal needs to be:

- specific
- measureable
- attainable
- completed within a specific timeframe

Setting an appropriate goal is one of the keys to successful teamwork. A goal should not be too large or ill defined. For example, for a team performing data analysis, "find a cure for cancer" is too large, unstructured, and unrealistic to be a successful goal. "Find data elements associated with recurrence of breast cancer" is a much more specific goal. It is also realistically achievable for this type of project.

Building a Team

Working as a team does not always come naturally in our society. As young children we are taught to strive to "be number one," to win, and to get ahead. But working as a team requires members to put the well-being and success of the team before personal gain. And the team leader must ensure that the individuals on the team understand and share this philosophy, and that they have the knowledge and qualifications to support the team's success.

As a leader, it is important to select the best-qualified people to serve on the team. Team members should:

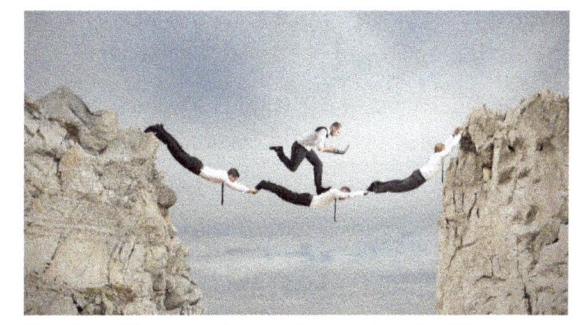

- be committed to achieving the goal
- have knowledge of the subject matter
- communicate professionally and effectively

Simply putting people together and saying "You are a team!" isn't enough. Successful teams go through several development stages.

Chapter 12   Management

Stages of Team Development

Once a team has been assembled and team members have agreed upon a well-defined goal, everything should go smoothly—right? Probably not. Simply putting people together and saying "You're a team" will not ensure success. To ensure a team's success, it is important to understand the dynamics of teamwork. During a project, a team goes through several stages of development. In 1965, psychologist Bruce Tuckman first described these stages of development as forming, storming, norming, and performing. Tuckman's process is still widely used today to develop high-performance teams.

Forming is the first stage of team development. Team members may experience excitement and a little bit of anxiety as they learn about the team's tasks and goals and their individual roles.

Storming, the second stage, can become uncomfortable for team members as they begin to assert themselves and try to define their individual roles. Anxiety levels may increase throughout this stage. Team members may question the validity of the team's goals or the way team members are approaching those goals. Team functionality is at a pivotal point during storming. The storming phase does not last long; sometimes this stage passes after one meeting. As a leader, you must quickly move the team through the storming stage while being careful to allow time for input from everyone. The leader must be made clear and be accepted at this stage. Consequently, this is the stage at which many teams fail.

Norming, which is the third stage, takes place when everyone is comfortable with his or her role on the team. Team members begin to develop relationships with each other, many times socializing together as they begin to focus on the goal at hand. Occasionally, storming may pop back up when, for example, a new task is introduced; however, the team members have developed trusting relationships at this stage, so this regression is not likely to last long.

Performing is the fourth stage. This is the easiest stage for a leader because everyone on the team has a shared vision of the team's goals and work is progressing. During this stage, trust is firmly in place. Trust is demonstrated when all team members exhibit consistent, open, and cooperative behavior.

The advancement of the team toward the goal should not solely depend on the leader. Each team member should be assigned specific duties. Every team includes certain key roles:

- The recorder is responsible for the agenda and minutes.
- The timekeeper keeps the discussion of each subject within the time allotted in the agenda.
- The parking lot attendant records issues that come up during discussions that are not currently on the agenda and ensures these items are placed on a future agenda and are not forgotten.
- The facilitator assists with problem solving and helps the team achieve consensus during difficult discussions.

Meetings

Meetings, whether conducted in person or virtually via telephone or computer conferencing, are necessary to provide key employee stakeholders a setting in which to discuss topics of mutual interest. (A *stakeholder* is someone who can affect or be affected by a decision.) Meetings can feel like a waste of time if clear objectives are not laid out in advance. Developing an agenda and defining team roles can help ensure a meeting goes smoothly and is efficient and productive.

The team leader should provide an **agenda** that lists the items to be discussed and any proposed actions. As shown in Example 12.1, an agenda should always include the start time and duration of the meeting and indicate the amount of time allotted for each discussion item. It is the responsibility of the timekeeper to inform the team leader when the time allotted for a topic is about to run out.

Example 12.1 Sample Agenda

HIM Scanning Team Meeting

Date | time 5/11/2015 1:00 PM | *Location* Conference A2

Meeting called by	Gabriela Ortiz
Duration of Meeting	1 hour
Facilitator	Quality Dept. Representative
Record Keeper	Kiara Johnson
Timekeeper	Samuel Gallagher

Attendees: Gabriela Ortiz, Kiara Johnson, Samuel Gallagher, Tyrone Brown, Emma Reed, Jasmine Flores

Guest: Mary Pat Mackey, Facilitator

Please read: Last month's meeting minutes

Please bring: Completed assignments

Ground Rules: Start and end on time; leave titles at the door; be respectful of others; cell phones off; no side conversations; all meeting content remains confidential

Topic	Presenter	Time allotted
☐ Call to order, approval of previous month's minutes	Gabriela	1M
☐ Agenda review, additions to new business	Gabriela	1M
Old Business:		
☐ Assignment report: number of scanned documents per day	All	10M
☐ Scanning labs from Mayo Clinic	Tyrone	20M
New Business:		
☐ Service agreements for scanners (moved from parking lot)	Emma	10M
☐ Scanning quality review schedule	Gabriela	10M

Assignments and next meeting:

Assignments	Gabriela	5M
Next meeting:	Gabriela	2M
Adjourn:	Gabriela	1M

The team members should agree on a set of ground rules during the first meeting and those ground rules should be included on all subsequent meeting agendas. **Ground rules** are the values and standards by which team members agree to abide to facilitate teamwork. Each team is unique and will need to develop ground rules to meet its specific needs.

Some basic ground rules include but are not limited to:

- Start and end on time.
- Leave titles at the door.
- Listen to the person talking; no side discussions.
- Decisions will be made by majority rule.
- Once a decision is made, all team members must publicly support the decision.
- Complete all assignments by the due date.
- Treat other team members with respect and dignity.

It is important to specify how the team will make decisions. The team leader, with assistance from the team facilitator, guides the team in all decision making. A variety of strategies exist to help teams facilitate decision making.

- Rank the issues and responses in order of importance.
- Use a flowchart to determine efficient workflow (see Example 12.2).
- Employ a cause-and-effect diagram, also known as a *fishbone diagram*, to illustrate the possible causes of a problem (see Example 12.3).

Using a Flowchart

A **flowchart** is a visual diagram used to illustrate the physical steps in a process. A flowchart can reveal problem areas, redundancies, and areas where standardization can be applied. It allows the viewer to see the process, revealing areas that need more investigation.

The four basic flowchart symbols are:

- ○ Start/stop
- □ Task/activity/step
- ◇ Decision point (yes/no)
- → Direction of process

The flowchart shown in Example 12.2 illustrates the steps necessary to retrieve and scan discharged patients' paper records.

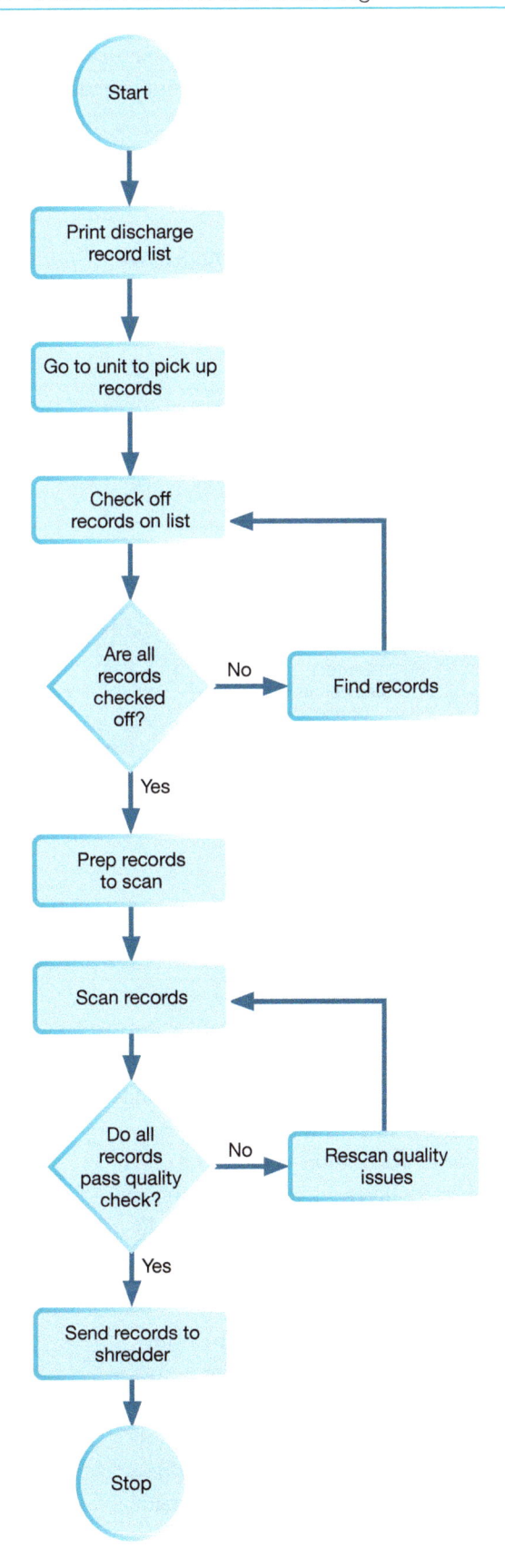

Example 12.2 Flowchart—Record Retrieval and Scanning

```
Start
  ↓
Print discharge record list
  ↓
Go to unit to pick up records
  ↓
Check off records on list ←─────────┐
  ↓                                  │
Are all records checked off? ──No──→ Find records
  │ Yes
  ↓
Prep records to scan
  ↓
Scan records ←──────────────────────┐
  ↓                                  │
Do all records pass quality check? ──No──→ Rescan quality issues
  │ Yes
  ↓
Send records to shredder
  ↓
Stop
```

Chapter 12 Management

A **fishbone diagram** examines the causes and effects of a problem in a process. In Example 12.3, the four branches that create the "fishbone" identify the four areas (equipment, policies/procedures, supplies, and people) that are causing the problem (effect). In this scenario, the records are not coded in a timely manner, which can result in delayed reimbursement.

Example 12.3 Fishbone Diagram—Cause-Effect

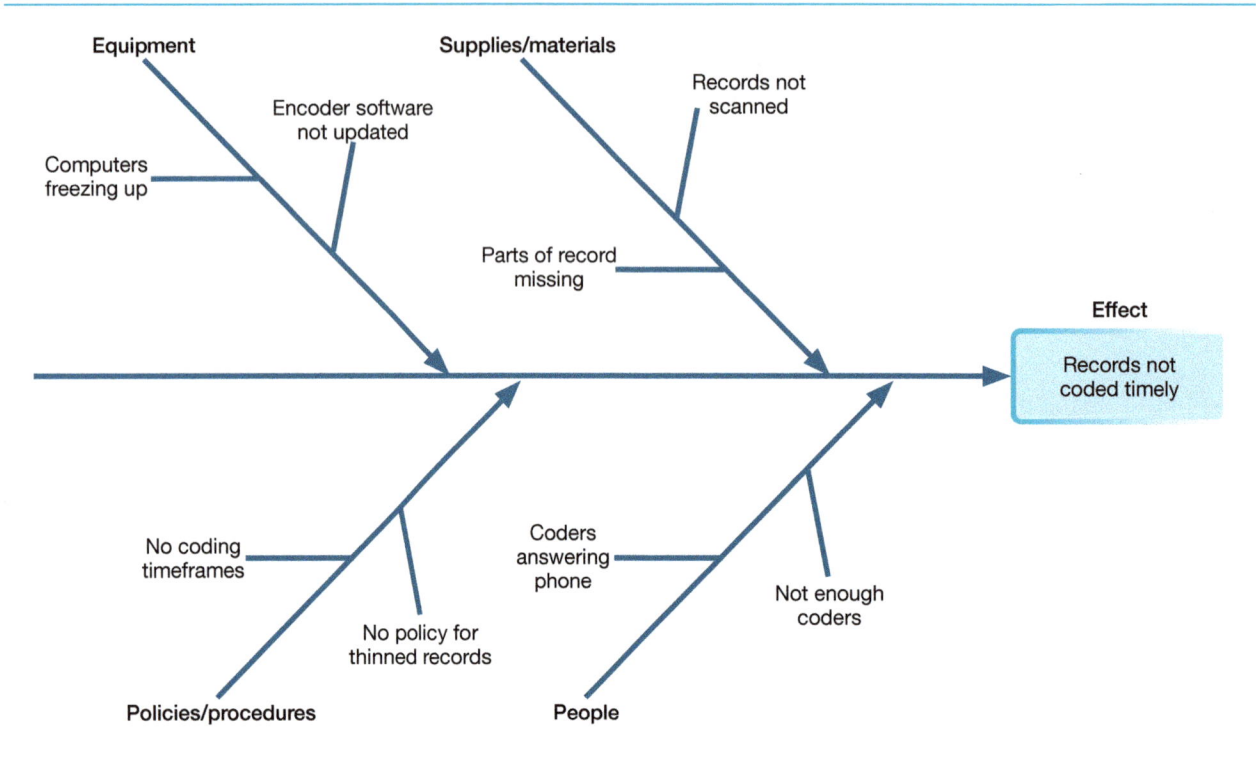

Equipment: Encoder software not updated; Computers freezing up

Supplies/materials: Records not scanned; Parts of record missing

Policies/procedures: No coding timeframes; No policy for thinned records

People: Coders answering phone; Not enough coders

Effect: Records not coded timely

Recognition and Rewards

The team leader collaborates with the team to establish dates for accomplishing tasks and interim goals and for completing the project (achieving the goal). The team should celebrate the completion of each milestone along the way. The type of celebration will depend on team members' preferences. A celebration can be large or small, and it should reflect the difficulty of the task and the time it took the team to achieve the goal.

Once the main goal has been met, the team should follow up to ensure everything is on track. Once this process is complete, the team will disband. This will be a time of major celebration, possibly mixed with a bit of sadness, because the team members may have become close and may miss working together.

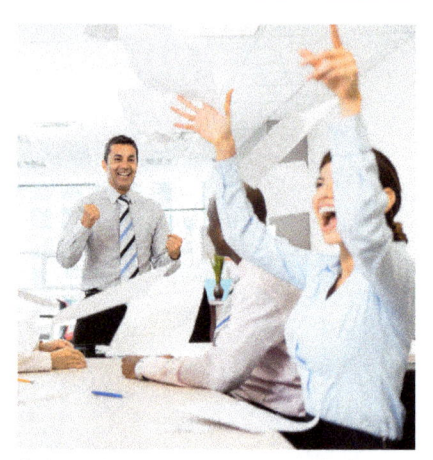

Celebrating smaller, interim goals or milestones can help sustain members' motivation until the team achieves its ultimate goal.

Project Management

As an HIM professional, you may be responsible for one or more projects at any given time. A **project** is a temporary endeavor designed to produce a specific product, service, or result. A project is also unique; it is not part of an individual's regular job duties. It is a specific, defined task that may bring together individuals from different parts of the organization as well as people from outside of the organization.

In its simplest form, a project typically includes three elements: a description outlining the scope of the project, a budget, and a deadline for completing the work.

When all three of these elements are in balance, the project is likely to be completed on time and within budget. There are many factors that can upset this balance, however. A project may take more than the allotted time to complete, the cost of completing the project may exceed the amount budgeted, or the scope of the project may shrink or grow. **Project management** is the process of planning, organizing, and guiding a project from start to finish. Effective project management requires someone with good organizational, communication, and problem-solving skills.

Simple and Complex Projects

Although every project is different, projects are generally broken down into two broad categories, simple and complex.

A **simple project** is limited in scope. It usually involves a defined number of tasks and may be completed in a few days or a few months. In general, simple projects do not include a large number of subprojects and do not require project management tools to organize and track the project.

One example of a simple project that might be developed by an HIM department is the creation of a computer database tool to make it easier and more efficient to track which physicians have delinquent records. The HIM department keeps an ongoing and detailed report of delinquent records and submits that data to the employee responsible for physician credentialing. Tracking physicians' delinquent records is an important HIM task because a physician with too many delinquent records may lose his or her hospital privileges.

Staffing for this relatively simple project would likely require a project manager and three to five additional HIM employees with knowledge of the delinquent records process. The budget for such a project can vary widely. No additional dollars may be needed if the project uses existing staff and software. If the project requires the purchase of new software and employee overtime, it could cost the department several thousand dollars.

In general, a **complex project** involves more people and resources than a simple project and requires more time and money to complete. There may be one goal or many goals. Complex projects often include multiple subprojects that must be completed either before the main project or simultaneously with it. With more interrelated and interdependent variables, the execution of complex projects is also more unpredictable; goals, resources, and the people involved may change as the project evolves. Complex projects often require project management tools to organize, track, and manage the tasks and subprojects that must be completed, each of which may have its own budget, staff, and deadline.

One example of a complex project that involves the HIM department is the selection and implementation of an electronic health record (EHR) system. As discussed in Chapter 7, in a hospital setting, an EHR system interacts with many other hospital computer systems. The purchase and implementation of an EHR system requires the collaboration of representatives from many hospital departments, the medical staff, and outside vendors and is both costly and time consuming.

The Project Management Process

The Project Management Institute (PMI), a nonprofit, professional membership association, suggests that successful project management involves five separate phases or processes: initiating, planning, executing, monitoring and controlling, and closing. These processes are often overlapping but may vary in intensity during different parts of the project.

The **initiation process** involves defining the scope of the project, determining the key participants, and outlining the goals and objectives.

The **planning process** may include identifying resources, developing a budget, creating a project schedule, and identifying potential problems that may arise during the course of the project.

The **execution process** begins when the project commences and continues until the project is complete. During this stage the management of the project is most complex, requiring the coordination of staff, resources, and deadlines.

Monitoring and controlling is also an ongoing process. It involves monitoring schedules and costs, making sure all projects objectives are met, and problem solving when things don't go according to the project plan.

Once a project is complete, there should be a formal process for closing the project. The **closing process** may involve paying vendors or contractors, evaluating the outcome against the project goals, and capturing lessons learned for the benefit of future projects.

Project Management Tools

Having a project manager with the right skills is important to the success of a project. Many types of project management tools and systems are available to make the job of managing a complex project easier. The manager must carefully consider the size and scope of the project in order to select the right tool(s) or system(s) to manage it.

One of the best tools for managing complex projects is a Gantt chart. A **Gantt chart** is a type of bar chart that can be used to outline and monitor a project, including establishing start and stop dates and task assignments. It allows the user to identify overlapping and critical tasks or phases of a project, as well as track the progress of the project and changes to the project plan. Read more about Gantt charts and view examples at http://IntroHIM.ParadigmCollege.net/Gantt.

Selecting and Evaluating Employees

The HIM manager is responsible for making sure that the department runs smoothly, efficiently, and reliably. Maintaining adequate staffing levels is an important part of that goal, which begins with interviewing, hiring, and training the right employees. Employees should receive ongoing feedback on their work, as required by the Joint Commission and other accrediting agencies.

Interviewing Potential Employees

When hiring a new employee, it may be tempting to look for a candidate who is the "perfect fit" and someone who is knowledgeable, experienced, and productive. However, these qualities may not be sufficient to ensure that a candidate is the best fit for the department or organization. Skills and experience are no longer the only qualities most employers look for in a new hire. Employers also want individuals who can think critically and behave professionally.

A survey conducted by the organization Leadership IQ found that 46 percent of new hires were fired, received poor performance reviews, or were written up within the first 18 months. The study, which looked at 20,000 employees hired over a three-year period, identified poor interpersonal skills as the chief reason new employees failed. These individuals could not be coached, ignored constructive feedback, resisted change, and lacked emotional intelligence and motivation.

The fact that these individuals were knowledgeable, experienced, and productive was not sufficient to overcome their lack of interpersonal skills. As a manager, it is important to be familiar with the job description and effective interview techniques and practices to quickly identify the best candidate for the job. In general, you will have only 30 to 60 minutes to interview a candidate and determine if that individual is a good fit for your organization.

Writing a Job Description

When recruiting a new employee, refer to the **job description**, which provides a broad, general statement of employee roles and responsibilities. The HIM management team should develop and regularly update job descriptions for each position in the department. Each organization will have its own format and content requirements; however, at a minimum, a job description should include these elements:

- job title
- reporting relationships (who is the supervisor)
- qualifications, including education, credentials, and experience requirements
- physical requirements, such as sitting, standing, traveling, or lifting (maximum pounds)
- essential duties and responsibilities

Having a clear and accurate job description helps to ensure the Human Resource (HR) Department drafts an accurate job placement advertisement and makes it easier

Think Ethics!

Hiring a family member is not necessarily illegal, but it may be considered unethical, particularly if that person will report directly to another family member. The practice of hiring or promoting a family member regardless of merit is called **nepotism** and is prohibited in many organizations.

to prescreen applicants. A full and accurate job description can also help protect an organization from a wrongful termination lawsuit. (View sample job descriptions in the Student eResources section of Navigator+.)

Telephone Screening

It is not uncommon for many applicants to apply for any one position. Start by reviewing résumés and select those individuals whose qualifications most closely match the job description. In-person interviews are time consuming. Many organizations use prescreening telephone interviews to further reduce the pool of applicants. Screening interviews can help eliminate candidates who are not interested in the position at the salary offered and those lacking sufficient experience or a particular skill. Basic screening questions may include:

- What type of job are you looking for?
- Are you willing to work rotating shifts, weekends, and holidays?
- Have you used _____ computer software before?
- What type of salary are you looking for?

Interview Questions

Once the final pool of applicants has been identified, it is time to think about the interview process. Conducting an effective interview is essential for finding and selecting the right candidate. Most of us have been in interviews in which the questions seem predictable and routine. Familiar questions such as, "Tell me about yourself" and "What are your strengths and weaknesses?" do not go deep enough. The first question may be a good ice-breaker, but what do these questions really reveal? Interview questions should be open-ended and situational. Ask the candidate to describe how he or she would behave in a given situation. Some questions can bring out more in-depth information about a candidate's personality and work ethic.

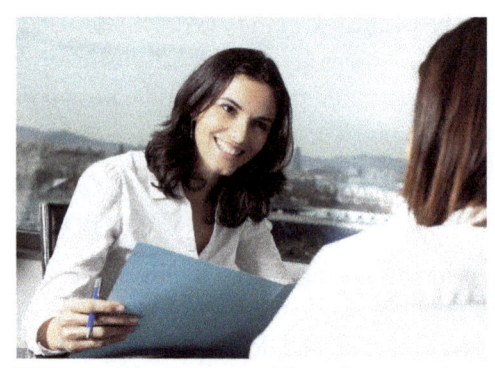

When interviewing potential employees, ask open-ended questions.

Questions like these reveal a candidate's ability to deal with difficult situations.

Tell me how you would deal with an angry physician who is yelling and refusing to complete his or her records.

Tell me what you would do if a coworker was interrupting you and putting you down during a team meeting.

Responses that should raise red flags include, for example, "I would go to my supervisor," or "I would yell and tell the person off."

Other questions can demonstrate a candidate's ability to research and problem solve.

Tell me how you would find an unusual code for a rare diagnosis.

If you are given a new task and you cannot remember how to do it, what would you do?

The individual should describe how he or she would independently solve the problem, referring to coding research materials or procedure manuals.

Certain questions can help an employer evaluate a candidate's ability to plan and organize.

Tell me how you plan your day.

How do you prioritize your work?

When a candidate makes an open-ended comment or vague statement in response to a question, it is important to ask a follow-up question. Consider what the following exchange reveals about this candidate.

Interviewer: *What type of person do you like to work for?*

Candidate: *A nice and understanding person.*

Interviewer: *Please tell me what you mean by "nice and understanding."*

Candidate: *Well, I have a lot of personal problems and I tend to be late a lot.*

Based on this exchange, this candidate would not be selected for employment. Asking follow-up questions often provides more detailed information that can help to identify undesirable candidates.

Illegal Interview Questions

Federal and state laws prohibit employers from asking discriminatory questions during a job interview. In general, it is illegal to ask questions related to a job seeker's:

- political or religious affiliation
- illness or disability
- marital status or pregnancy
- age, race, or place of birth
- sexual orientation

Prehire Assessments

After selecting a candidate for the position, it is important to contact the candidate's professional references. Employers are sometimes reluctant to discuss former employees out of concern for potential legal repercussions. However, the candidate should provide references who will speak openly about his or her past work history. Much like in an interview, when speaking with a candidate's references, use open-ended questions.

Tell me about the employee's attendance record over the last year.

Can you tell me about a time when the employee handled a difficult customer situation?

In what area would you say this employee could improve? ("None" is not a sufficient answer.)

Would you hire this employee again? Please explain.

Individuals who work in health care can expect to undergo additional screening. Many healthcare employees provide patient care or have access to confidential patient information. Organizations often require employees to undergo a full background check, including employment, criminal history, drug screening, a review of the candidate's social media profile, and, in some cases, personality testing.

An offer of employment should not be made until all pre-hire assessments have been completed and the results are satisfactory.

Employee Feedback

Providing an employee with constructive feedback on his or her job performance is essential to keeping communication open between the manager and employee, which helps the employee gauge how well he or she is meeting the manager's expectations. Feedback is more informal than a performance evaluation. It can be all positive, all negative, or a little of both. What is important is that feedback is given regularly (e.g., weekly) and is accurate and concise.

Conversations about an employee's performance must take place in private. If a situation requires correction, always discuss the situation, behavior, or task instead of the person or his or her personality. If the employee has difficulty communicating or accepting criticism, ask another manager to sit in on the discussion. The witness should be at or above the level of the manager in the organizational structure; a nonmanagerial employee should never be asked to participate.

TAKE THE CHALLENGE

You are the manager of Mercy Hospital's HIM department and need to speak to a scanning technician about her low productivity. You have discussed this issue with the employee before and documented the discussion as a verbal warning in the employee's file. During these discussions, the employee has become defensive and argumentative, accusing you of discriminating against her. She argues that there are others in the department not producing at the required level and that she is the only one being singled out.

Outline your concerns. Explain in detail how you would handle your next meeting with this employee.

Performance Evaluations

A manager or consultant will use a **performance evaluation** to examine and evaluate the work of an employee against preset standards. These evaluations can help to determine when an employee requires additional training, to evaluate employees for promotions, merit increases, or bonuses, and to determine whether an employee should be counseled or fired. Every organization has its own employee evaluation format and policies governing its use. Some organizations evaluate employees every 90 days, although most companies conduct annual evaluations. The Joint Commission requires accredited organizations to conduct an annual performance evaluation for every employee. Some organizations have adopted an evaluation process called **360-degree feedback**. This process collects data from "all around" an employee, including assessments by supervisors, peers, subordinates, team members, and customers. Regardless of how an organization structures the evaluation process, every performance evaluation should follow some general rules, including:

- Information presented in an evaluation should never be a surprise to the employee. An employee should be able to anticipate what will be on the evaluation from ongoing conversations and meetings with a supervisor.

- Evaluations should be process-, behavior-, and data-driven.

- The evaluation should accurately assess the employee's accomplishments and identify opportunities for improvement.

- As part of the process, the manager and employee should establish goals for the employee for the following year.

- The evaluation should be documented in writing and signed by the employee and manager.

Motivation

First-time HIM managers often fall victim to visions of grandeur. As a manager, it is common to think that you can increase productivity and efficiency by motivating staff to work harder. The reality is a little more complex.

Motivation is the reason people do things. There are two types of motivation: intrinsic and extrinsic. **Intrinsic motivation** comes from inside the individual ("I want to be a good employee" or "It makes me feel good"). **Extrinsic motivation** comes from an outside source, for example, the opportunity to earn money or a promotion. A good HIM leader uses extrinsic motivation, such as providing a pleasant work environment, listening to employees with genuine interest, developing trust, and involving employees in decisions that affect them, to ensure that employees are fully engaged with, emotionally committed to, and involved in the work.

Managers who use fear, intimidation, or both as motivation are not likely to earn employees' respect or loyalty. Although some short-term increase may be seen in production, the long-term commitment from employees will be lost.

A leader must demonstrate strong personal ethics by being honest and trustworthy and acting with integrity. As discussed earlier in this chapter, a good leader is someone people want to follow, not just the person in charge. An HIM leader must share his or her vision with others in the department, recognize the importance of every task, show appreciation, and encourage employees to share their ideas.

IT REALLY HAPPENS

A patient unexpectedly died while intubated for anesthesia in the operating room. The hospital chief executive officer instructed the HIM director to secure the patient's medical record in a locked file in her office. The next day, the director noticed that the interoperative nursing documentation was missing. The director asked several employees to help look for the documentation. One of the department's informal leaders stood up and shouted, "Everybody, our director needs help!" All of the members of the department began to help look for the file. After the documentation was recovered, the employee who found it was rewarded with a paper crown with the words "Queen for the Day" printed on it.

Training

Whether orienting new employees, addressing a performance evaluation issue, or introducing a new system, training is another responsibility of an HIM manager. **Training** is the act of coaching or teaching a behavior or process through specific instruction and practice. Providing employees with high-quality training improves employee and customer satisfaction, increases productivity, decreases errors, and provides the organization with a financial return on investment (ROI). Time and money invested in employee training can increase employee retention and reduce absenteeism, which can result in lost productivity. Improving employee retention reduces the need to recruit, hire, and train new employees. The cost of hiring a new employee is estimated to be between 50 and 150 percent of an employee's annual salary.

> "Tell me, I'll forget; show me, I may remember. But involve me, and I'll understand."
> — Chinese Proverb

Training and Orientation

Individuals learn differently. Some people absorb information best by reading, while other people need to hear the information presented verbally, either in one-on-one conversation or in a lecture. Some people need information presented in more than one way to fully understand it. Therefore, it is important for a manager to know which learning style is most effective for an individual or group. Many employees enjoy hands-on training. **Hands-on training** involves the employee in the new activity and provides practical experience. Inputting data into a physician deficiency system and running a report of delinquent records are examples of tasks that can be learned through hands-on training.

Employee training can begin during the interview process. In fact, asking a potential employee how she or he learns best is a good interview question. Talk with the candidate about the culture, values, success indicators, work ethic, and expectations of the job.

Once hired, the employee should go through an orientation process. During **orientation**, the employee tours the new company and department, meets coworkers and his or her immediate supervisor, and learns about the policies, procedures, and culture of the workplace. The benefits of providing a thorough orientation include:

- reduced anxiety
- an increased understanding of and commitment to the organization
- clear performance expectations
- a better understanding of what to expect from the organization

After an employee has completed the orientation process, he or she will begin training for a specific job. Training materials should be easy to read, complete, and concise. New employees should receive a copy of all policies that apply to that position. If possible, training should be conducted away from an employee's workspace in a quiet location where there will be no interruptions. Training should be interactive. Encourage the employee to ask questions during the training session. Take breaks. Breaks can help the employee avoid information overload, and give the employee time to process the new information. Use a check list to ensure that all aspects of the training are covered. At the end of the session, administer a competency test, such as the one shown in Example 12.4, to ensure the employee is proficient in the new process.

Example 12.4 Sample Competency Test

Competency Test

Chart Deficiency Analysis and Deficiency Data Entry

Summary: HIM analysis technicians review discharged patient records for completeness. When a deficiency is identified, the HIM technician flags the item and records the data in the deficiency system.

Records must be accurate. A physician with delinquent records could lose surgical and admitting privileges.

Ask the employee to analyze 10 new discharged medical records.

Check each record for accuracy based on established policies and procedures.

If the employee achieves 100 percent accuracy, provide a permanent computer login and password for the deficiency system.

If the employee achieves less than 100 percent accuracy, ask the employee to analyze 10 more records. Continue the process until the employee achieves 100 percent accuracy.

Cross-Training

The HIM manager is also responsible for ensuring the department continues to function smoothly if an employee is ill, is on vacation, or leaves the organization. One way to ensure adequate staffing is to cross-train employees. **Cross-training** involves training employees to do tasks normally performed by coworkers. Don't be like Ted in the Dilbert cartoon below.

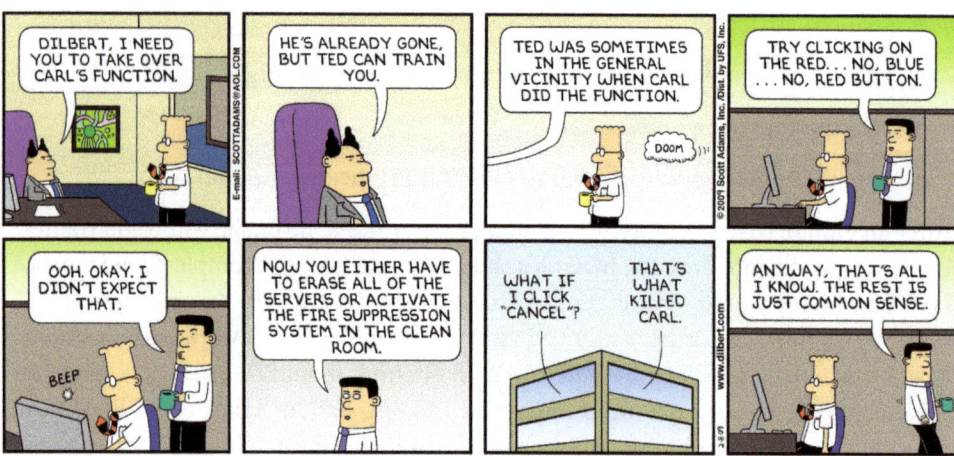

DILBERT © 2009 Scott Adams. Used By permission of UNIVERSAL UCLICK. All rights reserved.

Provide employees with opportunities to learn new skills through cross-training, on-the-job training, continuing education, and formal coursework. As a manager, you should get to know employees' long-term occupational goals and offer training to help them achieve those goals. Cross-training reduces backlogged work and can eliminate the need and expense of temporary employees.

Recognition and Reward

Acknowledging an employee who has done good work, showing appreciation for an employee's efforts, and letting employees know how their work contributes to the value to the organization are all good ways to motivate employees. Not everyone responds to the same type of motivation. Some people want a challenge, some want to feel like part of a team, some like to work toward future promotion, and some are motivated to provide for their family. Therefore, it is important to understand what motivates each employee.

Money is a short-term motivator. It does not sustain employee satisfaction if other issues on the job are discouraging. As long as employees are paid fairly and in a timely manner, money will not be an effective motivator in the long term or a sustainable form of reward or recognition. If employees are not being paid at the same rate as others in the same position at other organizations in the area, then the issue should be brought to the attention of the HR department. HR personnel can pull data from similar businesses to gauge the range of pay for a particular position. Be sure to compare similar jobs with similar duties. As discussed in Chapter 1, many job titles are interchangeably used in HIM. The same job title does not necessarily include the same duties or responsibilities from one organization to another.

Another way to learn about pay and job responsibilities at other organizations is to conduct an informal telephone survey of managers or supervisors at those organizations. Ask about the salary range and job duties for a particular title and the required education and credentials. This information may be helpful when discussing and comparing findings with HR staff.

Employees should receive rewards and recognition for specific accomplishments, rather than for simply "doing their job." After all, that is what they are paid to do. A reward should be given within one week for doing something extra without being asked, for going "above and beyond." For example, if an employee handled a difficult situation involving a customer and stayed late into the evening to resolve the customer's issue, then that employee provided exceptional customer service worthy of recognition. How should the manager reward that employee? By doing something that is meaningful to that individual. As a manager, it is important to know what motivates each employee.

For example, do not give a box of chocolates to an employee who is always dieting. If an employee enjoys public recognition, then congratulate and reward that person during an upcoming staff meeting. For someone who does not appreciate public recognition, the manager should congratulate the employee privately. Not only will the employee appreciate the respect for her privacy, but staff members will also learn that being called into the manager's office does not always mean that something is wrong! Rewards should be timely and given immediately or within one week.

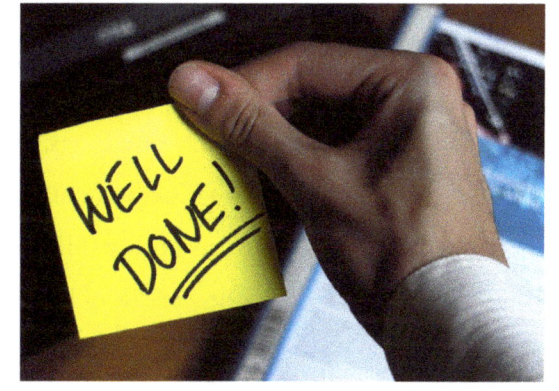

Recognition need not be limited to an employee's effort in the workplace. Recognize and reward the individual who helped another employee change a flat tire after work, for example.

Policies and Procedures

The HIM manager is responsible for overseeing day-to-day operations and workflow, regularly reviewing and updating policies and procedures, establishing budget parameters, and monitoring expenditures.

Policies and procedures are important organizational documents that provide employees with information needed to meet the organization's expectations. **Policies** are the principles, rules, and guidelines that govern the organization. Some policies are written to ensure the organization is meeting legal requirements, such as those outlined in HIPAA. **Procedures** describe an ordered series of steps or actions taken to complete a task. HIM department procedures outline the necessary steps to perform tasks such as coding, release of information, and physician analysis. Procedures help to ensure the tasks are completed in a consistent and accurate manner, particularly when more than one person is performing the same task. They also are a "go-to" reference for training or retraining employees.

Policies

As a manager in the HIM department, you may be asked to develop a policy for the department or the entire organization. A policy provides employees with direction on how to proceed in certain situations. Policies are based on laws and on the mission, ethics, and values of the organization.

HIM departments may have policies regarding:

- attendance
- customer service
- coding inpatient records
- notice of delinquent records to physicians

The HIM department manager may be asked to develop organizational policies for a variety of subjects, including:

- confidentiality
- privacy (HIPAA)
- release of health information over the telephone
- record retention

Procedures

Written procedures are instructions that describe how a job should be performed. Anyone who has tried to assemble a new toy or piece of furniture knows that products are easier to assemble if the directions are easy to read. Of course, it helps if the instructions include all the steps! Visual aids, including diagrams, illustrations, and photographs, are helpful, whether you're assembling furniture or reviewing records for short-term hospital stays. When writing a new procedure, keep a few basic guidelines in mind:

- Keep it simple, straightforward, and concise.
- Use bullet points to separate each step.
- Include screen captures, sample forms, pictures, and other visual aids.
- Begin each sentence with a verb to ensure an action is taken at every step.
- Designate the individual (by job title) responsible for each step.

Once the procedure is complete, test it: ask someone who has never performed the task to attempt to follow the procedure. Then ask the tester the following questions: Was the procedure easy to follow? Were you able to successfully complete the task?

Example 12.5 is a sample procedure used by the HIM and case management departments to verify that patients hospitalized for less than 24 hours are assigned the appropriate status.

Example 12.5 Status Review of Inpatient Records

Community General Hospital

Policy Name:	Status Review of Inpatient Records
Date:	January 2, 2014
Review/Revision Date:	1/2013, 1/2014
Policy number:	HIM205.12

Policy: It is the policy of the HIM Department of Community General Hospital to ensure that each patient's hospital status (inpatient vs. outpatient) is correctly assigned prior to coding a medical record.

Person responsible	Procedure
Coder	Retrieve records from to do list
	Identify inpatient records with length of stay less than 24 hours
	Place records in Case Manager queue in chart locator system
Case Manager	Review each record against criteria for inpatient status
	If no changes are required
	Return record to coder queue
	If changes are required
	Obtain a corrected telephone order from the admitting physician
	Document corrected order in record
	Send email to admitting department to change status in billing system to outpatient
	Place in coder queue
Admitting Clerk	Change status in billing system to outpatient
Coder	Change record status in locator system
	Code record using guidelines for designated coding status
	Place in Analysis Tech queue
Analysis Tech	Flag new order (telephone or verbal) on chart and update deficiency system
	Place in physician queue for completion

Budgeting

Every business or business unit in an organization, regardless of size, develops and maintains a budget. This important planning tool is used to track the financial health of the business, monitor trends, and provide financial data for decision making.

There are two types of budgets: operating budgets and capital budgets.

Operating Budget

A manager in an HIM department may be asked to submit an **operating budget** that includes projections for revenue and expenses, such as payroll, supplies, and services, which are required for the day-to-day running of a department. An operating budget generally spans a **fiscal year**, which is the legal accounting period for an organization.

> **BE AWARE**
>
> The HIM department is considered non-revenue producing because it does not generate much income (known as *hard dollars*). However, the department plays a crucial role in ensuring that the organization receives proper reimbursement for the charges submitted through accurate and timely coding. Coding provides cash flow—without cash, no one in the facility would be paid, including the president of the company. The importance of the HIM department to the overall financial success of the organization cannot be overstated, and it is an important factor in justifying the HIM department's budget requests.

The fiscal year may follow the calendar year and begin in January or it may follow a different 12-month period. For example, the federal government's fiscal year runs from October 1 through September 30.

In most healthcare departments, the operating budget has two parts: revenue and expenses. **Revenue** is money received for services provided or for products sold. Examples of revenue in the HIM department include fees paid by attorneys, insurance companies, and patients for copies of medical records. HIM departments do not typically bring in much revenue compared with departments that provide patient care and submit charges for those services.

An **expense** is money the organization pays to an individual or company (third party) in exchange for goods and services purchased. The following list includes the most common categories used in an HIM department budget.

Payroll Salaries; employer-paid contributions to Medicare, Social Security, and workers' compensation; benefits, including vacation, holiday, and sick pay; and the employer's contribution to health insurance or retirement accounts. To calculate the full cost of an employee, including employer contributions to salary and benefits, multiply the employee's base salary by 15 percent to 25 percent.

Supplies Basic desk supplies, including pens, note pads, staples, and, if the department staff uses a paper or hybrid medical record system, folders. These folders are made of heavy-duty material and come with special fasteners to accommodate the extreme weight of a medical record. Folders can be quite expensive and are often the costliest supply used by employees in the HIM department. Other supplies may include paper and printer toner for copying records.

Contract services Work performed by an outside company or contractor. Tasks may include transcription, coding, auditing, and consulting services. The cost of temporary staff is also budgeted here.

Software licensing Software used exclusively by the HIM department, including encoder software, chart deficiency/analysis software, transcription software, and release-of-information software is included in this category.

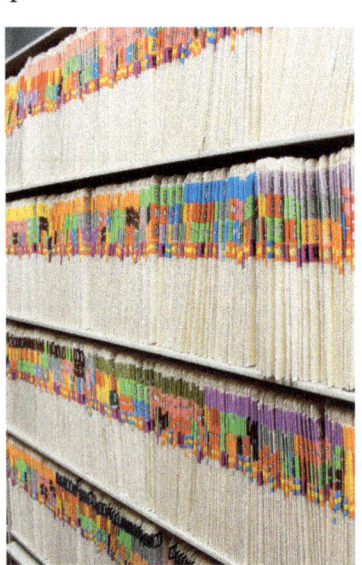

Paper folders are one of the most expensive supplies that an HIM department uses.

Minor equipment An item priced below $500 that does not qualify as a basic supply should be categorized as minor equipment. Examples of minor equipment include printers, desk lamps, and office chairs.

Dues and subscriptions Professional organizations, such as the American Health Information Management Association (AHIMA), are sometimes paid for by the employer. Annual subscriptions to magazines and online resources, such as the American Medical Association's *Coding Clinic*, which is an essential resource for all coders, are included in this category.

Education Continuing education necessary for employees to remain current in their field and to maintain professional credentials, as well as education for new software implementation, should be budgeted in this category.

Travel Mileage, hotel, airfare, and other travel-related expenses.

Postage The cost of postage to send copies of medical records to requestors should be budgeted in this category.

Miscellaneous Unique items that do not fit elsewhere should be categorized as miscellaneous. This is a good area to budget for employee recognition (e.g., pizza parties, awards).

Example 12.6 is a sample of a monthly budget report for a typical HIM department. It is one of 12 monthly columns that, when added together, make up the department's annual budget.

Example 12.6 Monthly Budget Report

HIM Department Budget Report– April 2017

	April 2017			YTD 2017			
	Budget	Actual	Difference	Budget	Actual	Difference	% Difference
Revenue	1,000.00	2,000.00	1,000.00	4,000.00	3,753.00	(247.00)	(1.1)
Revenue Total	1,000.00	2,000.00	1,000.00	4,000.00	3,753.00	(247.00)	(1.1)
Payroll	46,800.00	47,259.00	(459.00)	187,200.00	179,441.00	7,759.00	1.1
Supplies	8,500.00	7,949.00	551.00	34,000.00	36,254.00	(2,254.00)	(0.9)
Contract Services	12,000.00	11,087.00	913.00	48,000.00	44,348.00	3,652.00	1.1
Software licensing	2,300.00	2,322.00	(22.00)	9,200.00	9,288.00	(88.00)	(1.0)
Minor Equipment	100.00	259.00	(159.00)	400.00	534.27	(134.27)	(0.75)
Dues & Subs.	50.00	0.00	50.00	200.00	50.00	150.00	4.0
Education	185.00	50.00	135.00	740.00	125.00	615.00	6.0
Travel	45.00	15.94	29.06	180.00	100.00	80.00	1.8
Postage	25.00	32.00	(7.00)	100.00	102.00	(2.00)	(0.9)
Misc.	125.00	72.12	52.88	500.00	326.00	174.00	1.5
Expenses Total	70,130.00	69,046.06	1,083.94	280,520.00	270,568.27	9,951.73	1.04
Budget Total			2,083.94			9,704.73	

When preparing to submit a budget, it is important to include documentation to justify all budget requests. **Justification** is the circumstance, fact, or explanation that proves an expense is reasonable or necessary.

At the beginning of the budget process each year, the HIM manager should contact the major suppliers, service contractors, and software vendors to obtain a price quote for the upcoming fiscal year. This is a good opportunity to negotiate pricing. After the price has been agreed upon, the manager will request a price estimate from the vendor and attach it to the budget as proof of the dollars needed. Obtaining an estimate in writing may protect the organization from a midyear price increase.

Capital Budget

A **capital budget** is a predetermined amount of money set aside to purchase fixed assets. This budget is established, reviewed, and approved in a separate process from the operating budget. The capital budget is for high-dollar investments and purchases, such as buildings, medical equipment, and computer systems, including the facility's EHR system. Staff from the HIM department may request, for example, capital approval for department construction, remodeling, or both, or for a new computer-assisted coding system. Typically, the HIM department competes with other departments for capital budget funding. The organization's capital budget contains a set amount available for the entire organization; equipment for patient care that produces new or additional revenue may be funded first.

Productivity

A time to assess staffing needs for the upcoming year is during the annual budget review process. Staffing requests for new or replacement employees, referred to as **full-time equivalents** (FTEs), must be justified. Typically, FTEs work 40 hours each week, or 2,080 hours per year. For budgetary purposes, add approximately 10 percent to 12 percent more work-hours for each FTE to cover the cost of education, sick leave, and vacation time. The best way to justify this expense is to provide data on the amount of work assigned to the department, along with an estimate of the number of employees needed to complete the work. Monitoring employee **productivity**, which is the ratio of inputs (time and labor) to outputs (work produced), can provide this information.

Take the challenge below to see if you can calculate how many FTEs the Good Samaritan Hospital will need next year.

TAKE THE CHALLENGE

Good Samaritan Hospital projects it will serve 12,500 inpatients during the year. As the HIM manager, you have calculated that an employee can process an average of five in-patient charts per hour.

How many FTEs will be needed to process in-patient records next year?

Data gathered by monitoring employee productivity can be used for other purposes, including:

- employee performance evaluations
- staffing and workflow decision making
- evaluating the effectiveness of process changes

A **production log** is a useful tool to monitor employee productivity. It should be designed to reflect the specific job duties of each employee. Example 12.7 shows how an employee lost production on Tuesday after leaving early, followed by an unexplained absence for 30 minutes on Thursday that also resulted in reduced production.

Example 12.7 Health Information Technology Production Log

Sample HIT Tech Production Log - Small hospital

Name: Anthony Peco
Week of: 10/6/17 – 10/12/17

	Sun	Mon	Tue	Wed	Thur	Fri	Sat	Total	Comments
Dates:	10/6	10/7	10/8	10/9	10/10	10/11	10/12		left early Tue, headache
Hours worked:	8	8	3.5	8	7.5	off	off	35	

Scanned:

	Sun	Mon	Tue	Wed	Thur	Fri	Sat	Total	Comments
Admits	10	25	20	35	18				
Updates		1		2	1				
Discharges	25	25							

Processed:

	Sun	Mon	Tue	Wed	Thur	Fri	Sat	Total	Comments
Folders made for discharge	25	25		35	10				
Assembled	15	30		30	0				
Analyzed									

Physician incomplete:

	Sun	Mon	Tue	Wed	Thur	Fri	Sat	Total	Comments
Charts re-analyzed									
# of letters sent				125	20				
# of reminder calls				20					

Filing/Pulling:

	Sun	Mon	Tue	Wed	Thur	Fri	Sat	Total	Comments
Folders to Perm									
Loose sheets (inches)									
# of charts pulled									
# of charts purged									
# of thinned charts made/filed									

Transcription:

	Sun	Mon	Tue	Wed	Thur	Fri	Sat	Total	Comments
# of reports corrected	1	4	2	5	1				
# of reports posted on units									
# of reports filed in incomplete record									

Release of Information:

	Sun	Mon	Tue	Wed	Thur	Fri	Sat	Total	Comments
# of faxes to physicians/healthcare providers	1								
# of requests									
# semi-processed									
# completed									

| Meetings/Education (time spent) | | | | 30 min. | | | | |

It is the HIM department manager's responsibility to determine what constitutes a reasonable level of productivity for each job duty. There are several ways to estimate productivity levels, including:

- Research professional journals or contact other similar organizations for production standards (known as *benchmarking*).
- Do the work yourself (but you may not be as fast as the employees who perform the function daily).
- Calculate the average rate of productivity of all employees doing the same task (use an average; some employees will be fast, while others will be slow).

Collecting accurate productivity data is important. Employees should be required to complete a weekly production log. Computerized reports, if available, can provide easy access to production statistics without requiring employees to count and track individual process numbers. The manager should review the data collected with each employee on a weekly basis to ensure that:

- the information collected is complete and accurate
- the employee is maintaining productivity standards
- the work is not becoming backlogged
- the employee is not performing any additional or unnecessary work without informing a manager

It is important to monitor productivity and also to assess the quality of the work process. **Process reengineering**, sometimes called *process redesign* or *process improvement*, is a systematic evaluation and modification of an existing process. Process reengineering is used to simplify and eliminate wasted effort (i.e., to identify ways to complete a task in fewer steps). Process reengineering may be initiated for several reasons, including:

- Staff productivity is low.
- New responsibilities or systems were added to a process.
- A team has reviewed the process to achieve its goal.
- Staff size is being reduced.
- A manager new to the process uses reengineering as a way to learn the workflow.

When reengineering a process, the first step is to see how the process is currently accomplished. The manager should observe employees while they perform the work, ask questions, and document each step of the process. Then the manager can review the process and identify any redundant or unnecessary steps. Putting the steps into a flowchart, like the one shown in Example 12.2 on page 351, may also help identify inefficiencies.

IT REALLY HAPPENS

A new manager in the HIM department noticed that an employee was printing information from the computer and then copying that same information by hand into five separate notebooks. The manager asked the employee why she was hand copying information already in the computer. The employee answered, "Because we've always done it that way."

The manager then asked whom the notebooks were for, but the employee did not know. The manager looked into the matter and discovered that the notebooks had been used by a quality manager who had left the facility more than 10 years ago! After analyzing the process, the manager eliminated this manual, time-consuming, and unnecessary step.

Chapter Summary

There is nothing more exciting or challenging than managing people or processes. As a manager in the field of health information management (HIM), you will have opportunities to help employees develop skills and talents and, in many cases, assist them in reaching their career goals. Taking on the responsibilities of management may not always be easy, but studying and applying current techniques and strategies in leadership and management can provide a foundation for success.

As an HIM professional, you may be responsible for one or more projects at any given time. In its simplest form, a project typically includes three elements: a description outlining the scope of the project, a budget, and a deadline for completing the work. Although every project is different, projects are generally broken down into two broad categories, simple and complex. A simple project is limited in scope, involves a defined number of tasks, and may be completed in a few days or a few months. A complex project involves more people and resources than a simple project and requires more time and money to complete. A complex project may have one goal or many goals. Successful project management involves five separate phases or processes: initiating, planning, executing, monitoring and controlling, and closing. These processes are often overlapping but may vary in intensity during different parts of the project.

Careful hiring and training is an important part of a manager's job. It is essential to keep communication open between the management team and the employees by providing employees with timely feedback and recognizing those employees who go above and beyond with rewards and recognition. Well-written policies and procedures can enhance employee job satisfaction and improve productivity. Extrinsic motivators, such as providing a supportive work environment, can improve employee morale. Process reengineering is an effective way to highlight inefficiencies and improve workflow.

Every healthcare organization develops and maintains a budget to track the financial health of the business, monitor trends, and provide financial data for decision making. There are two types of budgets: operating budgets and capital budgets. An operating budget includes projections for revenue and expenses, such as payroll, supplies, and services, which are required for the day-to-day running of a department. A capital budget is a predetermined amount of money set aside to purchase fixed assets such as building and renovation, medical equipment, computer systems, and equipment needed for patient care.

As the HIM profession continues to evolve, there will be a growing need for highly skilled and effective managers who demonstrate the necessary expertise and leadership abilities to meet the changes to come.

HIM Review

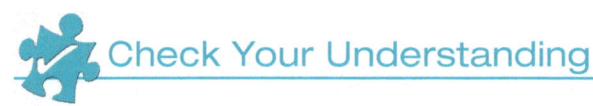

Check Your Understanding

Test your understanding of the material covered in this chapter by completing the following multiple-choice questions. For each question, select the best answer from the choices provided.

1. A(n)_____ involves choosing a course of action from among the available alternatives.

    a. agenda

    b. change agent

    c. performance evaluation

    d. decision

2. When selecting members for a team, a team leader would not select members who_____

    a. have good communication skills.

    b. do not know the subject matter.

    c. would be committed to achieving the goal.

    d. can effectively express themselves.

3. For a goal to be achievable, it must be _____

    a. attainable.

    b. specific.

    c. measureable.

    d. All of the choices are correct.

4. _____ are guiding principles that direct the actions of an organization.

    a. Procedures

    b. Goals

    c. Policies

    d. Production logs

5. The _____ is the legal accounting period for an organization.

    a. operating budget

    b. fiscal year

    c. revenue

    d. justification

6. Productivity data may be used for _____

    a. making a decision.

    b. risk-taking.

    c. average length-of-stay calculations.

    d. delinquent record calculations.

7. Which of the following is not an appropriate interview question?

    a. How do you plan your day?

    b. Can you work weekends and holidays?

    c. I see you use a cane; are you able to use the stairs?

    d. What are your salary expectations?

8. A _____ is a visual diagram that illustrates the actual events of a project.

    a. flowchart

    b. cause-and-effect diagram

    c. fishbone diagram

    d. budget

9. A good written procedure _____

    a. always starts each sentence with a noun.

    b. may omit simple steps.

    c. always starts each sentence with a verb.

    d. should never have pictures.

10. Which of the following choices is not a duty performed by a team member?

    a. recorder

    b. celebration planner

    c. parking lot attendant

    d. leader

Think Critically

Consider the following real-world scenario and draft a response.

Due to rising costs and reduced patient stays at Good Samaritan Hospital, the hospital's president has announced that each department must eliminate one full-time equivalent position and reduce other expenses by 5 percent. You are the manager of the HIM department. How would you cut one FTE position and keep the department optimally functioning? How and where would you cut 5 percent of your other expenses? Use the sample budget provided in Example 12.6 on page 367 to answer this question.

Sharpen Your Comprehension

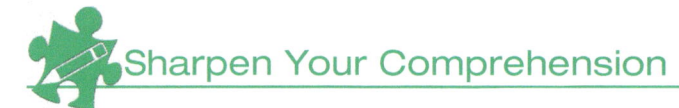

Complete the following matching exercise by selecting, from the list provided, the answer that best matches each of the numbered statements. For each statement, only one answer is correct.

a. capital budget
b. performance evaluation
c. job description
d. performing
e. informal leader
f. manager
g. money
h. change agent
i. project
j. storming

1. _____ A temporary endeavor designed to produce a specific product, service, or result
2. _____ Is used by a manager or consultant to examine and evaluate an employee's work against preset standards.
3. _____ Plans, organizes, and delegates tasks.
4. _____ The stage when team members begin to assert themselves and try to define their individual roles.
5. _____ Does not hold a position of authority or power but can influence the decisions and actions of others.
6. _____ Provides a broad, general statement of employees' roles and responsibilities.
7. _____ The stage when the team members have a shared vision of the team's goals and work is progressing.
8. _____ Assists individuals, teams, and organizations in moving from the current state to a desired future state.
9. _____ A predetermined amount of money set aside to purchase fixed assets.
10. _____ Cannot sustain employee satisfaction if other issues on the job are discouraging.

Connect Theory to Practice

To help translate the concepts presented in this chapter to the workplace, complete the following exercise.

Go to http://IntroHIM.ParadigmCollege.net/Change and read the article "Ten Ways to Help Employees Adapt to Change" by Christine Corelli. For each of the 10 tips, write a detailed paragraph describing how you would use the tip to manage changing the role of HIM assembly and file clerks to HIM scanning technicians.

Student eResources

*To enhance your comprehension of the chapter material, go to **Navigator+** and complete the additional practice items as advised by your instructor.*

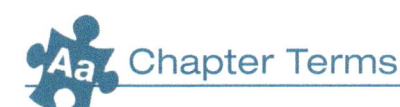

Chapter Terms

360-degree feedback
agenda
capital budget
change agent
closing process
complex project
cross-training
decision
delegating
execution process
expense
extrinsic motivation
fiscal year
fishbone diagram
flowchart
forming
full-time equivalent
Gantt chart
goal
ground rules
hands-on training
informal leader
initiation process
intrinsic motivation
job description
justification
leader
manager
monitoring and controlling
motivation
nepotism
norming
operating budget
orientation
performance evaluation
performing
planning process
policy
procedure
process reengineering
production log
productivity
project
project management
revenue
risk taker
simple project
storming
teamwork
training

Appendix A

Acronyms and Abbreviations

Acronym or Abbreviation	Meaning
A&C	adults and children
AAAHC	Accreditation Association for Ambulatory Health Care
AACN	American Association of Colleges of Nursing
ACA	Affordable Care Act or Patient Protection and Affordable Care Act
ACDIS	Association of Clinical Documentation Improvement Specialists
ACO	accountable care organization
ACS	American College of Surgeons
ADC	average daily census
ADLs	activities of daily living
ADT	admission, discharge, and transfer
AHA	American Hospital Association
AHC	Allied Health Careers
AHDI	Association for Healthcare Documentation Integrity
AHIMA	American Health Information Management Association
AHRQ	Agency for Healthcare Research and Quality
AJCC	American Joint Committee on Cancer
ALC	alternative level of care
ALOS	average length of stay
AMA	American Medical Association
AMIA	American Medical Informatics Association
AOD	accounting of disclosures
APC	ambulatory payment classification
ARLNA	Association of Record Librarians of North America
ARRA	American Recovery and Reinvestment Act
ASC	ambulatory surgery center
BA	business associate
BC	Blue Cross

Acronym or Abbreviation	Meaning
BCBS	Blue Cross Blue Shield
BMI	body mass index
BoK	HIM Body of Knowledge
BP	blood pressure
BS	Blue Shield
BUN	blood urea nitrogen
C&S	culture and sensitivity
CAC	computer-assisted coding
CAH	critical access hospital
CAHIIM	Commission on Accreditation for Health Informatics and Information Management Education
CARF	Commission on Accreditation of Rehabilitation Facilities
CBC	complete blood count
CCA	certified coding associate
CCHIIM	Commission on Certification for Health Informatics and Information Management
CCS	certified coding specialist
CCS-P	certified coding specialist-physician-based
CCU	cardiac care unit
CD	compact disc
CD-R	compact disc, recordable
CD-ROM	compact disc, read only memory
CD-RW	compact disc, rewriteable
CDC	Centers for Disease Control and Prevention
CDI	clinical documentation improvement
CDIP	certified documentation improvement practitioner
CDR	clinical data repository
CDS	clinical decision support
CE	continuing education
CEO	chief executive officer
CfCs	Conditions for Coverage
CFO	chief financial officer
CHAP	Community Health Accreditation Program
CHDA	clinical health data analyst
CHDS	certified healthcare documentation specialist
CHF	congestive heart failure
CHIP	Children's Health Insurance Program
CHPS	certified in healthcare privacy and security
CHRO	chief human resources officer
CHTS	certified healthcare technology specialist
CHTS-CP	clinician/practitioner consultant
CHTS-IM	implementation manager
CHTS-IS	implementation support specialist

Acronym or Abbreviation	Meaning
CHTS-PW	practice workflow and information management redesign specialist
CHTS-TR	trainer examination
CHTS-TS	technical/software support staff
CIO	chief information officer
CLL	chronic lymphocytic leukemia
CMI	case mix index
CMO	chief medical officer
CMS	Centers for Medicare & Medicaid Services
CNO	chief nursing officer
CNS	clinical nurse specialist
CoC	Commission on Cancer
COO	chief operating officer
CoPs	Conditions of Participation
CORF	comprehensive outpatient rehabilitation facility
CPC	certified professional coder
CPOE	computerized provider order entry
CPR	cardiopulmonary resuscitation
CPT	Current Procedural Terminology
CPU	central processing unit
CQI	continuous quality improvement
CRNA	certified registered nurse anesthetist
CT	computerized tomography
CTR	certified tumor registrar
DBMS	database management system
DC	doctor of chiropractic
DDS	doctor of dental surgery
DLP	data loss prevention
DME	durable medical equipment
DNR	do not resuscitate
DO	doctor of osteopathic medicine
DOB	date of birth
DOD	Department of Defense
DOS	disk operating system
DPM	doctor of podiatric medicine
DRG	diagnosis-related group
DSM-5	*Diagnostic and Statistical Manual of Mental Disorders, Fifth Edition*
DSS	decision support system
ECG	electrocardiogram
ED	emergency department
EHR	electronic health record
EKG	electrocardiogram

Acronym or Abbreviation	Meaning
eMAR	electronic medication administration record
EMR	electronic medical record
EMT	emergency medical technician
EOB	Explanation of Benefit
EP	eligible professional
ePHI	electronic protected health information
eRx	e-prescribing
FACTA	Fair and Accurate Credit Transactions Act
FDA	Food and Drug Administration
FORDS	*Facility Oncology Registry Data Standards*
FTE	full-time equivalent
GB	gigabyte
GCP	good clinical practice
GEMs	General Equivalency Mappings
GFR	glomerular filtration rate
GHz	gigahertz
GI	gastrointestinal
GINA	Genetic Information Nondiscrimination Act of 2008
H&P	history and physical
HAI	hospital-acquired infection
HCPCS	Healthcare Common Procedure Coding System
HCUP	Healthcare Cost and Utilization Project
HDD	hard disk drive
HEDIS	Healthcare Effectiveness Data and Information Set
HFMA	Healthcare Financial Management Association
HHS	US Department of Health and Human Services
HIE	health information exchange
HIM	health information management
HIMSS	Healthcare Information and Management Systems Society
HIPAA	Health Insurance Portability and Accountability Act of 1996
HIPPS	Health Insurance Prospective Payment System
HIT	health information technology
HITECH	Health Information Technology for Economic and Clinical Health
HL7	Health Level Seven International
HMO	health maintenance organization
HR	human resource
HSP	human subject protection
HTML	Hypertext Markup Language
HTTP	Hypertext Transfer Protocol
ICD	International Classification of Diseases
ICD-9-CM	International Classification of Diseases, Ninth Revision, Clinical Modification

Acronym or Abbreviation	Meaning
ICD-10-CM	International Classification of Diseases, Tenth Revision, Clinical Modification
ICD-10-PCS	International Classification of Diseases, Tenth Revision, Procedure Coding System
ICD-O	International Classification of Diseases for Oncology
ICD-O-3	International Classification of Diseases for Oncology, Third Edition
ICU	intensive care unit
IG	information governance
IIS	immunization information systems
IP	inpatient or Internet Protocol
IRB	institutional review board
IS	intensity of service
ISMP	Institute for Safe Medication Practices
IT	information technology
JC	Joint Commission
KB	kilobyte
LAN	local area network
LOINC	Logical Observation Identifiers, Names, and Codes
LOS	length of stay
LPN	licensed practical nurse
LTAC	long-term acute care hospital
LTC	long-term care
LVN	licensed vocational nurse
MB	megabyte
MD	doctor of medicine
MDS	Minimum Data Set
ME	medical examiner
MHz	megahertz
MI	myocardial infarction
MIS	management information systems
MPI	master patient index
MR	medical record
MRI	magnetic resonance imaging
MRN	medical record number
MRSA	methicillin-resistant Staphylococcus aureus
MS-DRG	Medicare Severity Diagnosis Related Group
NB	newborn
NCBDDD	National Center on Birth Defects and Developmental Disabilities
NCDB	National Cancer Data Base
NCQA	National Committee for Quality Assurance
NCRA	National Cancer Registrars Association
NCVHS	National Committee on Vital and Health Statistics
NHAMCS	National Hospital Ambulatory Medical Care Survey

Acronym or Abbreviation	Meaning
NHCS	National Hospital Care Survey
NHDS	National Hospital Discharge Survey
NIS	National (Nationwide) Inpatient Sample
NP	nurse practitioner
NPCR	National Program of Cancer Registries
NVSS	National Vital Statistics System
OB	obstetrics
OCR	Office for Civil Rights
OHRP	Office for Human Research Subjects Protection
OIG	Office of the Inspector General
ONC	Office of the National Coordinator for Health Information Technology
OP	outpatient
OPD	outpatient department
OPPS	Outpatient Prospective Payment System
OS	operating system
PA	physician assistant
PACS	picture archiving and communication system
PB	petabyte
PCP	primary care physician
PDR	*Physicians' Desk Reference*
PhD	doctor of philosophy
PHI	protected health information
PHR	personal health record
PI	performance improvement
PIN	personal identification number
PKU	phenylketonuria
PMI	Project Management Institute
PMS	practice management system
PNA	pneumonia
POA	Present on Admission
POC	point of care
POMR	problem-oriented medical record
POS	point of service
PPO	preferred provider organization
PPS	prospective payment system
PROMIS	problem-oriented medical information system
QI	quality improvement
RAC	Recovery Audit Contractor
RAM	random access memory
RHDS	registered healthcare documentation specialist
RHIA	registered health information administrator

Acronym or Abbreviation	Meaning
RHIT	registered health information technician
RN	registered nurse
ROI	release of information or return on investment
ROM	range of motion or rupture of membranes
RUG	resource utilization group
SE	sentinel event
SEER	*Surveillance, Epidemiology, and End Results*
SI	severity of illness
SNOMED CT	Systematized Nomenclature of Medicine—Clinical Terms
SOAP	subjective, objective, assessment, and plan
SOB	shortness of breath
SPA	state plan amendment
SSI	Supplemental Security Income
TB	terabyte
TCP	Transmission Control Protocol
TNM	tumor, lymph node, metastasis
TPO	treatment, payment, or operations
UICC	Union for International Cancer Control
URL	uniform resource locator
UTI	urinary tract infection
VA	Department of Veterans Affairs
VBP	value-based purchasing
VPN	virtual private network
WAN	wide area network
WAP	wireless access point
WBC	white blood cell
WHO	World Health Organization
WLAN	wireless local area network
WWW	World Wide Web

Appendix B

Glossary

360-degree feedback an evaluation process that collects data from all around an employee, including assessments by supervisors, peers, subordinates, team members, and customers

access speed the speed at which a request for data from a computer system is completed; RAM is rated by access speed

accession number a unique eight-digit identifier assigned by a cancer registrar to each reportable cancer case

accountable care organization (ACO) a group of healthcare providers (primary care physicians, specialists, hospitals, and other healthcare facilities) working together to coordinate care of Medicare patients across care settings

accounting of disclosures a recording by covered entities of all disclosures of patient identifiable information, including the person or entity to whom the information was disclosed and what information was provided

accreditation certification granted to an organization that has met a set of predetermined standards following a peer review process conducted by an impartial, external accrediting organization

activities of daily living (ADLs) activities an individual could normally do in the course of daily living, such as eating, bathing, dressing, toileting, transferring (walking), and continence (the ability to control bladder and bowel functions)

acute care hospital a hospital that treats patients in the acute phase of an illness or a condition

acute illness an illness or injury with a rapid onset that is severe in nature but of short duration

adaptive skills behavior and daily living skills that demonstrate the job seeker's ability to fit into the organization's culture

administrative safeguards administrative actions undertaken to meet security standards

admission, discharge, and transfer (ADT) system a system that tracks patient movement during hospitalization and generates daily reports, including unit census reports and admission and discharge lists

adult day care an organized program of services for elderly or disabled individuals that provides social, physical, and emotional support and respite for the primary in-home caregiver

advance directive a legal document prepared by the patient with instructions regarding medical care in the event that the patient is unable to make such decisions

agenda a list of the items to be discussed in a meeting and any proposed actions

aggregate data data abstracted from a group of patient records for statistical reporting purposes in which no individual patient can be identified

AHIMA Foundation the charitable affiliate of the American Health Information Management Association that provides funding and resources for research, education, and career development

alerts warnings to providers about potential medication interactions

allowable costs charges for services and supplies covered under a health insurance plan

ambulatory care outpatient care delivered during a single day with no overnight stay

ambulatory payment classifications (APCs) groupings of services that set reimbursement rates for similar clinical services and apply to outpatient surgery, outpatient clinics, emergency department services, and observational services

American College of Surgeons (ACS) an association founded in 1913 to improve the quality of care for surgical patients through improved education and training

American Health Information Management Association (AHIMA) the professional membership organization for individuals interested in or involved in the field of health information management

American Hospital Association (AHA) a national professional organization that represents hospitals and healthcare networks, advocating for its members on issues of healthcare policy and regulation

American Medical Association (AMA) a professional association for physicians

American Recovery and Reinvestment Act (ARRA) a federal law enacted in 2009 that provided financial incentives to encourage healthcare organizations to adopt and use certified electronic health records to improve the quality of patient care and the exchange of health information

analytics the systematic analysis of data or statistics, or the identification and communication of significant patterns in data

anatomic site relating to the structure of the body

anesthesia death rate the number of deaths directly attributable to anesthesia

application software a program or a group of programs designed to perform specific tasks

audit trail a computer-generated report that identifies who accessed a computer system or an individual record and the action taken

authentication a signature attesting to the validity of a document or report; for example, a handwritten signature is required to authenticate a paper record

authentication scheme industry-standard security and a strong password requirement

authorized release of information a form that must be requested and completed by the patient so that patient information may be released to others

average daily census (ADC) the average number of inpatients present each day during specified periods of time

average length of stay (ALOS) the average length of stay for all inpatients discharged during a specified period of time

behavior a term used to indicate whether a tumor is malignant, benign, in situ, or uncertain if benign or malignant

behavioral health care mental health care and substance abuse treatment

bell curve a symmetrical, bell-shaped line curve that represents a distribution of values, frequencies, or probabilities of a dataset

benchmark a standard or reference point for comparison or assessment

bereavement grief

biomedical research scientific investigation of the cause, prevention, and treatment of diseases

birth defects registry a registry of data used to investigate, monitor, and treat birth defects

bit the smallest unit of information on a machine; shorthand for *binary digit*

Blue Cross (BC) created in 1929 as one of the first health insurance programs in the United States; was created to address a patient's inability to pay his or her hospital bills

Blue Shield (BS) created in 1930 as a health insurance program that provided reimbursements for physicians' services

board of directors the group responsible for overseeing hospital management and appointing the hospital's chief executive officer (CEO)

body language nonverbal communication that sends a visual message to another person

breach an unauthorized use or disclosure of information protected under the Health Insurance Portability and Accountablity Act Privacy Rule

business associate (BA) a person or organization that acts on behalf of a covered entity and requires access to protected health information

business associate agreement a written contract that specifies the safeguards required to ensure the proper handling and disclosure of PHI

business record a record of medical care provided to a patient that is used to substantiate the care provided for legal purposes, most notably as evidence in court proceedings; also the legal health record.

cancer registrar/tumor registrar a specialist who reviews patient records for diagnoses and treatments related to cancer and then abstracts the cancer-related data into a database

cancer registry/tumor registry a registry that collects, stores, manages, and analyzes data on people diagnosed with and treated for malignant cancer and people diagnosed with certain benign yet aggressive tumors

cancer stage the severity of a patient's cancer based on tumor location, size, and histology, and how far the cancer has spread

capital budget a predetermined amount of money set aside to purchase fixed assets

care coordination care done in conjunction with a patient's insurance provider to evaluate the patient's progress toward treatment goals

case finding a process used to identify all reportable cancer diagnoses, inpatient or outpatient, that are diagnosed or treated at a facility

case management department a department in a hospital or other healthcare facility that plays a key role in ensuring that patients get the right care at the right time in the appropriate setting

case manager a person whose job is to evaluate the level of service provided to an individual patient to determine if the care meets the criteria for medical necessity

case mix a group or type of patient based on common traits such as age, insurance provider, diagnosis, or other criteria

case mix index (CMI) a number calculated by averaging the relative weights of a hospital's DRGs

Centers for Disease Control and Prevention (CDC) the US public health institute

Centers for Medicare & Medicaid Services (CMS) the federal agency that administers Medicare and Medicaid

central processing unit (CPU) the part of a computer where all calculations and processes take place

certification confirmation that a healthcare entity has demonstrated its compliance with the health and safety standards spelled out by the Centers for Medicare Services (CMS)

change agent a person who assists individuals, teams, and organizations in moving from the current state to a desired future state

charge capture and coding the process of capturing or identifying all services provided to a patient for the purposes of billing and reimbursement

chargemaster a comprehensive listing of all items billable to a patient or an insurance provider, including each medication, specific diagnostic test, minutes of anesthesia, etc.

chart analysis review of the paper record for completeness

chief executive officer (CEO) the hospital president; responsible for the overall success of the organization, its strategic vision, as well as ongoing and future hospital operations; reports to the board of directors

chief financial officer (CFO) the person responsible for the organization's financial stability and integrity

chief human resources officer (CHRO) the vice president of human resources who oversees recruitment, benefits, compensation, employee relations, and workers' compensation

chief information officer (CIO) a member of the executive leadership team who is responsible for overseeing the hospital's information technology and network infrastructure

chief medical officer (CMO) a licensed practicing physician who is responsible for the medical staff services department, medical staff education, quality management, and all of the medical directors employed by the organization

chief nursing officer (CNO) the vice president of nursing or patient care services

chief operating officer (COO) the person responsible for all hospital operations

Children's Health Insurance Program (CHIP) a Medicaid program specifically for children whose families earn too much to qualify for Medicaid but not enough to afford private insurance

chronic illness a long-developing, persistent illness that may have residual effects

claim submission the process of submitting a universal claim form documenting all billable fees to the third-party payer for reimbursement

classification system a system that organizes groups or terms into categories

clinical data repository (CDR) a central database that consolidates all of a patient's clinical information from separate sources into one location

clinical decision support (CDS) software used by the EHR to analyze patient-specific information and generate reminders, alerts, clinical guidelines, diagnostic support, and relevant reference information

clinical documentation the capture and recording of clinical information

clinical documentation improvement (CDI) a program to improve the quality of patient-care documentation to ensure that it is complete, legible, timely, concise, clear, patient-centered, and accurate

clinical documentation improvement (CDI) specialist a specialist who works with physicians in an acute care setting to ensure that the documentation in the medical record supports all of the diagnoses and procedures provided to a patient

clinical information information used in making patient care decisions that includes the patient's medical history and physical exam, labs, and X-rays along with evaluations by the practitioner(s)

clinical (medical) terminology standard medical language

clinical services departments (such as laboratory, radiology, and pharmacy) that have direct patient contact and impact patient health

clinical trial a type of research study conducted to test the effectiveness of a new drug or treatment on human subjects

cloning copying and pasting information from the documentation of one episode of care into the documentation of another episode of care or from one note to another

closing process the process of closing a project once the project is complete

cloud computing storing and accessing data and programs over the Internet

cloud-based application an application that is stored on a site maintained by a third party and can be accessed from a web browser or mobile app

coinsurance a type of insurance in which the insured is required to pay a share of the cost of care, usually a percentage, after services are provided

collections a step in the revenue cycle management process that begins at the time of registration when any copayment or insurance payment is collected

Commission on Accreditation for Health Informatics and Information Management (CAHIIM) an independent accrediting organization that promotes and enforces accreditation standards for health information and health informatics education programs

Commission on Accreditation of Rehabilitation Facilities (CARF) an accrediting organization that evaluates the quality of care provided at facilities offering rehabilitative care for mental and behavioral health and aging services

community hospital a facility equipped and staffed to provide basic diagnostic services and treatment for injured or ill patients

comorbidities two or more coexisting medical conditions or disease processes that are present as additional diagnoses

complete record a record in which all required reports, signatures, and dates have been entered

complex project a project that may have more than one goal, may involve multiple subprojects, and may require the use project management tools to track and organize

compliance to act in accordance with established guidelines or requirements

compliant conforming to the rules

complications a disease or injury that arises during treatment for another condition

comprehensive outpatient rehabilitation facility (CORF) facilities that provide diagnostic, therapeutic, and restorative services for the rehabilitation of an injury, disability, or sickness

computer port a physical or virtual connection that provides a communication link between other computers or peripheral devices

computer-assisted coding (CAC) software that analyzes typed physician documentation and diagnostic test results to identify specific data elements and recommend the applicable diagnostic or procedural codes

computerized provider order entry (CPOE) medication ordering performed by the EHR system

concurrent review review of patient care documentation that is conducted while a patient is still undergoing treatment within the facility

Conditions for Coverage (CfCs) health and safety standards established by the Centers for Medicare and Medicaid Services (CMS) with which healthcare entities must demonstrate compliance

Conditions of Participation (CoPs) health and safety standards established by the Centers for Medicare and Medicaid Services (CMS) with which healthcare entities must demonstrate compliance

confidentiality keeping something secret or private

conflict of interest a situation or circumstance in which financial or other personal considerations have the potential to compromise an individual's professional judgment and objectivity

consent permission to proceed with a proposed medical intervention or treatment

consent form a form used to document a patient's approval, assent, or permission to receive care

consent for surgery a form the patient signs before a surgical procedure to indicate that he or she understands the specifics of the procedure and has been informed of the associated risks and of other treatment options

consultation a request by the attending physician for another physician to examine the patient health record and the patient and provide an opinion or a treatment recommendation in a written report

consultation rate the ratio of the number of patients who received consultation (multiplied by 100) over the number of patients who were discharged

continuing education (CE) educational requirements that a health information management professional must meet to maintain professional certification

continuous data data that it is measured on a continuous scale with an indefinite number of points along a continuum

continuous quality improvement (CQI) ensures care that is safe, effective, patient centered, timely, efficient, and equitable; also called *process improvement*

cookie a small file that attaches to an individual's computer when the user visits certain websites and tracks the user's information and activities, usually without his or her knowledge

copay a flat fee paid by the insured at the time services are provided

copy and paste function an electronic function that allows providers to copy information from one section of a patient record to another, much like copy and paste in a word processing document

core EHR system/central system the central computer system of an electronic health record that connects to and receives information from other hospital computer systems, including the admissions, clinical, and document management systems

core health data elements a list of 42 data elements developed by the National Committee on Vital and Health Statistics (NCVHS) to facilitate data sharing among providers and healthcare agencies

court order a decision or order issued by a judge during a court proceeding

covered entity (CE) any health plan, healthcare clearinghouse, or healthcare provider that electronically transmits any health information in connection with transactions for which HHS has adopted standards, usually for the billing and payment of services

creation the first stage in the record retention cycle; it includes all documentation entered into the record during a single inpatient stay or outpatient visit, from the time of admission through the course of treatment

critical access hospital (CAH) small hospitals that are most often located in rural areas that provide limited outpatient and inpatient hospital services

critical thinking the intellectually disciplined process of thinking that is clear, rational, open-minded, and supported by evidence

cross-training training employees to do tasks normally performed by coworkers

Current Procedural Terminology (CPT) codes that identify medical, surgical, and diagnostic procedures provided in an outpatient setting

custodian the person receiving a *subpoena duces tecum* who will be required to swear to the authenticity of the patient health record in court proceedings

daily impatient census the number of inpatients present in the facility at the time the census is taken, plus any inpatients who were admitted and discharged the same day but are not present when the census is taken

data a single fact, number, letter, statistic, code, or item that can be collected and stored in a database and, when processed by a computer, becomes information

data collection the process of gathering data for a study

data dictionary identifies the individual data elements recorded by each professional in a health record

data element a single fact with a single meaning, defined for the purpose of data processing

data elements units of data that may be recorded in an independent system and downloaded to the EHR or typed directly into the EHR, such as date of birth, sex, weight, and height

data field the physical unit of storage in a computer record

data integrity data or information that has not been altered or destroyed in an unauthorized manner

data integrity analyst a professional who provides oversight and supervision of all of the electronic processes related to the EHR system and HIM systems, record processing functions, and electronic master patient index processes related to ePHI

data loss prevention (DLP) software software used to defend against computer threats

data mining searching through and analyzing large amounts of data

database a collection of related data stored on a computer system that is organized so that its contents can easily be accessed, managed, updated, and extracted

database management system (DBMS) a group of programs that manages the access and retrieval of information from a database

dataset data elements with uniform definitions that are grouped together for a particular use

de-identified information data from which all identifying information has been removed

decision choosing a course of action from among the available alternatives

decision support software embedded within the EHR that provides physicians with the most current information about diseases and treatments

decision support system (DSS) an interactive computer application that generates data to facilitate decision making

Declaration of Helsinki a statement of ethical principles for medical research involving human subjects, including research on identifiable human material and data

deductible the amount of out-of-pocket costs the insured is responsible for each year, usually a percentage of the cost of care to be paid in full before the insurance company will provide payment for care

delegating assigning responsibility and authority for a particular task or role to another person or group

delinquent record a record that is incomplete after 30 days

deposition sworn oral testimony given before trial by a witness or a party in a criminal or civil proceeding

designated record set composed of all protected health information, including the legal health record, billing records, the information used to support care decisions, and established protocols

destruction the final stage in the record retention cycle, which occurs when the timeframe for keeping the record has been met and the information is no longer needed

diagnosis-related group (DRG) categories of similar treatments and procedures in which the reimbursement-rate amount reflects the level of treatment for an average patient in each category

diagnostic findings the results of testing conducted to aid in the diagnosis and treatment of a medical condition

dictation system a digital or other recording device into which the physician dictates his or her submission

dictionary-driven encoder an encoder-software program that requires the coder to enter a keyword or code and then responds with a list of likely codes, definitions, and explanatory information in a format that is similar to the information provided in a printed coding book

digital certificate a public key certificate attached to an electronic message that provides identifying information about the sender, allowing companies and organizations to exchange information securely over the Internet while protecting data and computer systems

digital imaging the capture (scanning) and digital storage of information from text

disaster an event that occurs suddenly and that may cause great loss of life, damage, or hardship

disaster recovery plan a business continuity plan to protect and provide access to patient information during and after a natural disaster or other disruptive event

discharge days the sum of the lengths of stay for a group of inpatients discharged during a specific time period; also called *total length of stay*

discharge summary a summary of the patient's stay from admission to discharge

discrete data data that has finite values, such as number of days or number of tests, and is categorized into a classification and based on counts

disease index a listing of all diagnostic codes for diseases and procedures for all patients treated at a healthcare facility

do not resuscitate (DNR) a legal document instructing all providers not to provide cardiopulmonary resuscitation (CPR) or any other heroic measure to prolong life when the heart or breathing stops

document management system a system that manages pictures or images of scanned documents

documentation integrity documentation that is complete and accurate with no mistakes, errors, or inconsistencies

documentation redundancy when the same data elements are collected and saved more than once by the same or different healthcare providers during the same patient encounter

domain name a unique website identifier that often indicates the type of organization that purchased and owns the domain

downcoding coding that does not sufficiently capture the severity of a patient's condition or the intensity of services provided to the patient

due diligence taking action to meet the intent of a law or guideline

durable power of attorney for health care gives an individual designated by the patient the legal power to make decisions about care and treatment if the patient is unconscious or incapacitated

e-prescribing (eRx) the practice of physicians generating electronic prescriptions

EHR implementation coordinator and trainer an individual who assists in the selection and implementation of the electronic health record system, develops training materials, and trains users

electronic health record (EHR) a computerized record of all of a patient's health information for different episodes of care across time and healthcare organizations

electronic medication administration record (eMAR) an interface that documents the time, dosage, and administration route for every medication administered to a patient in the hospital; the process of documenting physician orders electronically instead of on paper

electronic protected health information (ePHI) health information that is held or transmitted electronically

electronic signature a digital facsimile of the provider's handwritten signature or a code consisting of letters, numbers, characters, and/or symbols that is executed as the individual's signature and used to authenticate an electronic record

emergency department (ED) a department within a hospital that provides emergency medical care

encoder software a program used by coders to aid in assigning the most appropriate code for a diagnosis or procedure

encounter a specific interaction with a healthcare provider that can be either an outpatient visit or an inpatient stay

encounter utilization review and case management the process of evaluating the necessity, appropriateness, and efficiency of medical care provided by a facility for each patient against established medical standards

Ethernet a system of wires and ports used to connect one computer to another or to a local network

ethics standards of behavior based on moral values

ethics committee a committee that reviews cases and provides guidance on the implementation of advance directives; its purpose is to provide guidance and support to providers and administrators with regard to ethical decisions and to assist in resolving conflicts

etiology the cause of a disease or a condition

evidence-based medicine an approach that integrates the provider's expertise with external evidence, such as medical research or clinical trials, to support clinical decision making

execution process a stage in the project management process that begins when the project commences and continues until the project is complete

expense money the organization pays to an individual or company (third party) in exchange for goods and services purchased

external hard drive a large-capacity, portable storage device that can be used to store an exact copy of a computer's hard drive

extrinsic motivation motivation that comes from an outside source, for example, the opportunity to earn money or a promotion

False Claims Act a federal law under which any person who submits a claim to the federal government that he or she knows (or should have known) is false, is liable for monetary damages and penalties

fee-for-service an insurance plan in which individuals pay a predetermined percentage of the cost of services provided, commonly from 15 to 20 percent, and the insurer pays the remaining cost

fetal death rate a rate that is calculated to determine the percentage of all births that result in fetal death

file/scanning and retrieval clerk an entry-level clerical position that involves preparing documents for final storage (filing paper records or scanning documents into the electronic health record system) and may include pulling paper records from storage or responding to customer requests for access to electronic records

firewall a program that protects computer networks and individual computers from viruses and security threats by blocking or limiting outside users' access to data and systems

fiscal year the legal accounting period for an organization, which may follow the calendar year and begin in January or may follow a different 12-month period

fishbone diagram a diagram that examines the causes and effects of a problem in a process

flash drive a small, rewritable, lightweight, high-capacity device that can store up to 1 terabyte of data; also called a *thumb drive* or *jump drive*

flowchart a visual diagram used to illustrate the physical steps in a process

follow up the process of tracking cancer status, including recurrence treatment provided and quality of life to calculate survival rates by cancer site and state

for-profit/investor-owned hospital a facility owned by private investors or public shareholders

forming the first stage of team development in which team members learn about the team's tasks and goals and their individual roles

formulary a list of medications for which the insurance plan will cover the cost

fraud wrongful or criminal deception intended to result in financial or personal gain

frequency distribution table a table that may be used to show numerical ranges rather than individual numbers

full-time equivalent a new or replacement employee who typically works 40 hours each week, or 2,080 hours per year

Gantt chart a type of bar chart that can be used to outline and monitor a project

gatekeeper a person whose role is to authorize access to medical care on behalf of a health insurance company; often a primary care physician (PCP)

gigahertz (GHz) access speed of at least 1 billion cycles per second

go-live date the date the electronic health record system becomes operational in a healthcare facility

goal a desired result, or an endpoint toward which effort is directed

grade a term used to classify tumors based on the abnormality of the cells (how different they look from normal cells)

gross autopsy rate a rate that compares the number of autopsies conducted by hospital medical staff to the number of inpatient deaths

gross death rate the proportion of hospital discharges that result in death

ground rules the values and standards by which team members agree to abide to facilitate teamwork

hands-on training training that provides practical experience

hard dollars actual cash payments or savings

hard drive a storage device where information is saved, usually the C drive of a desktop or laptop computer; sometimes called a *hard disk drive (HDD)*

hardware the physical components of a computer system: the computer processor and all of its parts, input devices (e.g., mouse and keyboard), monitor, printer, and storage devices (e.g., hard drive, flash drive, and disc)

health information exchange (HIE) the standardized process of data exchange that involves the sharing of health information electronically across state, regional, and local areas

health information management (HIM) the practice of maintaining, analyzing, and protecting confidential patient information contained in the health record

health information technology (HIT) a broad concept that encompasses an array of technologies to store, share, and analyze health information

Health Information Technology for Economic and Clinical Health (HITECH) Act a federal law enacted to stimulate the adoption of electronic health records and supporting technology

health insurance a type of insurance coverage that pays for all or a portion of an individual's medical and surgical expenses

health insurance exchange a government-run insurance marketplace that is intended to foster competition and improve the quality and affordability of health insurance by lowering premium costs and expanding choice

Health Insurance Portability and Accountability Act of 1996 (HIPAA) a broad federal act that includes multiple provisions governing insurance coverage and provides federal protection for individually identifiable health information held by covered entities and their business associates

Health Insurance Prospective Payment System (HIPPS) a reimbursement system for skilled nursing facilities, home health agencies, and inpatient rehabilitation facilities

Health Level Seven International (HL7) a committee of members from more than 55 countries that is the global authority on the standards and interoperability of health information technology

health maintenance organization (HMO) a health insurance organization that provides health care to its members through its own network of physicians and hospitals

health record a medical record into which the healthcare provider records the patient's medical information every time the provider assesses or treats the patient

Healthcare Common Procedure Coding System (HCPCS) a standard code set used by medical coders and billers when submitting requests for reimbursement for medical procedures, supplies, products, and services

Healthcare Effectiveness Data and Information Set (HEDIS) a set of standardized measures developed to facilitate employer efforts to assess health plan performance

healthcare proxy an individual legally designated to make medical decisions for the patient when the patient is unable to do so

healthcare registry a collection of data elements that correlate to specific diseases, conditions, or procedures

HIM technician a general clerical staff position in the HIM department; responsibilities may include record assembly and analysis, transcription processing and routing, physician completion activities, and release of information

home health care healthcare services provided to a patient in the home or other place of residence

hospice symptom and pain control provided to patients in the terminal phase of an illness, commonly defined as someone with a life expectancy of less than six months

hospital autopsy rate the total number of autopsies done by hospital staff

hospital medical coder a coding specialist who reviews documentation in the medical record and assigns each reportable diagnosis and procedure an alphanumeric code

hospital privileges privileges granted by a hospital to a physician indicating the physician is allowed to provide care in that hospital

hospital-acquired condition a condition that was not present on admission

hospital-acquired infection (HAI) an infection acquired during a patient's stay in the hospital

hospitalist a physician who provides general medical care to patients in the hospital

human subjects people who participate in medical research conducted to test the effectiveness of a new drug or treatment

hybrid record a patient medical record that combines both electronic and paper records

hypothesis a problem statement or topic, or a tentative assumption established for the purpose of giving direction to a study

immunization registry a registry containing information on patient immunizations

in camera review a hearing or discussion before a judge that is conducted in the judge's chamber or in a courtroom from which the spectators have been excluded.

incomplete record a medical record that is lacking some required documentation or signatures

indemnity plan a plan that reimburses either the patient or the provider for healthcare expenses when they are incurred; also referred to as fee-for-service plans

index a list arranged in an order (e.g., alphabetically, or by author, subject, or keyword)

individually identifiable health information information in the medical record that can be used to identify the patient, such as address or date of birth

infection-control committee a committee that reviews documentation related to hospital-acquired infections and is responsible for developing strategies to reduce infections

informal leader a person who does not hold a position of authority or power but who can influence the decisions and actions of others

information data that is processed into a group of like items, such as text documents, images, audio clips, and software programs

information governance (IG) the structures, the principles, and practices needed to standardize, manage, protect, access, and communicate data in a business environment

information technology (IT) the study, design, development, application, implementation, support, or management of computer-based information systems

informed consent a patient's verbal or written permission to proceed with treatment or care after receiving full disclosure of the risks and benefits

infrastructure hardware used to connect computers

initiation process a stage in the project management process that involves defining the scope of the project, determining the key participants, and outlining the goals and objectives

inpatient census a count of the hospital's patients at a given time

inpatient service day a measure of the services provided to one patient in one 24-hour period—from census-taking time to census-taking time

institutional review board (IRB) a formally appointed group that reviews and monitors biomedical research involving human subjects

intensity of service (IS) documentation in the medical record that demonstrates that a patient meets criteria or is "sick enough" to require acute inpatient hospitalization

interface 1. a software program that facilitates the exchange of data between the two systems; 2. a two-way communication exchange by which medical systems that communicate with EHR

intermediate care facility a facility that provides care to disabled and elderly individuals with nonacute chronic illness

International Classification of Diseases for Oncology, Third Edition (ICD-O-3) the code set used primarily in tumor or cancer registry programs

International Classification of Diseases, Ninth Revision, Clinical Modification (ICD-9-CM) a code system used in the United States to code inpatient and outpatient diagnoses and inpatient procedures

International Classification of Diseases, Tenth Revision, Clinical Modification (ICD-10-CM) an update of the ICD-9 code that greatly expands the number of available codes from 13,000 to more than 68,000, allowing for greater specificity and flexibility in adding codes for new diseases and diagnoses

International Classification of Diseases, Tenth Revision, Procedure Coding System (ICD-10-PCS) a list of codes for surgical procedures; replaces ICD-9-CM, volume 3, the index of procedural codes

Internet an open-access, global network of computer networks

interoperability the ability of different information technology systems and software applications to communicate within and across organizations, to exchange data, and to use the information that has been exchanged

interoperable unrelated computer systems and software programs from multiple vendors exchanging data

intranet a private communications network that is password protected and accessible only to employees or other authorized users

intrinsic motivation motivation that comes from within an individual

IT director the head of the IT department who oversees all hospital computer systems and infrastructure

job description a broad, general statement of employee roles and responsibilities

job skills skills gained through paid or volunteer work—including those skills developed and sharpened at home or in school

Joint Commission an independent, nonprofit organization that sets standards and evaluates the safety of thousands of healthcare organizations across the country through its voluntary accreditation process

jurisdiction the authority, power, or right to govern or legislate

justification in budgeting it is the circumstance, fact, or explanation that proves an expense is reasonable or necessary

late or loose documentation reports that have not yet been incorporated into the patient record

leader a person who inspires and motivates others

legal health record a record of medical care provided to the patient and used to substantiate the care provided for legal purposes, most notably as evidence in court proceedings

length of stay (LOS) the number of calendar days from the date of admission to the date of discharge

level one trauma center a hospital that has an emergency room equipped and staffed to care for the most severely injured or ill patients

license a permit that grants a healthcare facility the authority to operate or grants a healthcare provider the authority to practice within his or her scope of care

living will a legal document that outlines a patient's wishes regarding medical treatment if he or she is unable to make decisions

local area network (LAN) a network type that connects computers located in a limited geographical area, such as in a home, office building, or hospital

log sheets and flow sheets documentation that provides a graphic summary of changes in the patient's vital signs, health status, or treatment, such as changes in weight, blood pressure, treatment, or medications administered

logic-based encoder an encoder-software program that requires the coder to type in a keyword and then asks a series of questions to refine and identify a specific diagnostic or procedural code

Logical Observation Identifiers, Names, and Codes (LOINC) a universal coding system used for tests, measurements, and observations that provides a common language to facilitate the exchange of clinical data between providers and between countries

long-term acute care hospital (LTAC) a hospital that provides acute care to patients who require care long term; stays average more than 25 days, rather than the two- to four-day average stay for patients in an acute care facility

long-term care (LTC) a general term that describes supportive care provided to individuals who are no longer able to live independently at home

longitudinal record a record that incorporates all of the information from multiple sources gathered over a period of time

macros computer shortcuts that can produce words, sentences, paragraphs, or entire reports with a few keystrokes

maintenance the third stage in the record retention cycle, which refers to handling the record as it becomes inactive over time

malware a malicious software program that is installed on a computer or a system without authorization and is designed to gain access to the user's system to damage or disrupt data or programs or to steal sensitive information

managed care a general term used to define insurance plans that require participants to use a specific network of physicians, providers, and hospitals in exchange for lower premium costs

manager a person who plans, organizes, and delegates tasks

master patient index (MPI) a component of an admission, discharge, and transfer system that collects patient demographic information, including name, date of birth, address, phone number, and medical record number

maternal death a patient death directly linked to or exacerbated by pregnancy

maternal death rate a statistic hospitals use to calculate the percentage of maternal deaths compared to the total number of obstetric patients. The statistic is used to review the outcome of care.

mean the mathematical average of a group of numbers

meaningful use the use of certified EHR technology to meet identified goals for improving patient and public health

measures of variation the extent to which data points differ from each other, or the spread of a group of numbers

median the number that falls in the middle of a set of numbers when the set is arranged in ascending or descending order

Medicaid a federal health insurance program for low-income Americans

medical biller and coder a clerical staff position in a physician office or physician billing company that involves entering pre-coded information from a physician's charge ticket

medical coding editor a coder who reviews the output from a computer-assisted coding program for accuracy and makes changes as necessary

medical identity theft the act of stealing and using personal information to secure medical care, buy drugs, or falsify medical claims for payment

medical language editor a person who transcribes and edits medical documentation

medical necessity justification that the care provided to the patient is reasonable, necessary, and/or appropriate based on evidence-based clinical standards of care

medical record number (MRN) the unique identifier for each patient MPI record

medical referral a recommendation made by the primary care physician (PCP) that a patient see a physician specialist

medical scribe an unlicensed person who enters patient information into an electronic health record or the paper chart at the direction of a physician

medical staff bylaws organizational rules that dictate the governance and structure of the hospital medical staff

medical staff rules and regulations policies and procedures that govern the hospital medical staff practices

medical transcriptionist a healthcare documentation specialist or medical editor who transcribes physician dictation

Medicare a federal health insurance program, administered by the Centers for Medicare and Medicaid Services (CMS) that primarily serves elderly Americans age 65 and older

Medicare Part A Medicare hospital insurance plan that covers inpatient care provided in a skilled nursing facility, a critical access hospital, or another type of hospital

Medicare Part B Medicare coverage of outpatient care, physician services, physical and occupational therapy, and home health care

Medicare Part C/Medicare Advantage Plan Medicare coverage provided by a federally approved private insurance company, including both Parts A and B

Medicare Part D a menu of prescription drug plans

medication record a record that documents the administration of each drug each time it is given to the patient, including the date and the time of administration and the initials of the nurse who administered the medication

Medigap policy a supplemental insurance plan that individuals can choose to purchase from a private insurer to help cover out-of-pocket expenses that are not covered under Medicare

megahertz (MHz) access speed of at least 1 million cycles per second

memory chip a computer chip that stores data and information

microcomputer a small computer

microfiche a flat film on which images are mounted in a matrix format

microfilm film strips onto which paper images are copied in miniature form order to reduce the amount of space needed for file storage

microprocessor the area that contains the CPU and controls the logic of most digital devices

middle digit filing a filing system for paper medical records in which the middle two digits identify the primary location of the file (i.e., the section); the first two digits identify the subsection; and the last two digits identify the tertiary number

military hospital a hospital that is designated for use by active duty and retired military personnel, military dependents and survivors, and other groups under special circumstances

minimum necessary a requirement that covered entities provide the least amount of patient identifying information necessary to respond to a request for information

mode the value that occurs most frequently in a set of data

morbidity disease state or symptom

morphology a term used to identify the histology (type of cancer)

mortality state of being mortal, subject to death

motherboard the main circuit board of a microcomputer

motivation the reason people do things

multiple malignancy more than one primary cancer site

National Committee for Quality Assurance (NCQA) an independent nonprofit organization focused on improving the quality of patient care

National Patient Safety Goals goals established by the Joint Commission that are intended to protect patient safety and improve the quality of patient care

National Quality Strategy a part of the Affordable Care Act (ACA) that serves as a catalyst for quality improvement efforts

National Vital Statistic System (NVSS) a part of the Centers for Disease Control and Prevention (CDC) to which county, state, and local registrars report vital statistics data for future statistical and trend analysis publication

nepotism the practice of hiring or promoting a family member regardless of merit

net autopsy rate a rate that calculates the number of inpatient autopsies performed

net death rate the number of inpatient hospital deaths that occur more than 48 hours after admission

networking the practice of linking two or more computing devices together to share data

nomenclature a system for naming things within a particular group

nonprofit hospital a partially or fully tax-exempt organization that provides care to patients regardless of their ability to pay and provides community benefits in accordance with state and federal guidelines

norming the third stage of team development in which team members begin to focus on the goal at hand and become comfortable with their roles on the team

nosocomial infection a hospital-acquired infection

nosocomial infection rate the number of patients who acquired an infection while in the hospital compared with the total patient population

notice of privacy practices a legal notice explaining how the patient's protected health information may be used or disclosed, and the patients' rights with regard to the use of protected health information

Nuremberg Code a set of ethical principles developed after World War II governing research involving human subjects

nursing note a note made by a member of the nursing staff describing the patient's general condition

obligatory disclosures of information the mandatory release of patient records, often as part of a legal proceeding

off-site storage a storage facility for patient records located away from the main care facility

Office of the National Coordinator for Health Information Technology (ONC) a position within the US Department of Health & Human Services that supports the adoption of health information technology and promotes nationwide health information exchange to improve health care

operating budget projections for revenue and expenses, such as payroll, supplies, and services, that are required for the day-to-day running of a business or organization

operations/procedures index a list of all of the operations and procedures performed in a healthcare facility listed with the appropriate medical codes

operative report a narrative description of a surgical procedure

optional field a field in a database designated for the collection of optional information

organizational flowchart a diagram illustrating the departments, personnel, and lines of authority of a business or an organization

orientation a process of introducing a new employee to a company or facility, to other employees, and to the policies, procedures, and culture of the workplace

Original Medicare Plan the original Medicare fee-for-service plan that includes a deductible and a copay or coinsurance and consists of Medicare Parts A and B (hospital and medical insurance, respectively) with the option of adding a stand-alone Part D plan to cover prescription medications

ORYX a Joint Commission performance measurement used to evaluate a hospital for accreditation

osteopathic hospital a hospital in which doctors of osteopathic medicine (DOs) provide the majority of care, emphasizing the whole person, rather than the treatment of specific symptoms or conditions, and the relationship of one body system to another

outliers Medicare patients for whom the cost of providing care (the value) is much higher or much lower than most others in the DRG

outpatient surgery day surgery, ambulatory surgery, or same-day surgery

password a secret code assigned to or chosen by an individual user to limit access to information stored on a computer or computer system

password aging a procedure that requires users to change passwords frequently and on a regular basis, such as every 90 days

pathology report a detailed report of the findings from the analysis of specimens removed during surgery

patient care services the largest department in a hospital (also called the *department of nursing*) which includes nurses, technicians, therapists, and other employees who provide direct patient care

patient portal a secure website that provides patients with convenient, 24-hour access to physician notes, diagnostic results, physical examination results, medications, and other information

Patient Protection and Affordable Care Act/Affordable Care Act (ACA) a federal law enacted in 2010 that is intended to improve the quality of health care and lower the cost of care, to improve consumer protections, and to expand consumer access to health plans

patient record a medical record or health record that documents a patient's medical history and all care and services provided to the patient during one episode of care

payment posting and appeals and collections the process of collecting medical fees not covered by insurance from patients; may include setting up payment plans

percentage the number of parts of 100

percentage of occupancy the percentage of the facility's inpatient beds that are occupied

performance evaluation a process used by a manager or consultant to examine and evaluate the work of an employee against preset standards

performance improvement coordinator an individual who coordinates technical and analytical support for quality and performance improvement (PI) initiatives and medical peer-review activities

performing the fourth stage of team development in which team members have a shared vision of the team's goals and work is progressing

personal health record (PHR) a record created and maintained by the patient that is used to organize and store information about medications, treatments, and other health-related information

phishing sending fake emails designed to appear as if they are coming from a legitimate source with the purpose of deceiving users into surrendering private information, such as user names, passwords, and credit card information

physical safeguards the mechanisms required to protect electronic systems and equipment and the data they hold from environmental and human threats and damage

physician assistant (PA) a medical professional who is licensed by the state and works under the direction of a licensed physician, performing duties similar to a nurse practitioner

physician office manager the position responsible for the overall operations of the medical office, including hiring, assessing and training staff, negotiating insurance contracts, preparing and monitoring budgets, paying invoices, and monitoring billing and accounts receivable

physician orders written orders that communicate a physician's instructions for the care of a patient

picture archiving and communication system (PACS) a system that captures and stores radiology images and scans (such as CAT scans) and then interfaces with the core EHR to store the image

planning process a stage in the project management process that may include identifying resources, developing a budget, creating a project schedule, and identifying potential problems that may arise during the course of the project

point of care (POC) the location where services are delivered, such as an exam room or a hospital patient's bedside

point of service (POS) plan a health insurance plan in which members are required to select a network physician as their primary care physician (PCP) as their "point of service"

point of service registration counseling the collection of a comprehensive set of data elements that is required to establish a medical record number and satisfy regulatory, financial, and clinical requirements

policy a guiding principle that directs the actions of an organization

portability the transfer and continuation of health insurance coverage when an individual changes or loses a job

postoperative death rate the number of inpatient deaths that occur after a surgical procedure and within 10 days of the procedure

practice management system (PMS) a system used to manage a physician practice that includes programs for an MPI, scheduling, medical billing, insurance verification, and revenue cycle management

preferred provider organization (PPO) a type of insurance plan that contract directly with specific healthcare providers, called *preferred providers*

premium a set amount paid monthly or annually to cover the cost of insurance

present on admission (POA) illness, injury, or other medical condition that is present at the time the patient is admitted to the hospital

primary cancer the anatomical site where the cancer started

primary care physician (PCP) a medical professional who is usually licensed in family practice, internal medicine, or pediatrics and often provides preventive and sick care

privacy the right to prevent the nonconsensual disclosure of sensitive, confidential, or discrediting information

privacy officer a person whose job it is to establish policies and procedures to protect the confidentiality of protected health information (PHI), educate all facility personnel on the HIPAA Privacy Rule, audit PHI access, handle complaints related to privacy, and produce reports for internal use and governmental agencies

Privacy Rule a component of HIPAA that specifically outlines requirements for the protection of confidential patient information

private health insurance insurance purchased from for-profit entities or nonprofit organizations

problem list a list of conditions or problems for which the patient is seeking treatment or for which treatment should be considered

problem-oriented medical information system (PROMIS) a system developed by Dr. Lawrence L. Weed in the 1960s that established standardized documentation formats

problem-oriented medical record (POMR) a record or process developed by Dr. Lawrence L. Weed in the 1960s that could be used to input data electronically

procedure instructions that describe how a job should be performed

process improvement (PI) a methodology that is used to identify and implement necessary changes to advance the efficiency, effectiveness, and reliability of a process or a procedure

process reengineering a systematic evaluation and modification of an existing process, which is used to simplify and eliminate wasted effort

production log a useful tool to monitor employee productivity

productivity the ratio of inputs (time and labor) to outputs (work produced)

professionalism the conduct, aims (aspirations and intentions), and qualities that characterize or mark a professional person

project a temporary endeavor designed to produce a specific product, service, or result

project management the process of planning, organizing, and guiding a project from start to finish

progress note a note written by a provider documenting changes in the patient's condition

prospective payment system (PPS) a Medicare payment system that uses a per-case reimbursement mechanism under which inpatient admission cases are divided into diagnosis-related groups (DRGs)

protected heath information (PHI) any information about the health status, the provision of care, or the payment for health care that can be linked to or can identify a specific patient

protocol a clinical-care guideline or pre-established plan for a course of medical treatment that is grounded in evidence-based medicine

provider an individual or an institution that provides direct patient care

public health insurance health insurance offered by state and federal government to individuals who meet specific criteria, such as age or income

purging the removal of pages from a patient health record that are no longer actively needed for the provision of patient care

qualitative research research that is descriptive data collection; often includes interviews and focus groups

quality excellence as defined by the customer in meeting or exceeding desired outcomes

quality control operational techniques and activities used to regulate performance and prevent undesirable changes in a process

quality improvement (QI) a methodology that is used to identify and implement necessary changes to advance the efficiency, effectiveness, and reliability of a process or a procedure

quantitative research research that relies on counting and measuring and requires that the data be objective, quantitative, and statistically valid

random access memory (RAM) computer memory used to run programs and store data

range the difference between the largest and the smallest values in a set of values

rate a ratio that compares two quantities of different units of measure

ratio a comparison between two numbers or quantities, commonly displayed as two numbers separated by a colon

record analysis system an independent system that flags deficiencies in physician documentation in the health record

record retention cycle the health record life cycle, which begins at the time the patient checks in for an outpatient visit or is admitted to an inpatient facility and continues until the record is destroyed; the four major stages include creation, utilization, maintenance, and destruction

record retrieval pulling a record from storage in response to a request

Recovery Audit Contractor (RAC) a federal external auditor who may use patient information to identify and recover improper Medicare payments

recovery room report a report that documents a patient's condition during recovery from anesthesia

Red Flags Rule a rule intended to prevent medical identify theft by requiring businesses and organizations to develop theft detection and prevention programs

regulation rules created by a governmental agency to explain how the should be implemented

rehabilitation the process of restoring an individual's health and/or quality of life through therapy and education

release of information (ROI) a system that collects and stores information on all health records that have been requested, copied, and released

reliable when the same results are achieved on successive tests or calculations

remittance processing and rejections the posting or the applying of payments or payment adjustments, including denied claims, to the appropriate accounts

residential care/assisted living facilities facilities that provide support services to adults who cannot live alone but do not require skilled or intermediate care

resource management the process of evaluating the cost and efficiency of patient care services concurrently to control expenses, such as moving a patient from the intensive care unit (ICU) to a standard patient-care room once the patient is stable

resource utilization group (RUG) payment tiers based on the level of nursing care required, room considerations (including isolation), and minutes of therapy provided

respite care temporary institutional care of a dependent elderly, ill, or handicapped person to provide relief for their usual caregivers

restraint log a log maintained to document the use of restraints on a patient and monitoring of the patient by the staff

résumé a marketing tool that a job seeker uses to promote his or her skills and value to an organization

retrospective cost-based reimbursement a payment system in use when Medicare was introduced in 1965; no longer in use

retrospective review a review of a patient's discharge summary, including discharge instructions and final diagnosis, after the patient has been discharged

return on investment the ability of an investment to pay for itself over time and generate a profit

revenue money received for services provided or for products sold

revenue cycle management all administrative and clinical functions that contribute to the capture, management, and collection of patient service revenue

risk a situation involving exposure to danger, harm, or loss

risk management 1. the act of proactively preventing errors and injury to patients, staff, and visitors and mitigate financial losses if a problem occurs; 2. the department responsible for all medical malpractice and personal injury litigation brought against a healthcare facility

risk taker someone who chooses an action that offers an opportunity for gain but also has potential risk

rural hospital a hospital that typically offers basic health care; usually located in a small city or rural area at some distance from critical access hospitals

scheduling and preregistration the collection of patient registration information before the patient's arrival for inpatient or outpatient services, including eligibility, benefits, and authorizations

scheduling system a system that includes a calendar with dates and times allotted for each event, the name of the practitioner or physician, and the anticipated duration of the appointment

secondary data data abstracted from patient healthcare records that is used to track trends and identify patterns to improve the quality of patient care, in budgeting, and for planning purposes

security protecting information and information systems from unauthorized access

security incident the attempted or successful unauthorized access, use, disclosure, modification, or destruction of information or interference with system operations in an information system

Security Rule national standards developed by HIPAA for the protection of health information that is held or transmitted electronically in three broad areas

sentinel event (SE) an unexpected occurrence that results in a patient's death or in serious physical or psychological injury

serial numbering a file numbering system that requires that a patient file be renumbered each time the patient visits; files are shelved in chronological order so that individual records for a single patient are stored in multiple locations in the facility's file room

serial unit numbering a numbering system requiring that patient files receive a new number at every visit and records from previous visits be brought forward and filed with the current record

server many computers connected together

severity of illness (SI) documentation in the medical record required by insurers to determine the medical necessity of care provided

simple project a project that is limited in scope, usually involving a defined number of tasks that may be completed in a few days or a few months

skew to distort

skilled care facility a facility that provides nursing or rehabilitation care for patients in need of speech, physical, respiratory, psychological, or other therapy

SOAP note a format for organizing information documented in the patient record

soft dollars nonmonetary benefits and cost savings

software the programs and the instructions that run the hardware, manage computer resources, process data, and communicate or network with other computers

source-oriented medical record documentation that has information organized by source (where the information came from) or by category

specialist a physician who has advanced education and clinical training in a particular area of medicine

specialty clinic a facility that provides outpatient treatment of specific diseases and conditions

specialty unit an inpatient unit, such as psychiatry or neonatology, that is designated for the treatment of specific illnesses or conditions

standard deviation a calculation that indicates how closely the data points (values) in a set of data are grouped around the mean

statute of limitations a statute established by federal or state law that sets a time limit within which legal proceedings may be brought forward

storming the second stage of team development in which team members begin to assert themselves and try to define their individual roles

strategic plan a plan that documents an organization's goals, identifies the resources needed, and recommends the steps to take to achieve those goals

strong password a password that cannot be easily broken

subpoena a legal document issued by a judge ordering that a person, document, or record be produced in court

subpoena ad testificandum a type of subpoena that orders an individual to appear in court and testify

subpoena duces tecum a type of subpoena that is used to compel an individual to produce documentary evidence in court

supervisor/manager the position responsible for human resource activities such as hiring, counseling, firing, and training staff

system software software that controls the basic functions of a computer

Systematized Nomenclature of Medicine—Clinical Terms (SNOWMED CT) a comprehensive nomenclature of clinical terms and multilingual health terminology

teaching hospital a healthcare facility that provides medical students, interns, and residents with opportunities to observe and acquire hands-on training through interaction with patient populations having a wide variety of illnesses, injuries, and conditions

teamwork the cooperative effort by a group or team to achieve a common goal

technical safeguards automated processes that utilize software to protect and control access to data

templates fill-in-the blank features built into an EHR, or pretyped reports that require physicians to enter a few simple fill-in-the-blank answers from a drop-down screen

terminal digit filing a filing system for paper medical records in which the last two digits identify the primary location of the file (i.e., the section); the second two digits identify the subsection; and the first two digits identify the tertiary number.

third-party follow-up collecting payments from insurers after the initial claim has been filed

TNM staging system a tool that enables physicians to stage different types of cancers based on standardized criteria

topography a term used to identify the physical location of a tumor

total inpatient service days the sum of all inpatient service days during a select period

total length of stay the sum of the lengths of stay for a group of inpatients discharged during a specific time period; also called *discharge days*

training the act of coaching or teaching a behavior or process through specific instruction and practice

transcribed dictation typed into a medical record or document

transcription system an enhanced word processing system similar to Microsoft Word that has special capabilities such as an ADT interface, an EHR interface, medical spell-check, template design, and statistical tracking for staff production and physician document volume

transferable skills skills that can be transferred from one occupation to another

transfer record a record of patient information provided when a patient is transferred within the facility, or to or from another facility

transitional (discharge) planning the coordination of services for a patient after discharge from a hospital

trauma registry a registry that collects demographic and clinical information on all hospital trauma cases, such as injuries, falls, accidents, burns, and cuts

treatment, payment, operations (TPO) activities that a facility must do to carry out its operations, such as providing patient care and treatment, billing and reimbursement, risk management, and quality improvement

trend analysis the process of collecting and analyzing data to identify patterns or trends over time

Trojan horse malicious software that masquerades as a useful program

unbundling the practice of billing for multiple, individual items when services are grouped together as one

uniform resource locator (URL) a web address; each web page has a unique URL

unintended consequences side effects or complications that could occur during or as a result of the procedure

unit numbering a file numbering system in which the patient is assigned a patient/record number at the first visit, and all of the records related to that patient going forward are given the same number and maintained in a single file

unknown primary a description applied to metastatic cancer cells when the primary origin or site of the cancer cannot be determined

upcoding a fraudulent billing practice that involves the assignment of a higher-paying medical code to a treatment or procedure than is justified by the documentation in the medical record for the purpose of receiving increased reimbursement

urban hospital a hospital located in a large or midsized city equipped with sophisticated diagnostic equipment and a highly trained workforce

utilization the second stage in the record retention cycle, when the record is available to authorized personnel for internal and external uses during the patient stay or visit and afterward when access to the record is needed for insurance billing, committee review, and reporting to outside agencies

utilization management the process of evaluating the appropriateness of patient care care against objective criteria

valid statistics that have a sound basis in logic and are relevant to the purpose for which they are used

value-based purchasing (VBP) a payment methodology that rewards quality of care through payment incentives

variability the difference between a single value and every other value in a dataset

virtual private network (VPN) a secure computer network used by businesses to share data between users in remote locations, for example, between different branches of a bank or between different clinics in a health system

virus a computer program that is designed to spread from one file to another on a single computer to damage data and destroy files

vital signs temperature, pulse, respiration, and blood pressure

vital statistics quantitative data of specified population groups, such as the statistics collected on births and deaths used to monitor population trends

vital statistics clerk a clerical position that involves preparing birth and death certificates and submitting the information to the appropriate state agency

voice recognition software a computer program that allows the user to dictate into a microphone while the computer inputs the dictation

vulnerable subjects research study participants who might be subject to coercion or undue influence

warrant a written order directing law enforcement personnel to perform an act in support of the administration of justice

web browser a software application that is used to locate, retrieve, and display content on the web

website a related collection of one or more web pages, usually starting with a home page

whistle-blower someone who informs on a person or an organization engaged in illegal activity

wide area network (WAN) a network that uses telephone lines, fiber optic cables, and satellite links to connect computers and LANs located over a large geographical area, including across a country or around the world

Wi-Fi any wireless local area network (WLAN) technology that connects computers and other electronic devices to each other or to the Internet

wireless access point (WAP) allows computers to connect to a network or a device wirelessly

wireless local area network (WLAN) a technology that connects computers and other electronic devices to each other or to the Internet

workers' compensation insurance that covers employees injured on the job

World Health Organization (WHO) an organization that provides leadership on global public health issues and initiatives and works within the United Nations to coordinate and direct public health programs

worm a computer program designed to self-replicate and spread from one computer to another to damage data and destroy files

Appendix C

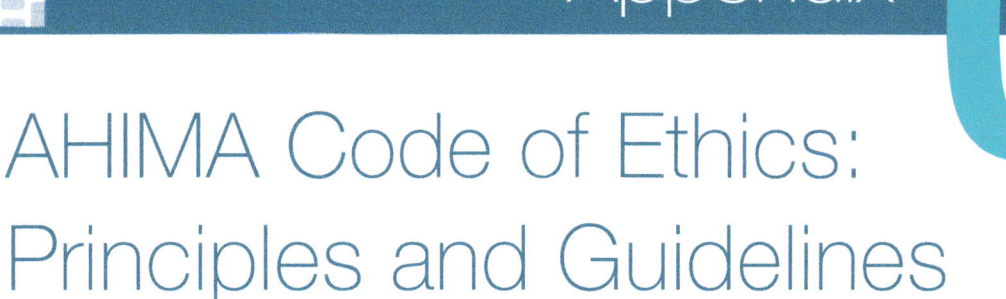

AHIMA Code of Ethics: Principles and Guidelines

The Code of Ethics and How to Interpret the Code of Ethics

Principles and Guidelines

The following ethical principles are based on the core values of the American Health Information Management Association and apply to all AHIMA members and certificants. Guidelines included for each ethical principle are a non-inclusive list of behaviors and situations that can help to clarify the principle. They are not meant to be a comprehensive list of all situations that can occur.

I. *Advocate, uphold, and defend the individual's right to privacy and the doctrine of confidentiality in the use and disclosure of information.*

A health information management professional **shall**:

1.1. Safeguard all confidential patient information to include, but not limited to, personal, health, financial, genetic, and outcome information.

1.2. Engage in social and political action that supports the protection of privacy and confidentiality, and be aware of the impact of the political arena on the health information issues for the healthcare industry.

1.3. Advocate for changes in policy and legislation to ensure protection of privacy and confidentiality, compliance, and other issues that surface as advocacy issues and facilitate informed participation by the public on these issues.

1.4. Protect the confidentiality of all information obtained in the course of professional service. Disclose only information that is directly relevant or necessary to achieve the purpose of disclosure. Release information only with valid authorization from a patient or a person legally authorized to consent on behalf of a patient or as authorized by federal or state regulations. The minimum necessary standard is essential when releasing health information for disclosure activities.

1.5. Promote the obligation to respect privacy by respecting confidential information shared among colleagues, while responding to requests from the legal profession, the media, or other non-healthcare related individuals, during presentations or teaching and in situations that could cause harm to persons.

1.6. Respond promptly and appropriately to patient requests to exercise their privacy rights (e.g., access, amendments, restriction, confidential communication, etc.). Answer truthfully all patients' questions concerning their rights to review and annotate their personal biomedical data and seek to facilitate patients' legitimate right to exercise those rights.

II. *Put service and the health and welfare of persons before self-interest and conduct oneself in the practice of the profession so as to bring honor to oneself, peers, and to the health information management profession.*

A health information management professional **shall**:

2.1. Act with integrity, behave in a trustworthy manner, elevate service to others above self-interest, and promote high standards of practice in every setting.

2.2. Be aware of the profession's mission, values, and ethical principles, and practice in a manner consistent with them by acting honestly and responsibly.

2.3. Anticipate, clarify, and avoid any conflict of interest, to all parties concerned, when dealing with consumers, consulting with competitors, in providing services requiring potentially conflicting roles (for example, finding out information about one facility that would help a competitor), or serving the Association in a volunteer capacity. The conflicting roles or responsibilities must be clarified and appropriate action taken to minimize any conflict of interest.

2.4. Ensure that the working environment is consistent and encourages compliance with the AHIMA Code of Ethics, taking reasonable steps to eliminate any conditions in their organizations that violate, interfere with, or discourage compliance with the code.

2.5. Take responsibility and credit, including authorship credit, only for work they actually perform or to which they contribute. Honestly acknowledge the work of and the contributions made by others verbally or written, such as in publication.

A health information management professional **shall not**:

2.6. Permit one's private conduct to interfere with the ability to fulfill one's professional responsibilities.

2.7. Take unfair advantage of any professional relationship or exploit others to further one's own personal, religious, political, or business interests.

III. *Preserve, protect, and secure personal health information in any form or medium and hold in the highest regards health information and other information of a confidential nature obtained in an official capacity, taking into account the applicable statutes and regulations.*

A health information management professional **shall**:

3.1. Safeguard the privacy and security of written and electronic health information and other sensitive information. Take reasonable steps to ensure that health information is stored securely and that patients' data is not available to others who are not authorized to have access. Prevent inappropriate disclosure of individually identifiable information.

3.2. Take precautions to ensure and maintain the confidentiality of information transmitted, transferred, or disposed of in the event of termination, incapacitation, or death of a healthcare provider to other parties through the use of any media.

3.3. Inform recipients of the limitations and risks associated with providing services via electronic or social media (e.g., computer, telephone, fax, radio, and television).

IV. *Refuse to participate in or conceal unethical practices or procedures and report such practices.*

A health information management professional **shall**:

4.1. Act in a professional and ethical manner at all times.

4.2. Take adequate measures to discourage, prevent, expose, and correct the unethical conduct of colleagues. If needed, utilize the Professional Ethics Committee Policies and Procedures for potential ethics complaints.

4.3. Be knowledgeable about established policies and procedures for handling concerns about colleagues' unethical behavior. These include policies and procedures created by AHIMA, licensing and regulatory bodies, employers, supervisors, agencies, and other professional organizations.

4.4. Seek resolution if there is a belief that a colleague has acted unethically or if there is a belief of incompetence or impairment by discussing one's concerns with the colleague when feasible and when such discussion is likely to be productive.

4.5. Consult with a colleague when feasible and assist the colleague in taking remedial action when there is direct knowledge of a health information management colleague's incompetence or impairment.

4.6. Take action through appropriate formal channels, such as contacting an accreditation or regulatory body and/or the AHIMA Professional Ethics Committee if needed.

4.7. Cooperate with lawful authorities as appropriate.

A health information management professional **shall not**:

4.8. Participate in, condone, or be associated with dishonesty, fraud and abuse, or deception. A non-inclusive list of examples includes:

- Allowing patterns of optimizing or minimizing documentation and/or coding to impact payment
- Assigning codes without physician documentation
- Coding when documentation does not justify the diagnoses or procedures that have been billed
- Coding an inappropriate level of service
- Miscoding to avoid conflict with others
- Engaging in negligent coding practices
- Hiding or ignoring review outcomes, such as performance data

- Failing to report licensure status for a physician through the appropriate channels
- Recording inaccurate data for accreditation purposes
- Allowing inappropriate access to genetic, adoption, health, or behavioral health information
- Misusing sensitive information about a competitor
- Violating the privacy of individuals

Refer to the AHIMA Standards for Ethical Coding for additional guidance.

4.9. Engage in any relationships with a patient where there is a risk of exploitation or potential harm to the patient.

V. *Advance health information management knowledge and practice through continuing education, research, publications, and presentations.*

A health information management professional **shall**:

5.1. Develop and enhance continually professional expertise, knowledge, and skills (including appropriate education, research, training, consultation, and supervision). Contribute to the knowledge base of health information management and share one's knowledge related to practice, research, and ethics.

5.2. Base practice decisions on recognized knowledge, including empirically based knowledge relevant to health information management and health information management ethics.

5.3. Contribute time and professional expertise to activities that promote respect for the value, integrity, and competence of the health information management profession. These activities may include teaching, research, consultation, service, legislative testimony, advocacy, presentations in the community, and participation in professional organizations.

5.4. Engage in evaluation and research that ensures the confidentiality of participants and of the data obtained from them by following guidelines developed for the participants in consultation with appropriate institutional review boards.

5.5. Report evaluation and research findings accurately and take steps to correct any errors later found in published data using standard publication methods.

5.6. Design or conduct evaluation or research that is in conformance with applicable federal or state laws.

5.7. Take reasonable steps to provide or arrange for continuing education and staff development, addressing current knowledge and emerging developments related to health information management practice and ethics.

VI. *Recruit and mentor students, staff, peers, and colleagues to develop and strengthen professional workforce.*

A health information management professional **shall**:

6.1. Provide directed practice opportunities for students.

6.2. Be a mentor for students, peers, and new health information management professionals to develop and strengthen skills.

6.3. Be responsible for setting clear, appropriate, and culturally sensitive boundaries for students, staff, peers, colleagues, and members within professional organizations.

6.4. Evaluate students' performance in a manner that is fair and respectful when functioning as educators or clinical internship supervisors.

6.5. Evaluate staff's performance in a manner that is fair and respectful when functioning in a supervisory capacity.

6.6. Serve an active role in developing HIM faculty or actively recruiting HIM professionals.

A health information management professional **shall not**:

6.7. Engage in any relationships with a person (e.g. students, staff, peers, or colleagues) where there is a risk of exploitation or potential harm to that other person.

VII. *Represent the profession to the public in a positive manner.*

A health information management professional **shall**:

7.1. Be an advocate for the profession in all settings and participate in activities that promote and explain the mission, values, and principles of the profession to the public.

VIII. *Perform honorably health information management association responsibilities, either appointed or elected, and preserve the confidentiality of any privileged information made known in any official capacity.*

A health information management professional **shall**:

8.1. Perform responsibly all duties as assigned by the professional association operating within the bylaws and policies and procedures of the association and any pertinent laws.

8.2. Uphold the decisions made by the association.

8.3. Speak on behalf of the health information management profession and association, only while serving in the role, accurately representing the official and authorized positions of the association.

8.4. Disclose any real or perceived conflicts of interest.

8.5. Relinquish association information upon ending appointed or elected responsibilities.

8.6. Resign from an association position if unable to perform the assigned responsibilities with competence.

8.7. Avoid lending the prestige of the association to advance or appear to advance the private interests of others by endorsing any product or service in return for remuneration. Avoid endorsing products or services of a third party, for-profit entity that competes with AHIMA products and services. Care should **also** be exercised in endorsing any other products and services.

IX. ***State truthfully and accurately one's credentials, professional education, and experiences.***

  A health information management professional **shall**:

   9.1. Make clear distinctions between statements made and actions engaged in as a private individual and as a representative of the health information management profession, a professional health information association, or one's employer.

   9.2. Claim and ensure that representation to patients, agencies, and the public of professional qualifications, credentials, education, competence, affiliations, services provided, training, certification, consultation received, supervised experience, and other relevant professional experience are accurate.

   9.3. Claim only those relevant professional credentials actually possessed and correct any inaccuracies occurring regarding credentials.

   9.4. Report only those continuing education units actually earned for the recertification cycle and correct any inaccuracies occurring regarding CEUs.

X. ***Facilitate interdisciplinary collaboration in situations supporting health information practice.***

  A health information management professional **shall**:

   10.1. Participate in and contribute to decisions that affect the well-being of patients by drawing on the perspectives, values, and experiences of those involved in decisions related to patients.

   10.2. Facilitate interdisciplinary collaboration in situations supporting health information practice.

   10.3. Establish clearly professional and ethical obligations of the interdisciplinary team as a whole and of its individual members.

   10.4. Foster trust among group members and adjust behavior in order to establish relationships with teams.

XI. ***Respect the inherent dignity and worth of every person.***

  A health information management professional **shall**:

   11.1. Treat each person in a respectful fashion, being mindful of individual differences and cultural and ethnic diversity.

   11.2. Promote the value of self-determination for each individual.

   11.3. Value all kinds and classes of people equitably, deal effectively with all races, cultures, disabilities, ages and genders.

   11.4. Ensure all voices are listened to and respected.

Reprinted with permission from the American Health Information Management Association. Copyright © 2014 by the American Health Information Management Association. All rights reserved. No part of this may be reproduced, reprinted, stored in a retrieval system, or transmitted, in any form or by any means, electronic, photocopying, recording, or otherwise, without the prior written permission of the association.

Appendix D

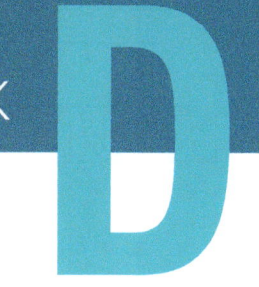

Sample Medical Forms

U.S. STANDARD CERTIFICATE OF LIVE BIRTH

LOCAL FILE NO. _____ BIRTH NUMBER: _____

CHILD
1. CHILD'S NAME (First, Middle, Last, Suffix): John Alan Ramos
2. TIME OF BIRTH (24 hr): 8:52
3. SEX: M
4. DATE OF BIRTH (Mo/Day/Yr): 6/23/2014
5. FACILITY NAME (If not institution, give street and number): Community Hospital
6. CITY, TOWN, OR LOCATION OF BIRTH: Enid, OK
7. COUNTY OF BIRTH: Ellis

MOTHER
8a. MOTHER'S CURRENT LEGAL NAME (First, Middle, Last, Suffix): Janet Marie Ramos
8b. DATE OF BIRTH (Mo/Day/Yr): 1/8/1989
8c. MOTHER'S NAME PRIOR TO FIRST MARRIAGE (First, Middle, Last, Suffix): Janet Marie McHale
8d. BIRTHPLACE (State, Territory, or Foreign Country): Oklahoma
9a. RESIDENCE OF MOTHER-STATE: Oklahoma
9b. COUNTY: Ellis
9c. CITY, TOWN, OR LOCATION: Enid
9d. STREET AND NUMBER: 104 Elm Drive
9e. APT. NO.: ___
9f. ZIP CODE: 73000
9g. INSIDE CITY LIMITS?: ☒ Yes ☐ No

FATHER
10a. FATHER'S CURRENT LEGAL NAME (First, Middle, Last, Suffix): Michael Alan Ramos
10b. DATE OF BIRTH (Mo/Day/Yr): 10/16/1987
10c. BIRTHPLACE (State, Territory, or Foreign Country): Colorado

CERTIFIER
11. CERTIFIER'S NAME: Albert Myers
TITLE: ☒ MD ☐ DO ☐ HOSPITAL ADMIN. ☐ CNM/CM ☐ OTHER MIDWIFE ☐ OTHER (Specify)
12. DATE CERTIFIED: 6/24/2014
13. DATE FILED BY REGISTRAR: 6/28/2014

INFORMATION FOR ADMINISTRATIVE USE

MOTHER
14. MOTHER'S MAILING ADDRESS: ☐ Same as residence, or: State: Oklahoma City, Town, or Location: Enid
Street & Number: 104 Elm Drive Apartment No.: ___ Zip Code: 73000
15. MOTHER MARRIED? (At birth, conception, or any time between) ☒ Yes ☐ No
IF NO, HAS PATERNITY ACKNOWLEDGEMENT BEEN SIGNED IN THE HOSPITAL? ☐ Yes ☐ No
16. SOCIAL SECURITY NUMBER REQUESTED FOR CHILD? ☒ Yes ☐ No
17. FACILITY ID. (NPI): 9999
18. MOTHER'S SOCIAL SECURITY NUMBER: 123 45 6789
19. FATHER'S SOCIAL SECURITY NUMBER: 123 67 4589

INFORMATION FOR MEDICAL AND HEALTH PURPOSES ONLY

MOTHER
20. MOTHER'S EDUCATION (Check the box that best describes the highest degree or level of school completed at the time of delivery)
- ☐ 8th grade or less
- ☐ 9th - 12th grade, no diploma
- ☐ High school graduate or GED completed
- ☐ Some college credit but no degree
- ☒ Associate degree (e.g., AA, AS)
- ☐ Bachelor's degree (e.g., BA, AB, BS)
- ☐ Master's degree (e.g., MA, MS, MEng, MEd, MSW, MBA)
- ☐ Doctorate (e.g., PhD, EdD) or Professional degree (e.g., MD, DDS, DVM, LLB, JD)

21. MOTHER OF HISPANIC ORIGIN? (Check the box that best describes whether the mother is Spanish/Hispanic/Latina. Check the "No" box if mother is not Spanish/Hispanic/Latina)
- ☒ No, not Spanish/Hispanic/Latina
- ☐ Yes, Mexican, Mexican American, Chicana
- ☐ Yes, Puerto Rican
- ☐ Yes, Cuban
- ☐ Yes, other Spanish/Hispanic/Latina (Specify)_____

22. MOTHER'S RACE (Check one or more races to indicate what the mother considers herself to be)
- ☒ White
- ☐ Black or African American
- ☐ American Indian or Alaska Native (Name of the enrolled or principal tribe)_____
- ☐ Asian Indian
- ☐ Chinese
- ☐ Filipino
- ☐ Japanese
- ☐ Korean
- ☐ Vietnamese
- ☐ Other Asian (Specify)_____
- ☐ Native Hawaiian
- ☐ Guamanian or Chamorro
- ☐ Samoan
- ☐ Other Pacific Islander (Specify)_____
- ☐ Other (Specify)_____

FATHER
23. FATHER'S EDUCATION (Check the box that best describes the highest degree or level of school completed at the time of delivery)
- ☐ 8th grade or less
- ☐ 9th - 12th grade, no diploma
- ☐ High school graduate or GED completed
- ☐ Some college credit but no degree
- ☐ Associate degree (e.g., AA, AS)
- ☒ Bachelor's degree (e.g., BA, AB, BS)
- ☐ Master's degree (e.g., MA, MS, MEng, MEd, MSW, MBA)
- ☐ Doctorate (e.g., PhD, EdD) or Professional degree (e.g., MD, DDS, DVM, LLB, JD)

24. FATHER OF HISPANIC ORIGIN? (Check the box that best describes whether the father is Spanish/Hispanic/Latino. Check the "No" box if father is not Spanish/Hispanic/Latino)
- ☐ No, not Spanish/Hispanic/Latino
- ☒ Yes, Mexican, Mexican American, Chicano
- ☐ Yes, Puerto Rican
- ☐ Yes, Cuban
- ☐ Yes, other Spanish/Hispanic/Latino (Specify)_____

25. FATHER'S RACE (Check one or more races to indicate what the father considers himself to be)
- ☐ White
- ☐ Black or African American
- ☐ American Indian or Alaska Native (Name of the enrolled or principal tribe)_____
- ☐ Asian Indian
- ☐ Chinese
- ☐ Filipino
- ☐ Japanese
- ☐ Korean
- ☐ Vietnamese
- ☐ Other Asian (Specify)_____
- ☐ Native Hawaiian
- ☐ Guamanian or Chamorro
- ☐ Samoan
- ☐ Other Pacific Islander (Specify)_____
- ☐ Other (Specify)_____

Mother's Name: Janet M. Ramos
Mother's Medical Record No.: 12345-14

26. PLACE WHERE BIRTH OCCURRED (Check one)
- ☒ Hospital
- ☐ Freestanding birthing center
- ☐ Home Birth: Planned to deliver at home? ☐ Yes ☐ No
- ☐ Clinic/Doctor's office
- ☐ Other (Specify)_____

27. ATTENDANT'S NAME, TITLE, AND NPI
NAME: Albert Myers NPI: 123
TITLE: ☒ MD ☐ DO ☐ CNM/CM ☐ OTHER MIDWIFE ☐ OTHER (Specify)_____

28. MOTHER TRANSFERRED FOR MATERNAL MEDICAL OR FETAL INDICATIONS FOR DELIVERY? ☐ Yes ☒ No
IF YES, ENTER NAME OF FACILITY MOTHER TRANSFERRED FROM:_____

REV. 11/2003

MOTHER

29a. DATE OF FIRST PRENATAL CARE VISIT: 11/04/2013 ☐ No Prenatal Care
29b. DATE OF LAST PRENATAL CARE VISIT: 06/15/2014
30. TOTAL NUMBER OF PRENATAL VISITS FOR THIS PREGNANCY: 11 (If none, enter "0".)

31. MOTHER'S HEIGHT: 5'6" (feet/inches)
32. MOTHER'S PREPREGNANCY WEIGHT: 135 (pounds)
33. MOTHER'S WEIGHT AT DELIVERY: 163 (pounds)
34. DID MOTHER GET WIC FOOD FOR HERSELF DURING THIS PREGNANCY? ☐ Yes ☒ No

35. NUMBER OF PREVIOUS LIVE BIRTHS (Do not include this child): 0
- 35a. Now Living: Number ___ ☒ None
- 35b. Now Dead: Number ___ ☒ None

36. NUMBER OF OTHER PREGNANCY OUTCOMES (spontaneous or induced losses or ectopic pregnancies):
- 36a. Other Outcomes: Number ___ ☒ None

37. CIGARETTE SMOKING BEFORE AND DURING PREGNANCY
Average number of cigarettes or packs of cigarettes smoked per day.
Time Period	# of cigarettes	OR	# of packs
Three Months Before Pregnancy	0	OR	
First Three Months of Pregnancy	0	OR	
Second Three Months of Pregnancy	0	OR	
Third Trimester of Pregnancy	0	OR	

38. PRINCIPAL SOURCE OF PAYMENT FOR THIS DELIVERY: ☒ Private Insurance ☐ Medicaid ☐ Self-pay ☐ Other (Specify)

35c. DATE OF LAST LIVE BIRTH: ___/___ MM/YYYY
36b. DATE OF LAST OTHER PREGNANCY OUTCOME: ___/___ MM/YYYY
39. DATE LAST NORMAL MENSES BEGAN: 09/21/2013
40. MOTHER'S MEDICAL RECORD NUMBER: 12345-14

MEDICAL AND HEALTH INFORMATION

41. RISK FACTORS IN THIS PREGNANCY (Check all that apply)
- Diabetes
  - ☐ Prepregnancy (Diagnosis prior to this pregnancy)
  - ☐ Gestational (Diagnosis in this pregnancy)
- Hypertension
  - ☐ Prepregnancy (Chronic)
  - ☐ Gestational (PIH, preeclampsia)
  - ☐ Eclampsia
- ☐ Previous preterm birth
- ☐ Other previous poor pregnancy outcome (Includes perinatal death, small-for-gestational age/intrauterine growth restricted birth)
- ☐ Pregnancy resulted from infertility treatment-If yes, check all that apply:
  - ☐ Fertility-enhancing drugs, Artificial insemination or Intrauterine insemination
  - ☐ Assisted reproductive technology (e.g., in vitro fertilization (IVF), gamete intrafallopian transfer (GIFT))
- ☐ Mother had a previous cesarean delivery If yes, how many ___
- ☒ None of the above

42. INFECTIONS PRESENT AND/OR TREATED DURING THIS PREGNANCY (Check all that apply)
- ☐ Gonorrhea
- ☐ Syphilis
- ☐ Chlamydia
- ☐ Hepatitis B
- ☐ Hepatitis C
- ☒ None of the above

43. OBSTETRIC PROCEDURES (Check all that apply)
- ☐ Cervical cerclage
- ☐ Tocolysis
- External cephalic version:
  - ☐ Successful
  - ☐ Failed
- ☒ None of the above

44. ONSET OF LABOR (Check all that apply)
- ☐ Premature Rupture of the Membranes (prolonged, ≥12 hrs.)
- ☐ Precipitous Labor (<3 hrs.)
- ☒ Prolonged Labor (≥ 20 hrs.)
- ☐ None of the above

45. CHARACTERISTICS OF LABOR AND DELIVERY (Check all that apply)
- ☐ Induction of labor
- ☐ Augmentation of labor
- ☐ Non-vertex presentation
- ☐ Steroids (glucocorticoids) for fetal lung maturation received by the mother prior to delivery
- ☐ Antibiotics received by the mother during labor
- ☐ Clinical chorioamnionitis diagnosed during labor or maternal temperature ≥38°C (100.4°F)
- ☐ Moderate/heavy meconium staining of the amniotic fluid
- ☐ Fetal intolerance of labor such that one or more of the following actions was taken: in-utero resuscitative measures, further fetal assessment, or operative delivery
- ☒ Epidural or spinal anesthesia during labor
- ☐ None of the above

46. METHOD OF DELIVERY
- A. Was delivery with forceps attempted but unsuccessful? ☐ Yes ☒ No
- B. Was delivery with vacuum extraction attempted but unsuccessful? ☐ Yes ☒ No
- C. Fetal presentation at birth
  - ☒ Cephalic
  - ☐ Breech
  - ☐ Other
- D. Final route and method of delivery (Check one)
  - ☒ Vaginal/Spontaneous
  - ☐ Vaginal/Forceps
  - ☐ Vaginal/Vacuum
  - ☐ Cesarean
    - If cesarean, was a trial of labor attempted?
    - ☐ Yes
    - ☐ No

47. MATERNAL MORBIDITY (Check all that apply) (Complications associated with labor and delivery)
- ☐ Maternal transfusion
- ☐ Third or fourth degree perineal laceration
- ☐ Ruptured uterus
- ☐ Unplanned hysterectomy
- ☐ Admission to intensive care unit
- ☐ Unplanned operating room procedure following delivery
- ☒ None of the above

NEWBORN INFORMATION

48. NEWBORN MEDICAL RECORD NUMBER: 12349-14
49. BIRTHWEIGHT (grams preferred, specify unit): 6/6/2 oz — ☐ grams ☒ lb/oz
50. OBSTETRIC ESTIMATE OF GESTATION: 36 (completed weeks)
51. APGAR SCORE:
- Score at 5 minutes: 8
- If 5 minute score is less than 6,
- Score at 10 minutes: ___
52. PLURALITY - Single, Twin, Triplet, etc. (Specify): Single
53. IF NOT SINGLE BIRTH - Born First, Second, Third, etc. (Specify): ___

Mother's Name: Janet M. Cames
Mother's Medical Record No.: 12345-14

54. ABNORMAL CONDITIONS OF THE NEWBORN (Check all that apply)
- ☐ Assisted ventilation required immediately following delivery
- ☐ Assisted ventilation required for more than six hours
- ☐ NICU admission
- ☐ Newborn given surfactant replacement therapy
- ☐ Antibiotics received by the newborn for suspected neonatal sepsis
- ☐ Seizure or serious neurologic dysfunction
- ☐ Significant birth injury (skeletal fracture(s), peripheral nerve injury, and/or soft tissue/solid organ hemorrhage which requires intervention)
- ☒ None of the above

55. CONGENITAL ANOMALIES OF THE NEWBORN (Check all that apply)
- ☐ Anencephaly
- ☐ Meningomyelocele/Spina bifida
- ☐ Cyanotic congenital heart disease
- ☐ Congenital diaphragmatic hernia
- ☐ Omphalocele
- ☐ Gastroschisis
- ☐ Limb reduction defect (excluding congenital amputation and dwarfing syndromes)
- ☐ Cleft Lip with or without Cleft Palate
- ☐ Cleft Palate alone
- ☐ Down Syndrome
  - ☐ Karyotype confirmed
  - ☐ Karyotype pending
- ☐ Suspected chromosomal disorder
  - ☐ Karyotype confirmed
  - ☐ Karyotype pending
- ☐ Hypospadias
- ☒ None of the anomalies listed above

56. WAS INFANT TRANSFERRED WITHIN 24 HOURS OF DELIVERY? ☐ Yes ☒ No
IF YES, NAME OF FACILITY INFANT TRANSFERRED TO: ___

57. IS INFANT LIVING AT TIME OF REPORT? ☒ Yes ☐ No ☐ Infant transferred, status unknown

58. IS THE INFANT BEING BREASTFED AT DISCHARGE? ☒ Yes ☐ No

U.S. STANDARD CERTIFICATE OF DEATH

1. **DECEDENT'S LEGAL NAME:** Jack William Jordan
2. **SEX:** M
3. **SOCIAL SECURITY NUMBER:** 987-65-4921
4a. **AGE-Last Birthday (Years):** 78
5. **DATE OF BIRTH:** 5-14-36
6. **BIRTHPLACE:** Chicago, Illinois
7a. **RESIDENCE-STATE:** Ohio
7b. **COUNTY:** Lancaster
7c. **CITY OR TOWN:** Columbus
7d. **STREET AND NUMBER:** 15321 S. 10th
7f. **ZIP CODE:** 70111
7g. **INSIDE CITY LIMITS?** ☒ Yes
8. **EVER IN US ARMED FORCES?** ☒ Yes
9. **MARITAL STATUS AT TIME OF DEATH:** ☒ Married
10. **SURVIVING SPOUSE'S NAME:** Linda Mae White
11. **FATHER'S NAME:** William James Jordan
12. **MOTHER'S NAME PRIOR TO FIRST MARRIAGE:** Sally Ann Schmidt
13a. **INFORMANT'S NAME:** Alice Jordan
13b. **RELATIONSHIP TO DECEDENT:** Daughter
13c. **MAILING ADDRESS:** P.O. Box 401, Denver, CO 68123
14. **PLACE OF DEATH:** ☒ Inpatient
15. **FACILITY NAME:** Our Hospital
16. **CITY OR TOWN, STATE, AND ZIP CODE:** Columbus, Ohio 70118
17. **COUNTY OF DEATH:** Lancaster
18. **METHOD OF DISPOSITION:** ☒ Burial
19. **PLACE OF DISPOSITION:** Willow Creek Cemetary
20. **LOCATION-CITY, TOWN, AND STATE:** Columbus, Ohio
21. **NAME AND COMPLETE ADDRESS OF FUNERAL FACILITY:** Sunset Funeral Home, 121 Main St Columbus
22. **SIGNATURE OF FUNERAL SERVICE LICENSEE OR OTHER AGENT:** Joe Nas
23. **LICENSE NUMBER:** X1234

ITEMS 24-28 MUST BE COMPLETED BY PERSON WHO PRONOUNCES OR CERTIFIES DEATH

24. **DATE PRONOUNCED DEAD:** 05/30/2014
25. **TIME PRONOUNCED DEAD:** 4:45 p.m.
26. **SIGNATURE OF PERSON PRONOUNCING DEATH:** Mylas Rodgers M.D.
27. **LICENSE NUMBER:** 2222
28. **DATE SIGNED:** 06/02/2014
29. **ACTUAL OR PRESUMED DATE OF DEATH:** 05/30/2014
30. **ACTUAL OR PRESUMED TIME OF DEATH:** 4:45 p.m.
31. **WAS MEDICAL EXAMINER OR CORONER CONTACTED?** ☒ No

CAUSE OF DEATH

32. **PART I.**
   a. **IMMEDIATE CAUSE:** Respiratory Failure — 1 day
   b. Congestive Heart Failure — 3 months
   c. **UNDERLYING CAUSE:** Chronic Obstructive Pulmonary Dis. — 5 yrs.

PART II. Other significant conditions contributing to death: Diabetes, hypertension

33. **WAS AN AUTOPSY PERFORMED?** ☒ No
35. **DID TOBACCO USE CONTRIBUTE TO DEATH?** ☒ Probably
37. **MANNER OF DEATH:** ☒ Natural

45. **CERTIFIER:** ☒ Certifying physician
Signature of certifier: Mylas Rodgers M.D.
46. **NAME, ADDRESS, AND ZIP CODE OF PERSON COMPLETING CAUSE OF DEATH:** 404 S. Grant St. Columbus, Ohio 70131
47. **TITLE OF CERTIFIER:** MD
48. **LICENSE NUMBER:** 2222
49. **DATE CERTIFIED:** 6/2/14
50. **FOR REGISTRAR ONLY-DATE FILED:** 6/5/14

51. **DECEDENT'S EDUCATION:** ☒ High school graduate or GED completed
52. **DECEDENT OF HISPANIC ORIGIN?** ☒ No, not Spanish/Hispanic/Latino
53. **DECEDENT'S RACE:** ☒ White

54. **DECEDENT'S USUAL OCCUPATION:** Truck driver
55. **KIND OF BUSINESS/INDUSTRY:** Commercial Food Supplier

REV. 11/2003

Appendix D Sample Medical Forms

METROPOLITAN MEDICAL CENTER

Informed Consent for Invasive, Diagnostic, Medical & Surgical Procedures

Patient Name __Walker, Marjorie__

Date of Birth __6/3/56__

Medical Record # __585120__

I hereby authorize __Dr. Stillwater__ and/or __—__ and/or such assistants and associates as may be selected by him/her/they to perform the following procedure(s)/treatment(s) upon myself/the patient

Procedure(s)/Treatment(s) __Excisional debridement, Left leg__

The procedure has been explained to me and I have been told the reasons why I need the procedure. The risks of the procedure have also been explained to me. In addition, I have been told that the procedure may not have the result that I expect. I have also been told about other possible treatments for my condition and what might happen if no treatment is received.

I understand that in addition to the risks describe to me and about this procedure there are risks that may occur with any surgical or medical procedure. I am aware that the practice of medicine and surgery is not an exact science, and that I have not been given any guarantees about the results of this procedure.

I have had enough time to discuss my condition and treatment with my health care providers and all of my questions have been answered to my satisfaction. I believe I have enough information to make an informed decision and I agree to have the procedure. If something unexpected happens and I need additional or different treatment(s) from the treatment I expect, I agree to accept any treatment which is necessary.

I agree to have transfusion of blood and other blood products that may be necessary along with the procedure I am having. The risks, benefits and alternatives have been explained to me and all of my questions have been answered to my satisfaction. If I refuse to have transfusions I will cross out and initial this section and sign a Refusal of Treatment form.

I agree to allow this facility to keep, use or properly dispose of, tissue, and parts of organs that are removed during this procedure.

__Marjorie Walker__   __3/18/12__
Signature of Patient or Parent/Legal Guardian of Minor Patient   Date

If the patient cannot consent for him/herself, the signature of either the health care agent or legal guardian who is acting on behalf of the patient, or the patient's next of kin who is asserting to the treatment for the patient, must be obtained.

_____   _____
Signature of Patient or Parent/Legal Guardian of Minor Patient   Date

_____   _____
Signature and Relationship of Next of Kin   Date

Witness:
I, _____, am a facility employee who is not the patient's physician or authorized health care provider named above and I have witnessed the patient or other appropriate person voluntarily sign this form

_____
Signature and Title of Witness

METROPOLITAN MEDICAL CENTER

METROPOLITAN MEDICAL CENTER

Walker, Marjorie
PT#1772571   MRN#585120
DOB: 06/03/1956   Age: 56   Sex: F
Physician: Chaplin, Patrick
Admit: 03/18/2012

Discharge Summary

Date of Discharge: 3/27/2012

Discharge Diagnosis:

1. Left leg wound, S/P MVA, left shin degloving injury
2. Anxiety
3. Hematoma, right thigh
4. Paroxysmal atrial fibrillation

History of Present Illness: This is a 56-year-old white female who on 2/23/12 was involved in a motor vehicle accident when she was driving from Florida to Cincinnati. She was admitted to a Chattanooga, Tennessee hospital and she had suffered multiple rib fractures and also suffered a left nondisplaced fibular fracture and an avulsion and degloving injury on the left shin. She also had possible suprapubic ramus fracture and a fracture of the sternum and a slight laceration of the liver and spleen and she was transfused 19 units of packed red blood cells for acute blood loss anemia. The patient was on Coumadin at the time for atrial fibrillation and she had to be reversed. She also went into a-fib with rapid rate needing Cardizem to reverse it.

She was then transferred to Northstar Medical Center and was pretty stable at the time. She had a lot of pain and then she was seen by Orthopedics for that left tib fib fracture and they said she was okay for weight-bearing and she was see by wound care, physical therapy and occupational therapy. The patient stayed in sinus rhythm throughout. She was maintained on Coumadin and her hemoglobin stayed in the 9 and 10 range and she had later complained of a lot of pain in the right leg and a Doppler had shown some small hematomas, however, the pain and hematomas resolved on their own.

The large wound on her left shin was treated by Dr. Stillwater, Plastic Surgeon. She underwent several debridements of this area and will later likely undergo a skin graft after the wound has healed more.

On the day of discharge, 31 minutes was spent on discharge planning and all medications were discussed with her in detail. Patient is discharged to home with home health care.

Dictated by: Patrick Chaplin, MD

NG
D: 3/27/12 1535
T: 03/28/2012 1124

METROPOLITAN MEDICAL CENTER

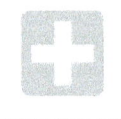

METROPOLITAN MEDICAL CENTER

Walker, Marjorie
PT#1772571   MRN#585120
DOB: 06/03/1956 Age: 56   Sex: F
Physician: Chaplin, Patrick
Admit: 03/18/2012

CONSULTATION REPORT
PLASTICS AND RECONSTRUCTIVE SURGERY

CHIEF COMPLAINT: Left leg wound

HISTORY OF PRESENT ILLNESS: This is a 56-year-old white female who on 2/23/12 was involved in a motor vehicle accident when she was driving from Florida to Cincinnati. She was admitted to a Chattanooga, Tennessee hospital and she had suffered multiple rib fractures and also suffered a left nondisplaced fibular fracture and an avulsion and degloving injury on the left shin. She also had possible suprapubic ramus fracture and a fracture of the sternum and a slight laceration of the liver and spleen and she was transfused 19 units of packed red blood cells for acute blood loss anemia. The patient was on Coumadin at the time for atrial fibrillation and she had to be reversed. She also went into a-fib with rapid rate needing Cardizem to reverse it.

PAST MEDICAL/SURGICAL HISTORY:
Significant for:
1. Hypertension
2. Rheumatoid arthritis
3. Depression
4. Osteopenia
5. Hyperlipidemia
6. History of perforated diverticulum, for which she required surgery and had a colostomy, and it was reversed.
7. History of hysterectomy
8. Hypothyroidism
9. Bilateral knee replacements
10. The patient does not report that she has congestive heart failure.
11. She does report that she had an angiogram for evaluation of atrial fibrillation, and she does not have any coronary artery disease.

ALLERGIES:
None

MEDICATIONS:
Prior to this accident included:
1. Methotrexate.
2. Misoprostol
3. Remicade
4. Methimazole

CURRENT MEDICATIONS:
That she was on when transferred from a Chattanooga, Tennessee hospital are as follows:
1. Keflex 500 mg every 8 hours for 5 days
2. Ipratropium as needed
3. Coumadin per pharmacy protocol
4. Lovenox 110 mg subcutaneously every twelve hours, to discontinue when INR is more than 2
5. Atenolol 50 mg every 12 hours
6. Vicodin 5/325 mg every four hours as needed for pain.
7. Paxil 20 mg daily

FAMILY HISTORY:
Positive for father dying of leukocytosis at age of 54. Mother had myocardial infarction at the age of 67. Sister has Parkinson disease and another sister died of colon cancer.

PHYSICAL EXAMINATION:

GENERAL:
She is awake, alert and oriented, in no acute distress.

VITAL SIGNS:
Stable. Her blood pressure this morning is 126/64, temperature 98.6, pulse 72.

HEAD, EYES, EARS, NOSE AND THROAT:
Shows pupils equal, round, and reactive to light and accommodation. Mucous membranes are moist.

NECK:
Shows no thyromegaly.

LUNGS:
Clear to auscultation.

HEART:
Regular rate and rhythm, a few missed beats.

ABDOMEN:
Shows no organomegaly.

EXTREMITIES:
Dorsalis pedis pulses bilaterally are 2+. There is a vacuum-assisted closure on the left upper skin extending to the knee. Large left lower leg wound with fairly well vascularized red granulation tissue in the bulk of the wound. There is a deep cavity on the medial aspect in the area of the recently evacuated hematoma. There are sutures in place which the patient was unaware and fibrin covering necrotic tissue on the lateral aspect of the wound space. There is no purulent discharge or evidence of infection. Remainder of the left lower extremity shows no other clinically significant lesions.

LABORATORY DATA:
From 3/17/12, her albumin was 2.4, total protein was 5.2. Her CBC from 3/16/12 shows a white cell count of 9.6, hemoglogin 9.7, platelets 252,000. INR was 1.4.

ASSESSMENT AND PLAN:
The patient needs protein repletion. She will ultimately need the sutures removed and the fibrinous exudate debrided from the lateral aspect of the wound. Would recommend resuming negative pressure wound therapy including packing, black GranuFoam dressing into the current hematoma cavity. The patient will ultimately require skin graft reconstruction.

It is always a pleasure seeing and treating your patients. We look forward to seeing and treating other patients in the future.

Dictated by Frank Stillwater, MD

KR
D: 03/20/12 1904
T: 03/20/12 23:50

METROPOLITAN MEDICAL CENTER

METROPOLITAN MEDICAL CENTER

Walker, Marjorie
PT#1772571 MRN#585120
DOB: 06/03/1956 Age: 56 Sex: F
Physician: Chaplin, Patrick
Admit: 03/18/2012

HISTORY AND PHYSICAL

HISTORY OF PRESENT ILLNESS:

History of Present Illness: This is a 56-year-old white female who on 2/23/12 was involved in a motor vehicle accident when she was driving from Florida to Cincinnati. She was admitted to a Chattanooga, Tennessee hospital and she had suffered multiple rib fractures and also suffered a left nondisplaced fibular fracture and an avulsion and degloving injury on the left shin. She also had possible suprapubic ramus fracture and a fracture of the sternum and a slight laceration of the liver and spleen and she was transfused 19 units of packed red blood cells for acute blood loss anemia. The patient was on Coumadin at the time for atrial fibrillation and she had to be reversed. She also went into a-fib with rapid rate needing Cardizem to reverse it.

She has been transferred to Northstar Medical Center and is stable at this time. Dr. Stillwater from Plastics will be consulted to address her wound on her left shin. PT, OT and Wound Care will be ordered. We will monitor her atrial fibrillation and labs for anemia.

PAST MEDICAL/SURGICAL HISTORY:

Significant for:

1. Hypertension
2. Rheumatoid arthritis
3. Depression
4. Osteopenia
5. Hyperlipidemia
6. History of perforated diverticulum, for which she required surgery and had a colostomy, and it was reversed.
7. History of hysterectomy
8. Hypothyroidism
9. Bilateral knee replacements
10. The patient does not report that she has congestive heart failure.
11. She does report that she had an angiogram for evaluation of atrial fibrillation, and she does not have any coronary artery disease.

ALLERGIES:

None

MEDICATIONS:

Prior to this accident included:

1. Methotrexate.
2. Misoprostol
3. Remicade
4. Methimazole

CURRENT MEDICATIONS:

That she was on when transferred from a Chattanooga, Tennessee hospital are as follows:

1. Keflex 500 mg every 8 hours for 5 days
2. Ipratropium as needed
3. Coumadin per pharmacy protocol
4. Lovenox 110 mg subcutaneously every twelve hours, to discontinue when INR is more than 2
5. Atenolol 50 mg every 12 hours
6. Vicodin 5/325 mg every four hours as needed for pain.
7. Paxil 20 mg daily

FAMILY HISTORY:

Positive for father dying of leukocytosis at age of 54. Mother had myocardial infarction at the age of 67. Sister has Parkinson disease and another sister died of colon cancer.

PHYSICAL EXAMINATION:

GENERAL:
She is awake, alert and oriented, in no acute distress.

VITAL SIGNS:
Stable. Her blood pressure this morning is 126/64, temperature 98.6, pulse 72.

HEAD, EYES, EARS, NOSE AND THROAT:
Sclerae are anicteric. Mucous membranes are moist.

NECK:
There is no carotid bruit.

LUNGS:
Clear to auscultation.

HEART:
Regular rate and rhythm, a few missed beats.

ABDOMEN:
Soft, nontender.

EXTREMITIES:
Dorsalis pedis pulses bilaterally are 2+. There is a vacuum-assisted closure on the left upper skin extending to the knee.

LABORATORY DATA:
From 3/17/12, her albumin was 2.4, total protein was 5.2. Her CBC from 3/16/12 shows a white cell count of 9.6, hemoglogin 9.7, platelets 252,000. INR was 1.4.

ASSESSMENT AND PLAN:
1. Status post MVA with multiple injuries. Pain control is an issue. Patient will be scheduled for PT and OT Therapy
2. Avulsion/degloving injury of the left shin with large wound. Plastic surgery will be consulted.
3. History of paroxysmal atrial fibrillation. Will follow and monitor.

Patrick Chaplin, MD

KK
Dictated: 3/18/12 14:45
Trans: 3/18/12 18:30

METROPOLITAN MEDICAL CENTER

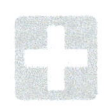

METROPOLITAN MEDICAL CENTER

Walker, Marjorie
PT#1772571   MRN#585120
DOB: 06/03/1956   Age: 56   Sex: F
Physician: Chaplin, Patrick
Admit: 03/18/2012

OPERATIVE REPORT

DATE OF OPERATION: 03/23/12

PREOPERATIVE DIAGNOSIS: Left leg wound

POSTOPERATIVE DIAGNOSIS: Left leg wound

PROCEDURE PERFORMED: Excision, necrotic tissue, left leg wound, 3.0 cm in length. Application of a Kerlix stack and less than 50 sq. cm negative pressure wound therapy dressing.

SURGEON: Frank Stillwater, MD

ASSISTANT: Karen Tweedle, MD

OPERATIVE PROCEDURE: The patient was properly prepped and draped under local sedation. A 0.25% Marcaine was injected circumferentially around the necrotic wound. A wide excision and debridement of the necrotic tissue taken down to the presacral fascia and all necrotic tissue was electrocauterized and removed. All bleeding was cauterized with electrocautery and then a Kerlix stack was then placed and a pressure dressing applied. The patient was sent to recovery in satisfactory condition.

Dictated by Frank Stillwater, MD

GR
D: 3/23/12 11:14
T: 3/23/12 15:10

METROPOLITAN MEDICAL CENTER

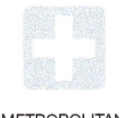

METROPOLITAN MEDICAL CENTER

Walker, Marjorie
PT#1772571   MRN#585120
DOB: 06/03/1956   Age: 56   Sex: F
Physician: Chaplin, Patrick
Admit: 03/18/2012

PHYSICIAN'S ORDERS

Date/Time		Nurse's Initials
3/18/12 9:30 AM	CBC, BMP in am PT/INR c a.m. labs *Patrick Chaplin MD*	
3/19/12 8 AM	U/A, C+S today *Patrick Chaplin MD*	
3/19/12 9 AM	D/C oxycontin Vicodin 5/500 mg i po q 4–6° prn pain. *Patrick Chaplin MD*	

METROPOLITAN MEDICAL CENTER

METROPOLITAN MEDICAL CENTER

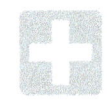

Walker, Marjorie
PT#1772571   MRN#585120
DOB: 06/03/1956   Age: 56 Sex: F
Physician: Chaplin, Patrick
Admit: 03/18/2012

Nurse's Notes (Include observations, medications, and treatment when indicated.)

Date/Time	
3/19/12 0816	Assessment complete as noted, sitting up in bed, IVPB infusing s̄ difficulty, dsg dry and intact, foley draining clear yellow urine, denies pain or SOB @ this time. Will continue to monitor wound care — B. Cullars, RN
3/19/12 1930	pt resting in bed. A+O x 3 VSS LSCTA per nurse assess. Foley draining clear yellow urine. Denies any further issues @ this time. SOB noted previously currently subsided. Will cont to monitor. Call light in reach. ——————
3/20/12 0730	VSS. Denies any pain or discomfort at this time. Assessment completed per flow sheet — no changes noted from previous shift. Able to make needs known. Call light in reach. Will monitor ———————

METROPOLITAN MEDICAL CENTER

METROPOLITAN MEDICAL CENTER

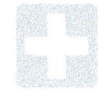

Walker, Marjorie
PT#1772571   MRN#585120
DOB: 06/03/1956   Age: 56 Sex: F
Physician: Chaplin, Patrick
Admit: 03/18/2012

Nurse's Notes (Include observations, medications, and treatment when indicated.)

Date/Time	
3/18/2012 @ 1300	Received pt via ACLS transport. Pt transferred from stretcher to bed. Pt did not bring any personal belongings. Admission assessment completed. VSS & WNL. Dr. Chaplin notified of pt's arrival - orders received. Pt informed of POC & instructed on safety to include use of call light & bed side controls. Will continue to monitor. D. Schmidt RN.
3/18/2012 2015	Assessment complete & charted. Pt is A+O x 4, lungs CTA, +BS x 4, no noted edema, heart sounds regular in rhythm. Pt has #20 @ FA dated 3/17 c̄ a dsg that is CD&I. VSS & hardly unchanged from admit. Pt has no needs or questions at this time & denies any pain. Call light left within reach, will continue to monitor. ──── S Salatn RN

Appendix D Sample Medical Forms

METROPOLITAN MEDICAL CENTER

Patient Continuum of Care Transfer Form

Patient label:
Walker, Marjorie
PT#1772571   MRN#585120
DOB: 06/03/1956   Age: 56   Sex: F
Physician: Chaplin, Patrick
Admit: 03/18/2012

Patient Last Name: Walker
Patient First Name: Marjorie
Transfer to: Spring Care
Attending Physician: Chaplin
Reason for Transfer: Wound Care
DATE/TIME: 3/18/12 6:50

- ☐ Attempted Treatment in SNF unsuccessful?
- ☒ Please list ALLERGIES (meds, dyes, food): Latex, Demerol
- ☐ NKA

Relative / Guardian Notified: Yes ☒ No ☐   Phone Number:
Name of Relative Notified: Jennifer DeCapua
Transfer Ambulance: Life Care

VITAL SIGNS TAKEN   Yes ☒ No ☐   Time Taken: 1230   AM ☐ PM ☒

Respirations: 24	Blood glucose: 118 Time: 1210
O2 Sat: 96%	VRE: Yes ☐ No ☒ Hx of ☐
Pulse: 84	MRSA: Yes ☐ No ☒ Hx of ☐
BP: 118/82	C. Diff: Yes ☐ No ☒ Hx of ☐
Temp: 99.2 (A)	ANY pending cultures? Yes ☐ No ☒
Height: 5'10"	If Yes, what?
Weight: 163 Lbs ☒ Kg ☐	MDRO?

ATTACHMENTS (Please check)
- ☒ Face Sheet
- ☒ History & Physical
- ☐ Discharge Summary
- ☒ MAR
- ☐ Wound Assessment & Tx Sheet
- ☒ Labs
- ☐ Code Status
- ☐ MD Orders
- ☒ X-rays
- ☐ MD Progress Notes
- ☐ Nurse's Notes (last 5 days)
- ☐ Other:
- ☐ Other:

ISOLATION PRECAUTIONS? Yes ☐ No ☒   **TYPE:** Contact ☐ Droplet ☐ Airborne ☐ Other: ☐

VACCINATION HISTORY
- Pneumococcal Vaccine: Yes ☒ DATE: 3-16-12 Refused ☐
- Flu Vaccine: Yes ☒ DATE: 11-7-10 Refused ☐
- Tetanus: Yes ☐ DATE: Refused ☐
- TB Skin Test: Negative ☐ Positive ☐ DATE:
- OR Chest X-ray ☒ Result Date: —
- Comments:

SKIN OR PRESSURE ULCER CONCERNS
- HIGH risk for skin breakdown **PLEASE TURN**   Yes ☐ No ☐
- Current Skin Breakdown: Yes ☐ No ☐
- Most Recent Treatment Time: AM ☐ PM ☐
- Please Treat at (time):   AM ☐ PM ☐
- Treat with (product name): Dakins Solution   orig BID
- To (what area): (B) LE

MEDICATION INFORMATION
- See Attached Medication Reconciliation
- Prefers meds with: applesauce
- Pain Meds in past 24 hours   Yes ☒ No ☐
- Level on **Pain Scale** at time of transfer:
  (Please circle level) 1 2 3 ④ 5 6 7 8 9 10

SAFETY CONCERNS
- History of Falls Yes ☐ No ☒   Risk for Falls Yes ☐ No ☒
- Behavior Issues Yes ☐ No ☒   Explain:
- RESTRAINT Use: Yes ☐ No ☒
- Type of Restraint Used:
- When Used:

DIET & FEEDING
- Current Diet: Diabetic 2000 kcal ADA
- Needs Assistance ☐   Feeds Self ☐   Feeding Tube ☐
- Thickened Liquid ☐ Consistency?
- Supplement ☐ If so, name:

ELIMINATION
- Bladder Incontinence ☐   DATE of UTI (within 14 days):
- Catheter: Yes ☐ No ☐   Date Inserted or Last Changed:
- Bowel Incontinence: Yes ☐ No ☐   Colostomy: Yes ☐ No ☐
- Date of Last BM:

IMPAIRMENTS/DISABILITIES: (Please check all that apply)
Speech ☐ Contractures ☐ Mental Confusion ☐ Vision ☒
Hearing ☐ Amputation ☐ Paralysis ☐ Language Barrier ☐
COMMENTS: wears glasses
Report Called to: Jane Elson RN

PATIENT EQUIPMENT/BELONGINGS: (Check all sent with resident)
None ☐   Right Hearing Aid ☐   Left Hearing Aid ☐
Glasses ☐   Upper Denture ☐   Lower Denture ☐
Jewelry ☐   Please list:
Other (i.e., prosthesis):

Nurse Name (Print): Karen Scheitlin RN
Nurse Signature: Karen Scheitlin RN
Phone #: 862-4444
Date/Time: 3/18/12 7:00

METROPOLITAN MEDICAL CENTER

METROPOLITAN MEDICAL CENTER

Walker, Marjorie
PT#1772571   MRN#585120
DOB: 06/03/1956   Age: 56   Sex: F
Physician: Chaplin, Patrick
Admit: 03/18/2012
Allergies: No Know Drug Allergy

Medication Administration Record

No:	Medication	Start/Stop	Adm	07:00 to 18:59	19:00 to 6:69	00:00 to 00:00
0286618	ATENOLOL 50 MILLIGRAM PO EVERY 12 HOURS ONE DOSE= 50 MILLIGRAM = 1 TABLETS TENORMIN (Atenolol Tab 50 MG) ****FLOOR STOCK****	03/18/2012 at 2200 03/27/2012 at 1000		1000	2200	
0286621	COZAAR 50 MILLIGRAM PO ONCE DAILY ONE DOSE= 50 MILLIGRAM = 1 TABLETS LOSARTAN (COZAAR) (Losartan Potassium Tab 50 MG) ****FLOOR STOCK****	03/18/2012 at 2200 03/27/2012 at 1000		1000		
0286631	DOCUSATE SODIUM 100 MILLIGRAM PO TWICE DAILY ONE DOSE= 100 MILLIGRAM = 1 CAPSULE USED FOR COLACE (Docusate Sodium Cap 100 MG) ****FLOOR STOCK****	03/18/2012 at 2200 03/27/2012 at 1000		1000	2200	
0286619	FLECAINIDE ACETATE 100 MILLIGRAM PO EVERY 12 HOURS ONE DOSE= 100 MILLIGRAM = 1 TABLETS USED FOR TAMBOCOR (Flecainide Acetate Tab 100 MG)	03/18/2012 at 2200 03/27/2012 at 1000		1000	2200	
0286630	LORazepam 0.5 MILLIGRAM PO TWICE DAILY ONE DOSE= 0.5 MILLIGRAM = 1 TABLETS ATIVAN (Lorazepam Tab 0.5 MG) ****FLOOR STOCK****	03/18/2012 at 2200 03/27/2012 at 1000		1000		
0286629	KLOR-CON M10 10 MILLIEQUIV PO ONCE DAILY ONE DOSE= 10 MILLIEQUIV = 1 TABLETS (Potassium Chloride Microencapsulated Crys CR Tab 10 mEq) ****FLOOR STOCK****	03/18/2012 at 2200 03/27/2012 at 1000		1000	2200	
0286628	FUROSEMIDE 40 MILLIGRAM PO ONCE DAILY ONE DOSE= 40 MILLIGRAM = 1 TABLETS LASIX 40MG TAB (Furosemide Tab 40 MG) ****FLOOR STOCK****	03/18/2012 at 2200 03/27/2012 at 1000		1000		
0286970	OXYCONTIN 10 MILLIGRAM PO EVERY EVENING ONE DOSE= 10 MILLIGRAM = 1 TABLETS (Oxycodone HCl Tab SR 12HR 10 MG) ****FLOOR STOCK****	03/18/2012 at 2200 03/27/2012 at 2200			2200	
0286627	PARoxetine HCL 20 MILLIGRAM PO ONCE DAILY ONE DOSE= 20 MILLIGRAM = 1 TABLETS PAXIL 20 MG TAB (Paroxetine HCl Tab 20 MG) ****FLOOR STOCK****	03/18/2012 at 2200 03/27/2012 at 1000		1000		

Signatures	Init	Shift	Signatures	Init	Shift
			Ryan Goldman RN Sylvia Yazzy RN		

Appendix D Sample Medical Forms

Index

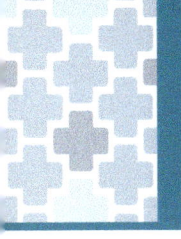

*Page numbers with *f* indicate figures; with *i* indicate illustrations; and with *t* indicate tables.

A

abbreviations in documentation, 322–323, 323*t*
abstracting, 333
access
   to patient information following discharge, 164*t*
   simultaneous, 164–165
access control, 179, 179*t*
accession number, 332
access speed, 140
   measuring, 140–141
accountable care organizations (ACOs), 3, 64
accounting, 179
accounting of disclosures (AODs), 187, 218
accreditation, 35–36
   for alternative care facilities, 44*t*
Accreditation Association for Ambulatory Health Care, 44
activities of daily living (ADLs), 43
acute care hospitals, 37–39
   classification of, 38–39
   documentation of care in, 80–82
   long-term, 40
acute care records, documentation standards for, 91–92, 92*t*
acute illness, 37
adaptive skills, 17
addendum notes, 95
administrative regulations, 201
administrative research, 300
administrative safeguards, 176, 177*t*
admission, discharge, and transfer (ADT) system, 160–161, 183–184, 184*f*, 279
admission forms, 80
adult day care, 43
advance directives, 80, 214
Affordable Care Act (2010), 29, 64, 72, 261, 319
   donut hole under, 34*i*
   implementation of value-based purchasing program, 320
   major provisions in, 30
Agency for Healthcare Research and Quality, 315
agendas, 349, 349*f*
aggregate data, 76, 143, 208
AHA Coding Clinic, 253

alerts, 158
Allied Health Careers (website), 18
allowable costs, 254
alphabetical filing, 113, 114*t*
alphabetic index, 250
alternative care facilities, 39
   accreditation for, 44*t*
ambulatory care facilities, 40–42
   patient records in, 74–75
ambulatory payment classifications, 255–256
ambulatory surgery, 40–41
American Association of Colleges of Nursing (AACN), 57
American Association of Medical Record Librarians, 3
American College of Surgeons (ACS), 3, 45
   cancer registries accredited by, 332, 335
American Health Information Management Association (AHIMA), xx, 1, 3, 9, 156, 366
   Career Assist Job Bank of, 18
   CHTS certifications offered by, 149, 149*t*
   Code of Ethics of, 19–20, 232
   Commission on Certification for Health Informatics and Information Management, 10
   credentials of, 10–11, 11*f*
   data quality management model of, 321
   e-HIM task force of, 206
   Foundation, 10
   Hill Day of, 9
   state chapters of, 18
American Hospital Association (AHA), 45
American Joint Committee on Cancer (AJCC), 334
American Medical Association (AMA), 29
   CPT codes and, 248
American Medical Informatics Association (AMIA), 10
American Medical Record Association, 3

American Recovery and Reinvestment Act (ARRA) (2009), 147, 174
analytics, 297
anatomic site, 246
anesthesia death rate, 288–289, 288–289*i*
anesthesia report, 85
Anti-Kickback Statute, 262
Apple Safari, 136
Apple's Mac OS® system, 135
application software, 135
artificial intelligence, 72
Association for Healthcare Documentation Integrity (CHDI), 15
Association of Clinical Documentation Improvement Specialists (ACDIS), 74
Association of Record Librarians of North America (ARLNA), 1, 3
audit logs, 220
audit trail, 166
authentication, 97, 179
   scheme for, 191
authorization, 179
authorized release of information, 224–226
autopsy, 289
autopsy rates, 289–291
   gross, 290, 290*i*
   hospital, 291, 291*i*
   net, 290–291, 290–291*i*
average daily census (ADC), 283
average length of stay (ALOS), 280–281, 281*i*
   use of, as benchmark, 285

B

bar chart, 294*i*, 294–295
battery, 211
Baylor Hospital, 29
bed control system, 185
behavior, 247
behavioral health care, 44
bell curve, 278, 278*i*
benchmark, 285
bereavement, 44
billing processes and procedures, 258–259

biomedical research, 303
birth certificate, 87
birth defects registry, 331
bit, 140
Blue Button technology, 72
Blue Cross (BC), 29
Blue Cross Blue Shield (BCBS) model, 29
Blue Shield (BS), 29
board of directors, 54
body language, 6
Braden, James H., 156
breach, 219
    notification of, 219–221
budgets/budgeting, 365–368, 366i, 367i
    capital, 368
    operating, 365–367
Bush, George W., 174
business associates, 218
    agreement between, 218
business continuity plan, 124
business records, 206

C

cancer registrar, 14, 332
cancer registry, 189, 332
cancer stage, 334
capital budget, 368
capturing, 260
cardiac surgeon, 59
cardiologist, 59
cardiology, 41–42
cardiovascular surgeon, 59
Cardozo, Benjamin, 199
care coordination, 326
careers
    cancer registrar, 14
    clinical analyst, 148
    clinical application coordinator, 148
    clinical documentation improvement specialists, 13–14
    data, application, or systems analyst, 148
    data architect, 148
    EHR implementation coordinator and trainer, 15
    file/scanning and retrieval clerk, 12
    in health information technology, 146–147
    HIM supervisor/manager, 12
    HIM technician, 12
    hospital medical coder, 12–13
    implementation support specialist, 148
    information security officer, 148
    medical biller and coder, 13

medical transcriptionist, 14–15
    performance improvement coordinator, 15–16
    physician officer manager, 16
    privacy officer, 15
    project manager, 148
    registered health information technician xx, xx
    vital statistics clerk, 12
case finding, 332–333
case law, 201
case management, 326–328, 327t, 328t
case management department, 326
case manager, 326
case mix, 257
case mix index (CMI), 257–258
cause-and-effect diagram, 350
cell phones, 134
Centers for Disease Control and Prevention (CDC), 297, 313
    compilation of National Hospital Discharge Survey, 330
    National Program of Cancer Registries of, 332
Centers for Medicare & Medicaid Services (CMS)
    on acute care patient records, 91, 92, 92t
    Conditions for Coverage (CfCs), 36
    Conditions of Participation (CoPs), 36–37, 96, 98
    on decision making, 169
    delinquent records and, 98, 98i
    on electronic health record documentation, 94, 96
    General Equivalency Mappings, 255
    on medical documentation, 165
    on paper record destruction, 123
    quality improvement and, 315
central processing unit (CPU), 135
central system, 160
certification, 36–37
certified coding associate (CCA), 11f
certified coding specialist (CCS), 11f
certified coding specialist-physician based (CCS-P), 11
certified documentation improvement practitioner (CDIP), 10
certified healthcare documentation specialist (CHDS), 15
certified healthcare technology specialist (CHTS), 10
certified in healthcare privacy and security (CHPS), 10

certified registered nurse anesthetist, 57
change agents, 346
charge capture and coding, 260
chargemaster, 261
charts. *See also* graphs
    analysis of, 119–120
    bar, 294i, 294–295
    flow, 350, 351f
    Gantt, 354
    pie, 296, 296i
chief executive officer (CEO), 54
    versus medical chief of staff, 64, 64t
chief financial officer (CFO), 54
chief human resources officer (CHRO), 54
chief information officer (CIO), 54
chief medical officer (CMO), 54–55
chief nursing officer (CNO), 54
chief operating officer (COO), 54
Children's Health Insurance Program (CHIP), 34
Chopra, Deepak, 53
chronic illness, 38
claim submission, 260
classification systems, 244–250
    comparing nomenclature and code systems, 249–250
    Current Procedural Terminology (CPT) codes, 248
    Diagnostic and Statistical Manual of Mental Disorders, Fifth Edition (DSM-5), 249
    Healthcare Common Procedure Coding System (HCPCS), 248–249
    International Classification of Diseases, 244–245
    International Classification of Diseases, Ninth Revision, Clinical Modification (ICD-9-CM), 245
    International Classification of Diseases, Tenth Revision, Clinical Modification (ICD-10-CM), 245
    International Classification of Diseases, Tenth Revision, Procedure Coding System (ICD-10-PCS), 245–247
    International Classification of Diseases for Oncology, Third Edition (ICD-O-3), 247–248
clinical data repository (CDR), 167
clinical decision support (CDS) software, 163
clinical documentation, 100–101
clinical documentation improvement, 101t, 264

clinical documentation improvement specialists, 13–14, 101
clinical health data analyst (CHDA), 10
clinical information, 100
clinical nurse specialist, 57
clinical pertinence, 324
Clinical Pharmacology, 253
clinical services, 55
clinical system, 161
clinical terminology, 242–243
clinical trials, 301
clinical vocabulary, 242
cloning, 169
closing process, 354
Clostridium difficile infections, 313
cloud-based applications, 190
cloud computing, 137
CMS. *See* Centers for Medicare & Medicaid Services (CMS)
coding, 188–189, 333–334, 365
   activities related to, 252–254
   comparing nomenclature and, 249–250, 250*t*
Coding Clinic for HCPCS, 253
coding references, 253–254
cognitive computing, 132
coinsurance, 31
collections, 259
colonoscopy, 42
Commission on Accreditation for Health Informatics and Information Management Education (CAHIIM), 11*f*
Commission on Accreditation of Rehabilitation Facilities (CARF), 35–36, 40, 44*t*
Commission on Cancer, 332
committees
   blood usage or transfusion, 122
   ethics, 214
   forms, 95–98
   infection-control, 320
   medical staff, 62, 63*t*
   pharmacy, 122
   quality improvement, 122
   requests for records, 122
common law, 201
communication, 4–8
   email, 5
   nonverbal, 6
   over the network, 138
   verbal, 6
   written, 5
Community Health Accreditation Program (CHAP), 44
community hospitals, 37
comorbidities, 245

complete records, 77
complex projects, 353–354
compliance, 233, 260–263
compliance monitoring, 303
complications, 245
comprehensive outpatient rehabilitation facilities (CORFs), 40, 44*t*
computer-assisted coding (CAC), 188–189, 253
computerized provider order entry (CPOE), 160
computer ports, 138
concurrent review, 320
confidentiality, 208–211
conflict of interest, 304
connecting to the network, 138–139
consent(s)
   express, 212, 212*t*
   forms for, 211
   implied, 212, 212*t*
   individual, 212, 212*t*
   informed, 212, 212*t*
   obtaining, 213
   for surgery, 84–85
   third-party/designee, 212, 212*t*
   types of, 212, 212*t*
constitutional law, 201
consultation, 293
consultation rate, 293, 293*i*
consultation report, 84
consultative evaluation, 76
consumer-based quality measures, 319–320
content for treatment, 211–213, 212*t*
continuing education, 11*f*
continuous data, 294
continuous quality improvement (CQI), 315, 316
contract services, 366
controlling, 354
cookies, 145
copays, 31
copy and paste function, 95
core EHR system, 160
core health data elements, 142
courtesy, 7–8
court order, 229
covered entities, 121, 216
Covey, Stephen R., 342
CPT Assistant, 253
CPT Physicians' Current Procedural Terminology, 248
CPT Physicians' Current Procedural Terminology: Specially Annotated for Hospitals: Hospital Outpatient Services, 248

creation stage in health record life cycle, 119
credentials, professional, 10–11, 11*f*
critical access hospitals (CAH), 38
critical thinking, 4
cross-training, 361–362
Current Procedural Terminology (CPT) codes, 13, 242, 248
custodian of the health record, 200

D

daily inpatient census, 281–282
data, 274
   aggregate, 76, 143, 208
   continuous, 294
   defined, 141
   discrete, 294
   financial, 162
   primary, 329
   secondary, 329
database management system (DBMS), 143
databases, 329
   defined, 143
   for reporting purposes, 329–330
data collection, 303
   case management and, 326–328, 327*t*, 328*t*
   databases in, 329–330
   registries and, 330–335
   risk management and, 328*i*, 328–329
data dictionary, 181
data display and presentation, 293–296
data elements, 141, 181
   core health, 142*t*
data integrity, 221, 321
data integrity analyst, 189
data loss prevention (DLP) software, 146
data management, 141–144
data mining, 144
data quality, characteristics of, 321
data security, 144–146
dataset, 143
data sharing, 167
data standardization, 142–143
data storage needs, calculating, 140, 140*t*
data table, 294
data threats, 145
Davidian, Marie, 273
day surgery, 40–41
death
   certifying a, 300
   pronouncing a, 300
death certificates, 299–300
death rates, 286–289

anesthesia, 288, 288–289*i*
  fetal, 287, 287*i*
  gross, 286, 286*i*
  maternal, 288, 288*i*
  net, 286–287, 286–287*i*
  postoperative, 289, 289*i*
decision, 345
decision matrix, 206–207, 207*t*
decision support software, 158
decision support system, 297
Declaration of Helsinki, 304
deductibles, 31
Defense, U.S. Department of, 39
de-identified information, 208–209
de-identified records, 76
delegating, 345
delinquent records, 98, 99*i*
deposition, 229
descriptive text, 249
designated record set, 205
designee consent, 212
destruction in health record life cycler, 119
diagnosis-related groups (DRGs), 255
Diagnostic and Statistical Manual of Mental Disorders, Fifth Edition (DSM-5), 249
diagnostic classifications, 249
diagnostic clinics, 41–42
diagnostic criteria sets, 249
diagnostic findings, 82
diagnostic index, 250
diagnostic payment system (PPS), 255
dictation system, 188
dictionary-driven encoder, 253
digital certificate, 146
digital imaging, 117
digital storage, 116
disaster, 124
disaster-preparedness and downtime procedures, 185–186
disaster recovery plan, 124
discharge, access to patient information following, 164–165, 164*t*
discharge days, 280
discharge summary, 84
discrete data, 294
disease index, 251–252
Dishman, Eric, 144
disk operating system (DOS), 135
documentation
  abbreviations in, 322–323
  incomplete, 324, 325*t*
  inconsistent, 324
  legible, 165, 165*f*, 322
  quality of, 169–172, 320–325

redundancy in, 180–182
  timeliness of, 321–322
documentation integrity, 169
document management system, 161
domain name, 136
do not resuscitate (DNR), 214
donut hole, 34*i*
Dorland's Illustrated Medical Dictionary, 253
downcoding, 261
downtime procedures, 186, 186*t*
Dr. Z's Interventional Radiology Coding Reference, 254
DRG Definitions Manual, 254
Drucker, Pater, 343
Drug Abuse Office and Treatment Act (1972), 227
due diligence, 233
dues, 366
duplicate records, 183
durable power of attorney for health care, 214

E

education, 367
  continuing, 11
EHR implementation coordinator and trainer, 15
electronic health records, 117–118, 157–191. *See also* patient care records
  adoption of, 108, 108*i*, 272
  advantages of, 162–167, 163*f*, 164*t*, 165*f*, 166*f*
  authority/responsibility for documenting, 96
  defined, 158
  disadvantages of, 167–173, 168*f*, 170*i*, 171*i*
  documentation requirements for, 94–98
  ensuring high quality documentation, 180–181
  evolution of, 173–176, 174*f*, 175*f*, 176*t*
  functions of, 158–159
  illegible documentation and, 322
  incomplete versus complete records, 97–98
  information flow from master patient index to, 182*f*
  organization of, 91
  role of health information management department in, 178–179
  security of, 176–179, 177*t*, 178*t*, 179*t*
  selection and maintenance, 180–181

  signature requirements, 97
  as system of systems, 159–162, 160*f*, 161*f*
    administrative, 160–161
    clinical, 161
    core, 160, 160*f*
    document management, 161, 161*f*
    financial systems, 162
  timelines and, 96
electronic medication administration record (eMAR), 161
electronic passport, 146, 146*t*
electronic prescribing, 166, 166*f*
electronic protected health information (ePHI), 176, 208
electronic signatures, 97, 163
email communication, 5
emergency departments, 41
  reasons for going to, 26
employee feedback, 358
employees, selecting and evaluating, 355–360
encoder, 188
encoder software, 252–253
encounter data, 142
encounters, 74, 210
encounter utilization review and case management, 259
endoscopy, 42
episode of care, 74
e-prescribing, 166, 166*f*
Esar, Evan, 272
esophagoscopy, 42
Ethernet, 137
ethics, 19–20
  defined, 231
  in health information management, 231–232
  in research, 304
ethics committee, 214
etiology, 246
Evans, David, 241
evidence-based medicine, 205
execution process, 354
exempt units, 58
expenses, 366
express consent, 211–213, 212*t*
external hard drive, 139
extrinsic motivation, 359

F

Facility Oncology Registry Data Standards (FORDS), 334
Fair and Accurate Credit Transactions Act (FACTA) (2003), 223
falls, 331*i*
False Claims Act, 262, 263

family numbering filing, 113, 114
federal quality standards, 319
Federal Trade Commission, Fair and Accurate Credit Transactions Act (FACTA) (2003), 223
feedback
   employee, 358
   360-degree
fee-for-service plans, 32, 34, 254
fetal death, 287
fetal death rate, 287, 287i
field, 141, 141f
file/scanning and retrieval clerk, 12
financial data, 162
firewall, 146
fiscal year, 365
fishbone diagram, 350, 352f
flash drive, 139
flowcharts, 350, 351f
   organizational, 55, 55t
flowsheets, vital signs, 82i, 82–83
forensic evidence, 290
forming in team development, 348
forms committee, 95–98
for-profit/investor-owned hospitals, 39
For the Record, 18
fraud, 261, 262
frequency distribution table, 294
full-time equivalents, 368

G

Gantt chart, 354
gastroscopy, 42
gatekeepers, 32
Gates, Bill, 132
Genetic Information Nondiscrimination Act (2008), 227
Giffords, Gabrielle, 220
gigahertz, 141
goals, 347
go-live date, 115
Google Chrome, 136
Google Glass, 72
grade, 247
graphs. *See also* charts
   bar, 294i, 294–295
   line, 295–296
gross autopsy rate, 290, 290i
gross death rate, 286, 286i
ground rules, 350

H

Halsted, William Stewart, 52
hands-on training, 360
hard disk drive (HDD), 139
hard dollars, 168
hard drive, 139
hardware, 135

health care
   access to quality, 72
   behavioral, 44
   calculating statistics, 279–293
   as data-driven field, 314
   evolution of, in the U.S., 28–30
   history of, 199
   home, 42–43
   information technology in, 133–149
      access speed in, 140–141
      basics of, 134–136, 135i
      consumer informatics in, 144
      data management in, 141–144, 141f, 142t
      data measurement in, 140t
      data security in, 144–146, 146t
      data standardization in, 142–143, 142t
      data storage needs in, 140, 141t
      defined, 134
      information access in, 136–137
      information storage in, 139–141
      information technology department in, 147i, 147–149, 148t, 149t
      networking in, 137–139, 138i, 140i
   provision of, 27
   statistical applications in, 274–276
healthcare benefits, 342
healthcare clearinghouses, 216
Healthcare Common Procedure Coding System (HCPCS), 242, 248–249
Healthcare Cost and Utilization Project (HCUP), 329–330
healthcare data systems, 182–185
   admission, discharge, and transfer system, 183–184, 184t
   bed control system, 185
   duplicate records, 183
   master patient index, 182, 182f
   practice management system, 185
   scheduling systems, 185
healthcare documentation specialist, 14
Healthcare Effectiveness Data and Information Set (HEDIS), 143, 319–320
healthcare facilities
   forms committee in, 95–98
   licensing of, 36, 36t
Healthcare Financial Management Association (HFMA), 10, 259
Healthcare Information and Management Systems Society (HIMSS), 10, 159

healthcare organizations, 37–38
   acute care hospitals as, 37–39
   ambulatory care facilities as, 40
   behavioral health care as, 44
   diagnostic clinics as, 41–42
   emergency departments as, 41
   home health care as, 42–43
   hospices as, 43–44
   long-term acute care hospitals as, 40
   long-term care as, 43
   observational services as, 41
   outpatient surgery centers as, 40–41
   physician offices as, 42
   rehabilitation care facilities as, 40
healthcare providers, 216
health-care proxy, 214
healthcare registry, 330
healthcare regulation, 35–37
   accreditation in, 35–36
   certification in, 36–37
   licensing in, 36, 36t
healthcare research, 300
healthcare technology specialist (CHTS), 149
health information
   individually identifiable, 203
   privacy and security of, 216–221
   protected, 158
   storage and release of protected, 3
health information exchange (HIE), 167
health information management (HIM), xx, 1–20, 156
   changing roles for staff, 189
   compliance and, 233
   decision support system and, 297
   decor-keeping and, 77
   defined, 2
   disaster planning and, 125
   in EHR security, 178–179
   essential skills in, 4–8
   ethics and, 19–20, 231–232
   versus health information technology, 16–17, 16t
   history of, 3
   job opportunities in, xx, 2, 12–16
   job search in, 17–18
   legal aspects of, 199–233
      advance directives, 214
      compliance and, 233
      do not resuscitate order, 214
      durable power of attorney for health care, 214
      ethical issues in, 231–232
      Health Insurance Portability and Accountability Act and, 215–216

identity theft in, 221*i*, 221–223
legal health record, 205–213, 205*t*, 207*t*, 209*f*, 212*t*
legal system in, 201–204
living wills in, 214
other documents in, 213–214
ownership of health record in, 204–205, 205
privacy and security of health information in, 216–221
release of information in, 223–225, 225*t*, 226*f*, 227–228
releases for legal purposes in, 229, 230*f*, 231
statute of limitations in, 115, 201
manners and courtesy in, 7–8
as nonrevenue producing, 365
paper records in, 110, 111, 115, 117, 119, 120, 122, 123
personal appearance and, 8
professionalism in, 7, 7*t*, 10–11
professional organizations in, 9–10
quality of documentation and, 322, 324
release of information and, 223–228
releases for legal purposes, 229–231
in research, 300–302
retrospective review of documentation and, 321
roles in, 3–4
software and, 135–136
systems used in, 187–189
  cancer registry (tumor registry), 189
  coding, 188–189
  record analysis, 187
  release of information, 187
  transcription and speech recognition, 187–188
vital statistics and, 297–299
work sites of, 4
health information technology (HIT), 12
career opportunities in, 148–149, 148*t*, 149*t*
defined, 134
hardware in, 135
versus health information management (HIM), 16–17, 16*t*
interoperability in, 159
software in, 135–136
Health Information Technology for Economic and Clinical Health (HITECH) Act (2009), 120, 174, 203

health insurance, 30–31
coinsurance in, 31
deductibles in, 31
defined, 30
private, 31–32
provider in, 31
public, 33–35
health insurance exchanges, 31
Health Insurance Portability and Accountability Act (HIPPA) (1966)
on access to patient records, 120, 121
breach notification and, 219–220
business associate agreements and, 218
compliance and, 233
designated record set and, 205
on destruction of patient records, 123
disaster preparedness and, 124, 185
encounters in, 210
health information not protected under, 210
patient privacy and, 166
privacy officers and, 217
Privacy Rule, 15, 121, 176, 203, 204, 213, 215, 216, 218, 220, 301
on release of information, 223–228
release of information and, 223–228
release of protected health information and, 200
Security Rule, 145, 176, 203, 215, 216, 218–219
Health Insurance Prospective Payment System (HIPPS), 256
HealthIT.gov, 72, 134
Health Level Seven International (HL7), 138, 181
health maintenance organization (HMO), 32
health plans, 216
health records, 2, 74. See also patient records
custodian of, 200
digital imaging and, 117
disaster recovery planning and, 124, 124*i*, 125*t*
electronic (See electronic health records)
elimination of lost or misplaced, 166
filing systems for, 113, 114–115*t*, 115

hybrid, 74, 117, 117*i*, 172, 206
legal, 205–214
life cycle for, 118–125, 118*f*, 119*i*, 121*t*
microfilm and digital storage of, 116
numbering of, 111–113, 112*i*
ownership of, 204–205
paper, 110–116
personal, 190–191
storage of, 110–116, 111*i*, 113*i*
heart monitoring, 133
HIM supervisor/manager, 12
positions that report to, 12
HIM technician, 12
HIPPA. See Health Insurance Portability and Accountability Act (HIPPA) (1966)
histogram, 295, 295*i*
home health care, 42–43, 44*t*
hospices, 43–44, 44*t*
hospital(s), 37*i*
acute care, 37–39
community, 37
critical access, 38
departments in, 55, 56*t*, 57
emergency department in, 41
facts on largest, 53
for-profit/investor-owned, 39
as level one trauma center, 37
licensing of, 36, 36*t*
long-term acute care, 40
medical services in, 79
medical staff of, 59–64, 60*t*, 61*t*, 63*t*, 64*t*
military, 39
newborn services in, 79, 79*i*
nonprofit, 39
nursing in, 57, 57*t*
obstetrical services in, 79
organization of, 54–59, 55*t*
osteopathic, 39
rural, 38
specialty clinics in, 59, 59*t*
specialty units in, 58, 58*t*
strategies for success, 52
surgical services in, 79
teaching, 39
urban, 39
hospital-acquired infections, 256, 313, 314–315
hospital autopsy rates, 291
hospitalists, 60
hospital medical coder, 12–13, 13*t*
Hospital Outpatient Prospective Payment System (OPPS), 255
hospital president, 54

434

Index

hospital privileges, 61–62, 61t
hospital records, 79
H&P (history and physical), 80–81, 81i
human resources, 136
human subjects, 303
hybrid health records, 74, 117, 117i, 172, 206
Hypertext Markup Language (HTML), 136
Hypertext Transfer Protocol (HTTP), 136–137, 139
hypothesis, 302
   developing a, 302

I

identification, 179
identity theft, 221–223
   medical, 221
illness
   acute, 37
   chronic, 38
immunization registry, 331
immunizations, 331i
implied consent, 212, 212t
Improving America's Hospitals: The Joint Commission's Annual Report on Quality and Safety, 318
in camera review, 229
incident reports, 231
incomplete records, 98
Indeed.com, 18
indemnity plans, 32
index, 244
   case mix, 257–258
Indiana Health Information Exchange, 273
indices, 250–252
individual consent, 212, 212t
individually identifiable health information, 203
infection-control committee, 320
infections
   central line-associated bloodstream, 313
   Clostridium difficile, 313
   hospital-acquired, 256, 313, 314–315
   methicillin-resistant Staphylococcuss aureus (MRSA) staph, 313
   nosocomial, 78, 276, 292, 313
   surgical-site, 313
   urinary tract, 313, 315, 315t
informal leaders, 345
information
   defined, 141
   release of, 223–228

information access, 136–137
information governance, 99–100
information storage, 139–141
Information Technology Association of America, 134
information technology department, 147–149
information technology in health care, 133–149
   access speed in, 140–141
   basics of, 134–136, 135i
   consumer informatics in, 144
   data management in, 141–144, 141f, 142t
   data measurement in, 140t
   data security in, 144–146, 146t
   data standardization in, 142–143, 142t
   data storage needs in, 140, 141t
   defined, 134
   information access in, 136–137
   information storage in, 139–141
   information technology department in, 147i, 147–149, 148t, 149t
   networking in, 137–139, 138i, 140i
informed consent, 212, 212t
   for surgery, 84–87, 85i
infrastructure, 147
initiation process, 354
inpatient census, 281
   daily, 281–282
inpatient hospital setting, patient records in, 75
inpatient records, standards/guidelines for documenting, 96, 97t
inpatient service day, 282–283
Institute for Medicine, 73
Institute for Safe Medication Practices (ISMP), 323
   list of error-prone abbreviations an, 323
institutional review board (IRB), 303
intake, 83
intensity of service, 326
interface, 138, 161
intermediate care facility, 43
International Classification of Diseases, 242, 244–245
International Classification of Diseases, Ninth Revision, Clinical Modification (ICD-9-CM), 245, 245t
International Classification of Diseases, Tenth Revision, Clinical Modification (ICD-10-CM), 13, 245, 245t

International Classification of Diseases, Tenth Revision, Procedure Coding System (ICD-10-PCS), 13, 245–247, 246t
International Classification of Diseases for Oncology (ICD-O), 189, 333
International Classification of Diseases for Oncology, Third Edition (ICD-O-3), 247–248, 248t
Internet, 136
Internet Explorer, 136
Internet Protocol (IP), 138
interoperability, 159
interoperable, 138
interview questions in hiring employees, 356i, 356–357
intranet, 137
intrinsic motivation, 359
inventory control, 136
IT director, 147

J

job description, writing, 355–356
job skills, 17–18
Johns Hopkins Hospital, 52
Joint Commission, 35
   on access to patient records, 120
   accreditation of alternative care facilities, 40, 44t
   on acute care record, 92t
   Core Measure Solution Exchange and, 318
   on destruction of patient records, 123
   disaster preparedness and, 185
   documentation requirements for acute care patient records, 91, 92
   Do Not Use abbreviations list of, 323
   electronic health record documentation requirements, 94, 96, 97, 98
   on H&P, 80
   Improving America's Hospitals: The Joint Commission's Annual Report on Quality and Safety, 318
   on legibility of documentation, 165, 165f, 322
   on medical documentation, 165
   on operative reports, 86
   ORYX, 317–318, 317t
   on the patient record, 74, 78, 91
   performance evaluations and, 359
   on physician privileges, 62

quality improvement and, 314, 315
requirement for chief nursing officer, 54
restraint logs and, 83
safety and regulatory standards and, 316–3617
sentinel events and, 318–319, 319i
setting of National Patient Safety Goals, 317
statistics and, 276
use of abbreviations and, 322–323, 323t
use of hospital performance data, 276
jump drive, 139
jurisdiction, 202
justification, 367

K
Kelly, Howard A., 52
Kloss, Linda, 1

L
laboratory clinics, 41
late documentation, 119–120
laws
  case, 201
  common, 201
  constitutional, 201
  of least action, 53
  statutory, 201
leaders, 344, 346
  informal, 345
leadership, management and, 344–346
Leadership IQ, 355
legal aspects of health information management, 199–233
  advance directives, 214
  compliance and, 233
  decision matrix in, 206–207, 207t
  do not resuscitate order, 214
  durable power of attorney for health care, 214
  ethical issues in, 231–232
  Health Insurance Portability and Accountability Act and, 215–216
  identity theft in, 221i, 221–223
  legal health record, 205–213, 207t, 209f, 212t, 205t
  legal system in, 201–204
  living wills, 214
  other documents, 213–214
  ownership of health record, 204–205, 205
  privacy and security of health information, 216–221

release of information, 223–225, 225t, 226f, 227–228
releases for legal purposes, 229, 230f, 231
statute of limitations in, 115, 201
legal documents in the health records, 213–214
legal health record, 205–213
legal purposes, release of information for, 229–231
length of stay, 279–280
level one trauma center, 37
liability, 222
licensed practical nurse (LPN), 57t
licensed vocational nurse (LVN), 57t
licensing, 36, 36t
line graph, 295–296, 296i
literature, reviewing in research, 302
living wills, 214
local area network (LAN), 137
log and flow sheets, 82i, 82–83
Logical Observation Identifiers, Names, and Codes (LOINC), 243–244, 243t
logic-based encoder, 252
logs, 211
longitudinal record, 158
long-term acute care hospitals, 40, 44t
long-term care, 43
loose documentation, 119–120
Louis, Thomas A., 273

M
macros, 170
Mahan, Julie, 109
maintenance stage in health record life cycle, 119
malware, 145
managed care, 32
management, 343–370
  budgeting and, 365–368, 366i, 367i
  fishbone diagrams and, 352, 352f
  flowcharts and, 51f, 350
  leadership and, 344–346
  meetings and, 349i, 349–352
  motivation and, 359
  policies and procedures and, 363–364, 365i
  productivity and, 368–370
  project, 353–354
  recognition and reward and, 362–363, 363i
  selecting and evaluating employees, 355–360
  teamwork and, 347i, 347–348
  training and, 360–362, 361i, 362i
management by walking around, 342

management information systems (MIS), 136
managers, 344, 345
manners, 7–8
master patient index, 160, 182, 182f, 250, 251
  admission, discharge, and transfer system, 183–184, 184t
  duplication of records and, 183
material management, 136
maternal death, 288
maternal death rate, 288
MCG, 326
McKesson's InterQual, 326
mean, 276–277
meaningful use, 120, 121, 175, 175t, 176t
  incentives for, 175–176
measures of central tendency, 276–277
measures of frequency, 277–278
measures of variation, 278–279
median, 277
Medicaid, 29, 34
  reimbursement rates for, 254
medical biller and coder, 13t
medical chief of staff versus chief executive officer (CEO), 64, 64t
medical coding editor, 188
medical editor, 14
medical history, 80
medical identity theft, 221
medical language editor, 188
medical necessity, 261, 326
medical practice management system, 185
medical protocols, 64
medical record number (MRN), 182
medical records, 2, 74. *See also* patient records
  problem-oriented, 87–89, 89t
  source-oriented, 89
medical record technicians, 156
medical referrals, 59
medical research, 300
medical services, 79
medical specialties, 60, 60t
medical staff, 59–64, 60t, 61t, 63t, 64t
  bylaws for, 62
  committees of, 62, 63t
  departments of, 63–64
  organization of, 62
  rules and regulations, 62
medical terminology, 242–243
medical transcriptionist, 14–15
Medicare, 29, 33–34, 72
  costs of, 254

fraud and abuse with, 262
Part A, 33
Part B, 33
Part C, 33, 34
Part D, 33, 34
reimbursement rates for, 254
rising costs of, 255
Medicare Advantage Plan, 33
Medicare Conditions of Participation (CoPs)
on access to patient records, 120
on destruction of patient records, 123
Medicare Severity Diagnosis Related Groups (MS-DRGs), 255, 257t
medication records, 83i, 83–84
Medigap policy, 3
meetings, 349–352
agendas for, 349, 349f
fishbone diagrams for, 352, 352f
flowcharts for, 350, 351f
ground rules for, 350
recognition and rewards and, 352, 352i
megahertz (MHz), 140–141
memory chip, 135
Merck Manual of Diagnosis and Therapy, 254
methicillin-resistant Staphylococcus aureus (MRSA) staph infections, 313
methodology, 303
microcomputers, 135
microfiche, 116
microfilm, 116, 116i
microprocessor, 135
Microsoft Office, 135
Microsoft Windows®, 135
middle digit filing, 113, 114t
military hospitals, 39
Minimum Data Set for long-term care, 167
minimum necessary, 218
minor equipment, 366
misfiles, 118
mode, 277
monitoring, 354
morbidity, 245, 276
morphology, 247
mortality, 245, 276
Mosby's Diagnostic and Laboratory Test Reference, 254
motherboard, 135
motivation, 359
extrinsic, 359
intrinsic, 359
Mozilla Firefox, 136
multiple malignancy, 333

N

National Association for Healthcare Quality, 312
National Cancer Data Base (NCDB), 167, 333
National Center for Ethics in Health Care at the Department of Veterans Affairs, 312
National Commission for the Protection of Human Subjects of Biomedical and Behavioral Research, 303
National Committee for Quality Assurance (NCQA), 44t, 91, 143, 319–320
National Committee on Vital and Health Statistics (NCVHS), 142
National Death Index, 330
National Hospital Ambulatory Medical Care Survey (NHAMCS), 330
National Hospital Care Survey, 330
National Hospital Discharge Survey (NHDS), 330
National (Nationwide) Inpatient Sample, 329
National Institutes of Health, on ethics in use of human subjects in research, 304
National Patient Safety Goals, 317
National Program of Cancer Registries (NPCR), 332
National Quality Strategy, 319
National Vital Statistics System (NVSS), 297
natural disasters, 185–186
nepotism, 355
net autopsy rate, 290–291
net death rate, 286–287, 287i
networks, 137–139
communication over the, 138
connecting to the, 138i, 138–139, 139i
newborns
forms for, 87
services for, 79, 79i
nomenclature, 241, 243
comparing code systems and, 249–250, 250t
nonacute care sites, 39
nonprofit hospitals, 39
nonverbal communication, 6
norming in team development, 348
nosocomial infections, 78, 276, 292, 313
notice of privacy practices, 213
Nuremberg Code, 304
nurse practitioners, 57t

nursing, 57
nursing credentials, 57t
nursing notes, 83

O

Obamacare. *See* Affordable Care Act (2010)
obligatory disclosures of information, 229
observational survives, 41
obstetrical patients
forms for, 86–87
services for, 79
Office for Civil Rights (OCR), 216
Office of the National Coordinator for Health Information Technology (ONC), 174
off-site storage, 116
operating budget, 365–367
operating system, 135
operations, 121
operations/procedures index, 250, 251–252
operative reports, 86
optional field, 189
orientation, 360–362
Original Medicare Plan, 33–34
ORYX, 317–318
Osler, William, 52
osteopathic hospitals, 39
outliers, 255
outpatient surgery, 40–41
outpatient surgery centers, 40–41
output, 83
outsourcing of release of information, 228

P

paperless referrals and prescriptions, 166
paper records. *See* patient care records
password, 146
aging of, 146
strong, 146t
pathology reports, 86
patient care records, 74–75, 82–83. *See also* health records
access to, 120
in ambulatory care facilities, 74–75
clinical documentation and, 100–101
color coding, 113i
committee requests for, 122
complete, 77
destruction of, 123
digital imaging and, 117
digital storage and, 116–117
disaster planning and, 124, 124i, 125t

electronic (*See* electronic health records)
elimination of lost of misplaced, 166
external uses of, 78
falsification of, 221
filing systems for, 113, 114–115*t*, 115
forms committee and, 95–98
forms/information included in, 79–87
hybrid, 74, 117, 117*i*, 172, 206
information governance and, 99–100
internal uses of, 78
life cycle of, 118*i*, 118–125, 118*f*, 119*i*, 121*t*
microfilm and, 116, 116*i*
numbering of, 111–113, 112*i*
off-site storage of, 116
organization of, 87–91
paper storage, 110–116
primary uses of, 75–76, 110
purging, 122–123
purging of, 122–123
purpose of, 75–78
release of information, 121–122
required documentation in the, 91–95
retrieval of, 111, 113, 120–121
secondary uses, 76–77
standards/guidelines for documenting inpatient, 96, 97*t*
storage of, 110–116
patient care services, 55
patient engagement, improved, 167
patient identification numbers, 111
patient information, access to, following discharge, 164–165, 164*t*
patient portal, 120, 167, 204
Patient Protection and Affordable Care Act (2010). *See* Affordable Care Act (2010)
payment, 121
payment methodologies
 ambulatory payment classifications, 254–256
 diagnostic-related groups, 255
 present on admission, 256–257
payment posting and appeals and collections, 260
payroll, 136, 366
percentage, 277
percentage of occupancy, 284
performance evaluations, 358–359
performance improvement coordinator, 15–16

performing in team development, 348
personal appearance, 8
personal/enrollment data, 142
personal health record (PHR), 190–191, 208
 applications of, 191
 benefits of, 190–191
 versus a provider record, 191
pharmaceutical drug trials and research studies, 305
phishing, 145
physical exams, 80–81, 81*i*
physical safeguards, 176, 177*t*
physician assistants (PAs), 57
physician officer manager, 16
physician orders, 82
physicians
 designations, 61, 61*t*
 employment of, 64
 offices of, 42, 42*i*
 primary care, 32, 59
 problem list for, 88, 89*t*
Physician Self-Referral Law, 262
picture archiving and communication system (PACS), 161
pie chart, 296, 296*i*
planning process, 354
point of care (POC), 163, 244
point of service (POS) plan, 32
point of service registration counseling, 259
policies, 363–364
population-based research, 300
portability, 215
postage, 367
postoperative death rate, 289, 289*i*
postoperative evaluation and follow-up, 86
practice management system, 185
precertification process, 326
predictive analytics, 272
preferred provider organizations (PPOs), 32
preferred providers, 32
prehire assessments, 357–358
premiums, 31
preregistration, 259
prescriptions, paperless, 166
Present on Admission (POA) indicator, 256–257, 257*t*
preventable medical errors, 292
primary cancer, 332
primary care physicians (PCP), 32, 59
primary data, 329
privacy
 defined, 215
 enhanced, 166

of health information, 216–221
privacy officer, 15, 217
private health insurance, 31–32
problem list, 88
problem-oriented medical information system (PROMIS), 173
problem-oriented medical records (POMR), 87–89, 89*t*, 173
procedures, 363, 364, 365*i*
process improvement (PI), 315, 370
process redesign, 370
process reengineering, 370
production log, 368–369, 369*i*
productivity, 368–370, 369*i*
professional credentials, 10–11, 11*t*
professionalism, 7, 7*t*
professional organizations, 9–10. *See also specific by name*
progress notes, 83
project management, 353–354
 process of, 354
 tools in, 354
Project Management Institute (PMI), 354
projects, 353
 complex, 353–354
 simple, 353
protected health information (PHI), 158, 208
 documentation of, 210–211
 storage and release of, 3
protocols
 evidence-based medicine and, 205
 Internet, 138
 medical, 64
 treatment, 75
providers, 31
 direct care, 31
 preferred, 32
psychiatrists, 61
psychologists, 61
public health insurance, 33–35
public key certificate, 146
purchasing, value-based, 320
purging of patient records, 122–123

Q

qualitative research, 303
quality, 315
 of documentation, 320–325
quality control, 315
quality improvement (QI), 210, 315
quality management
 documentation quality and, 320–325
 safety and regulatory standards and, 316–320
quality review/improvement

documents, 231
quantitative research, 303
questions, interview, 356*i*, 356–357
quorum, 62

R

radiology, 41
random access memory (RAM), 140
range, 278
rate, 278
ratios, 278
recognition, 352, 362–363
record analysis, 187
record filing systems, 113, 114–115*t*, 115
record retention cycle, 118–125
record retrieval, 111, 113
record storage, reduced, 167
Recovery Audit Contractor (RAC), 78
recovery room reports, 86
redact, 208
Red Flags Rule, 223
regional cost estimates, 329
registered health information administrator (RHIA), 10, 11*t*
registered health information technician (RHIT), xx, 4, 10, 11*t*
registered nurses, 57*t*
registries, 330–335
    abstracting and, 333
    birth defects, 331
    cancer, 332
    case finding and, 332–333
    coding and staging, 333–335
    immunization, 331
    trauma, 331
regulations, 202
rehabilitation, 40
rehabilitation care facilities, 40, 44*t*
reimbursement rates, 31
release of information, 121–122, 187, 223–228
    authorized, 224–226
    for legal purposes, 229–231
    outsourcing of, 228
reliability, 276
remittance processing and rejections, 260
research, 300*i*, 300–304
    administrative, 300
    biomedical, 303
    conducting, 303
    developing hypothesis in, 302
    ethics in, 304
    healthcare, 300
    medical, 300
    population-based, 300
    qualitative, 303
    quantitative, 303
    reviewing data in, 303
    reviewing literature in, 302
    role of health information management in, 300–302
    steps in, 302–303
    submitting for publication, 303
research methodology, 301
residential care/assisted living facilities, 43
resource management, 326–327
resource utilization group (RUG), 256
respite care, 44
restraint logs, 83
résumé, 17
    skills to include on, 18*t*
    writing effective, 17–18
retrospective cost-based reimbursement system, 254
retrospective review, 321
return on investment, 168
revenue, 366
revenue cycle management, 259–260, 260*f*
    charge capture and coding, 260
    claim submission, 260
    collections, 259
    encounter utilization review and case management, 259
    payment posting and appeals and collections, 260
    point of service registration counseling, 259
    remittance processing and rejections, 260
    scheduling and preregistration, 259
    third party follow-up, 260
review of systems form, 80*i*
rewards, 352, 362–363
risk, 328
risk management, 222, 328*i*, 328–329
risk taker, 346
rural hospitals, 38

S

safety and regulatory standards, 316–320
same-day surgery, 40–41
scheduling, 136, 185, 259
Schloendorff v. Society of New York Hospital, 199
secondary data, 329
security
    enhanced, 166
    of health information, 216–221
security incidents, 216
security threats, prevention of, 146
sentinel events, 318–319, 319*i*
serial numbering, 111–112, 112*i*
serial unit numbering system, 112*i*, 112–113
servers, 135
service assignment, 79
severity of illness, 326–327
Shalala, Donna E., 26
signatures, electronic, 97
simple projects, 353
simultaneous access, 164–165
skew, 277
Snake Oil Liniment, 28
SOAP (subjective, objective, assessment, and plan) notes, 88, 90
    components of, 90*t*
Social Security Act, 262
Society of Hospital Medicine, 60
soft dollars, 168
software, 135–136
    clinical decision support, 163
    decision support, 158
    encoder, 252–253
    licensing of, 366
    operating, 135
    system, 135
Solzhenitsyn, Aleksandr, 231
source-oriented medical records, 89
specialists, 59
specialty clinics, 59, 59*t*
specialty units, 58, 58*t*
speech recognition technology, 157, 157*i*
staging, 333–335
stakeholders, 349
standard deviation, 279, 279*i*
Stark Law, 262
statistics, 274
    applications in health care, 274–276
    basic terms and calculations, 276–279
    calculating healthcare, 279–293
    common, 276–277
    reliability of, 276
    validity of, 276
statute of limitations, 115, 201
statutory law, 201
storming in team development, 348
straight numeric filing, 113, 114, 114*t*
strategic plan, 147
strong password, 146*t*
subject category filing, 113, 115*i*
subpoena, 229, 230*f*

subpoena ad testificandum, 229
subpoena duces tecum, 229
subscriptions, 366
success
    hospitals' strategies for, 52
    rules for, xx
supplemental insurance plan, 3
supplies, 366
surgery/surgical services, 79
    consent for, 84, 85*i*
    forms for, 84–87, 85*i*
    outpatient, 40–41
Surveillance, Epidemiology, and End Results (SEER) Summary Staging Manual, 334
Systematized Nomenclature of Medicine—Clinical Terms (SNOMED CT), 243, 243*t*
system output usability, 172
system software, 135

T

teaching hospitals, 39
teams
    building, 347
    developing, 348
teamwork, 347*i*, 347–348
technical safeguards, 178, 178*t*
telephone screening in hiring employees, 356
templates, 169
terminal digit filing, 113, 114*t*
third-party consent, 212, 212*t*
third party follow-up, 260
3-D printers, 134
360-degree feedback, 359
thumb drive, 139
timeliness of documentation, 321–322
TNM staging system, 334–335
topography, 247
total inpatient service days, 282–283
total length of stay, 280
training, 360–362

competency tests and, 361, 361*i*
cross-, 361–362
in electronic health record system, 168–169
hands-on, 360
transcription, 77, 187–188
transferable skills, 18
transfer records, 84
transitional (discharge) planning, 326
Transmission Control Protocol (TCP), 138
trauma registry, 331
travel, 367
treaties, 201
treatment, 121
    consent for, 211–213, 212*t*
    payment, or operations (TPO) activities, 218
    protocols in, 75
trend analysis, 297*i*, 297–298
Trojan horse programs, 145
Truman, Harry, 29
Tuckman, Bruce, 348
tumor grade, 247*i*
tumor registry, 189, 332

U

unbundling, 263
uniform resource locater (URL), 136–137
Union for International Cancer Control (UICC), 334
US Constitution, 201
US Criminal Code, 262
unit numbering system, 112*i*, 112–113
unknown primary, 332
upcoding, 171, 231, 260–261, 263
urban hospitals, 39
urinary tract infections, 313, 315, 315*t*
utilization management, 326
utilization stage in health record life cycle, 119

V

validity, 276
value-based purchasing, 320
variability, 278
verbal communication, 6
    mistakes to avoid in, 6
Veterans Affairs, U.S. Department of, 39
    National Center for Ethics in Health Care at the, 312
virtual private network (VPN), 137
viruses, 145
vital signs, 75
    flow sheet for, 82*i*, 82–83
vital statistics, 275, 297–299, 299*i*
vital statistics clerk, 12
vulnerable subjects, 304

W

warrant, 231
Watson, 132, 132*i*
web browser, 136
websites, 136
Weed, Lawrence L., 173
Welch, William H., 52
whistle-blower, 263
wide area network (WAN), 137
Wi-Fi, 137
wireless access point (WAP), 137
wireless local area network (WLAN), 137
Workers' compensation, 35
World Health Organization (WHO), 33, 45, 244, 292
World Medical Association, 304
World Wide Web (WWW), 136
worms, 145
written communication, 5

Photo credits

Page xx *top*, © iStockphoto/danleap; *bottom* © iStockphoto/digitalskillet; **1** © iStockphoto/Prykhodov; **6** *bottom left*, © Shutterstock/Sarah Cheriton-Jones; *bottom middle* © Shutterstock/Michal Kowalski; *bottom right* © Shutterstock/Maridav; **7** © Shutterstock/Warren Goldswain; **9** Photo by Leslie Anderson, © Paradigm Publishing, Inc.; **17** © Shutterstock/Cartoonresource; **19** © Shutterstock/travellight; **26** *top*, © Shutterstock/Andy Dean Photography; *bottom* © Shutterstock/Ilya Andriyanov; **27** *top*, © iStockphoto/fotostorm; *bottom* © Shutterstock/Everett Collection; **31** *top*, © Shutterstock/zimmytws; *bottom* © Shutterstock/Cartoonresource; **33** © Shutterstock/Keith Bell; **34** © iStockphoto/Kameleon007; **37** © iStockphoto/babyblueut; **40** © Shutterstock/Alexander Raths; **42** Photo by Leslie Anderson, © Paradigm Publishing, Inc.; **52** *top*, © iStockphoto/UmerPK; *bottom* © iStockphoto/dbencek; **53** © *top*, Shutterstock/s_bukley; *bottom* Shutterstock/Alexander Raths; **58** © Shutterstock/Cartoonresource; **59** © Shutterstock/wavebreakmedia; **72** *top*, Courtesy of The Ohio State University Wexner Medical Center; *bottom* © Shutterstock/Hasloo Group Production Studio; **73** Courtesy of US Department of Health & Human Services; **79** © Shutterstock/XiXinXing; **80** © iStockphoto/doublediamondphoto; **94** Photo by Leslie Anderson, © Paradigm Publishing, Inc.; **100** © iStockphoto/digitalskillet; **108** *top*, Courtesy of C-J Hsiao and E. Hing, National Center for Health Statistics; *bottom* © iStockphoto/koya79; **109** © Shutterstock/Lisa S.; **111** © iStockphoto/PixHouse; **113** © Shutterstock/val lawless; **116** *top*, Courtesy of Underground Vaults & Storage, Inc.; *bottom* © Shutterstock/jps; **117** © iStockphoto/Razvan; **118** © iStockphoto/onurdongel; **119** © iStockphoto/Frannyanne; **124** © iStockphoto/SteveDF; **132** *top*, © Shutterstock/JStone; *middle* © Shutterstock/Ovchinnkov Vladimir; *bottom* © iStockphoto/dra_schwartz; **133** *top*, © Shutterstock/Alexey Boldin; *bottom* © iStockphoto/amriphoto; **135** © Shutterstock/Oleksiy Mark; **138** © Shutterstock/krichie; **139** © Shutterstock/mr.Timmi; **147** *front*, © Shutterstock/Mckyartstudio; *back* © Shutterstock/Lightspring; **156** *top*, © R.J. Romero; *bottom* © iStockphoto/Spiderstock; **157** *top*, © Shutterstock/MC_Noppadol; *middle* © Shutterstock/Soundsnaps; *bottom left* © iStockphoto/Spiderstock; *bottom right* © Shutterstock/zphoto; **172** © R.J. Romero; **198** *top*, © iStockphoto/stuartbur; *bottom* © iStockphoto/AndreyPopov; **199** © iStockphoto/jgroup; **205** © iStockphoto/yongyuan; **215** © Shutterstock/megainarmy; **219** © Shutterstock/Maksim Kabakou; **221** © iStockphoto/bonniej; **223** © Shutterstock/Ljupco Smokovski; **240** *top*, © iStockphoto/DNY59; *bottom* iStockphoto/fotek; **241** *top*, © Shutterstock/WilleeCole Photography; *bottom* © iStockphoto/exdez; **246** © Shutterstock/Suzanne Tucker; **247** © Shutterstock/Alila Medical Media; **256** © Shutterstock/Image Point Fr; **258** © Shutterstock/JohnKwan; **261** © Shutterstock/Andrii Kondiuk; **263** © Shutterstock/Elnur; **272** *top*, © Shutterstock/Gregg Brekke; *bottom* Shutterstock/Novelo; **273** *top*, © iStockphoto/kertlis; *bottom* © Shutterstock/Manuel carmona carmona; **278** © Shutterstock/Ersin Kurtdal; **293** © Shutterstock/wavebreakmedia; **297** *top*, © Shutterstock/Sergey Nivens; *bottom* © iStockphoto/jpa1999; **300** © Shutterstock/KPG_Payless; **301** © Shutterstock/ra2studio; **312** © Shutterstock/nasirkhan; **313** © Shutterstock/Samuel Borges Photography; **318** © Shutterstock/askib; **319** © iStockphoto/tirc83; **328** © Shutterstock/R. Gino Santa Maria; **331** *top*, iStockphoto/SLRadcliffe; *bottom* © Shutterstock/JPC-PROD; **342** *top*, © Shutterstock/CoraMax; *bottom* © iStockphoto/STEEX; **343** © Shutterstock/violetkaipa; **347** © Shutterstock/alphaspirit; **352** Shutterstock/Andresr; **356** © Shutterstock/Adam Gregor; **362** DILBERT © 2009 Scott Adams. Used By permission of UNIVERSAL UCLICK. All rights reserved.; **363** © iStockphoto/glegorly; **366** © Shutterstock/val lawless.

CPSIA information can be obtained
at www.ICGtesting.com
Printed in the USA
LVHW061055271021
701491LV00001B/1